Lens and Cataract

Section 11
2012–2013

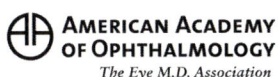

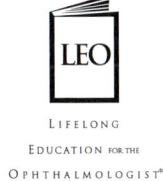

LIFELONG
EDUCATION FOR THE
OPHTHALMOLOGIST

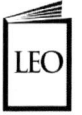 The Basic and Clinical Science Course (BCSC) is one component of the Lifelong Education for the Ophthalmologist (LEO) framework, which assists members in planning their continuing medical education. LEO includes an array of clinical education products that members may select to form individualized, self-directed learning plans for updating their clinical knowledge. Active members or fellows who use LEO components may accumulate sufficient CME credits to earn the LEO Award. Contact the Academy's Clinical Education Division for further information on LEO.

The American Academy of Ophthalmology is accredited by the Accreditation Council for Continuing Medical Education to provide continuing medical education for physicians.

The American Academy of Ophthalmology designates this enduring material for a maximum of 10 *AMA PRA Category 1 Credits*™. Physicians should claim only the credit commensurate with the extent of their participation in the activity.

The BCSC is designed to increase the physician's ophthalmic knowledge through study and review. Users of this activity are encouraged to read the text and then answer the study questions provided at the back of the book.

To claim *AMA PRA Category 1 Credits*™ upon completion of this activity, learners must demonstrate appropriate knowledge and participation in the activity by taking the posttest for Section 11 and achieving a score of 80% or higher. For further details, please see the instructions for requesting CME credit at the back of the book.

The Academy provides this material for educational purposes only. It is not intended to represent the only or best method or procedure in every case, nor to replace a physician's own judgment or give specific advice for case management. Including all indications, contraindications, side effects, and alternative agents for each drug or treatment is beyond the scope of this material. All information and recommendations should be verified, prior to use, with current information included in the manufacturers' package inserts or other independent sources, and considered in light of the patient's condition and history. Reference to certain drugs, instruments, and other products in this course is made for illustrative purposes only and is not intended to constitute an endorsement of such. Some material may include information on applications that are not considered community standard, that reflect indications not included in approved FDA labeling, or that are approved for use only in restricted research settings. **The FDA has stated that it is the responsibility of the physician to determine the FDA status of each drug or device he or she wishes to use, and to use them with appropriate, informed patient consent in compliance with applicable law.** The Academy specifically disclaims any and all liability for injury or other damages of any kind, from negligence or otherwise, for any and all claims that may arise from the use of any recommendations or other information contained herein.

Cover image courtesy of Karla J. Johns, MD.

Copyright © 2012
American Academy of Ophthalmology
All rights reserved
Printed in Canada

Basic and Clinical Science Course

Gregory L. Skuta, MD, Oklahoma City, Oklahoma, *Senior Secretary for Clinical Education*
Louis B. Cantor, MD, Indianapolis, Indiana, *Secretary for Ophthalmic Knowledge*
Jayne S. Weiss, MD, New Orleans, Louisiana, *BCSC Course Chair*

Section 11

Faculty Responsible for This Edition

James C. Bobrow, MD, *Chair,* Clayton, Missouri
Thomas L. Beardsley, MD, Asheville, North Carolina
Sharon L. Jick, MD, St Louis, Missouri
Lisa F. Rosenberg, MD, Chicago, Illinois
Michael N. Wiggins, MD, Little Rock, Arkansas
Joseph Reich, MD, *Consultant,* Toorak, Australia
Edward K. Isbey III, MD, Asheville, North Carolina
   Practicing Ophthalmologists Advisory Committee for Education

The Academy wishes to acknowledge Hilary A. Beaver, MD, *Committee on Aging,* for her review of this edition.

The Academy also wishes to acknowledge the American Society of Cataract and Refractive Surgery for recommending faculty members to the BCSC Section 11 committee.

Financial Disclosures

Academy staff members who contributed to the development of this product state that they have no significant financial interest or other relationship with the manufacturer of any commercial product discussed in this course or with the manufacturer of any competing commercial product.

The authors state that they have no significant financial interest or other relationship with the manufacturer of any commercial product discussed in the chapters that they contributed to this course or with the manufacturer of any competing commercial product.

The reviewers state the following financial relationships:

Dr Beaver: Genzyme, lecture fees

Recent Past Faculty

Mark H. Blecher, MD
David B. Glasser, MD
Kenneth B. Mitchell, MD

In addition, the Academy gratefully acknowledges the contributions of numerous past faculty and advisory committee members who have played an important role in the development of previous editions of the Basic and Clinical Science Course.

American Academy of Ophthalmology Staff

    Richard A. Zorab, *Vice President, Ophthalmic Knowledge*
    Hal Straus, *Director, Publications Department*
    Christine Arturo, *Acquisitions Manager*
    Stephanie Tanaka, *Publications Manager*
    D. Jean Ray, *Production Manager*
    Ann McGuire, *Medical Editor*
    Steve Huebner, *Administrative Coordinator*

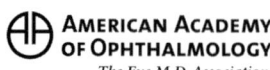

655 Beach Street
Box 7424
San Francisco, CA 94120-7424

Contents

General Introduction xiii

Objectives 1
Introduction 3

1 Anatomy 5
   Normal Crystalline Lens 5
      Capsule 7
      Zonular Fibers 7
      Lens Epithelium 8
      Nucleus and Cortex 8

2 Biochemistry and Physiology 11
   Molecular Biology 11
      Crystallin Proteins 11
      Membrane Structural Proteins and Cytoskeletal Proteins 12
      Increase of Water-Insoluble Proteins With Age 13
   Carbohydrate Metabolism 13
   Oxidative Damage and Protective Mechanisms 16
   Lens Physiology 17
      Maintenance of Lens Water and Cation Balance 17
   Accommodation and Presbyopia 19

3 Embryology and Developmental Defects 21
   Normal Development 21
      Lens Placode 21
      Lens Pit 21
      Lens Vesicle 21
      Primary Lens Fibers and the Embryonic Nucleus 22
      Secondary Lens Fibers 23
      Lens Sutures and the Fetal Nucleus 24
      Tunica Vasculosa Lentis 25
      Zonules of Zinn 25
   Congenital Anomalies and Abnormalities 26
      Congenital Aphakia 26
      Lenticonus and Lentiglobus 26
      Lens Coloboma 26
      Mittendorf Dot 27
      Epicapsular Star 27
      Peters Anomaly 27
      Microspherophakia 28

　　　　Aniridia 29
　　　　Congenital Cataract 30
　　Developmental Defects 35
　　　　Ectopia Lentis 35
　　　　Genetic Contributions to Age-Related Cataracts. 37
　　　　Ectopia Lentis et Pupillae. 38
　　　　Persistent Fetal Vasculature. 38

4 Pathology 39

　　Age-Related Lens Changes 39
　　　　Nuclear Cataracts 39
　　　　Cortical Cataracts 41
　　　　Posterior Subcapsular Cataracts 42
　　Drug-Induced Lens Changes 47
　　　　Corticosteroids 47
　　　　Phenothiazines 48
　　　　Miotics 49
　　　　Amiodarone 49
　　　　Statins 49
　　　　Tamoxifen 49
　　Trauma 50
　　　　Contusion 50
　　　　Perforating and Penetrating Injury. 51
　　　　Intralenticular Foreign Bodies 51
　　　　Radiation 51
　　　　Chemical Injuries 53
　　　　Metallosis 53
　　　　Electrical Injury. 54
　　Metabolic Cataract 55
　　　　Diabetes Mellitus 55
　　　　Galactosemia 56
　　　　Hypocalcemia 57
　　　　Wilson Disease 57
　　　　Myotonic Dystrophy. 57
　　Effects of Nutrition, Alcohol, and Smoking. 57
　　Cataract Associated With Uveitis 59
　　Cataracts Associated With Ocular Treatments 60
　　Cataracts and Hyperbaric Oxygen Therapy. 60
　　Exfoliation Syndrome 61
　　Cataract and Atopic Dermatitis 62
　　Phacoantigenic Uveitis 62
　　Lens-Induced Glaucoma. 63
　　　　Phacolytic Glaucoma 63
　　　　Lens Particle Glaucoma 63
　　　　Phacomorphic Glaucoma 63
　　　　Glaukomflecken 64
　　Ischemia. 64
　　Cataracts Associated With Degenerative Ocular Disorders 64

5 Epidemiology of Cataracts 65

6 Evaluation and Management of Cataracts in Adults 69
    Clinical History: Signs and Symptoms 69
        Decreased Visual Acuity 69
        Glare and Altered Contrast Sensitivity 70
        Myopic Shift 70
        Monocular Diplopia or Polyopia 70
        Decreased Visual Function 71
    Nonsurgical Management 71
    Indications for Surgery 72
    Preoperative Evaluation 73
        General Health of the Patient 73
        Pertinent Ocular History 75
        Social History 75
    Measurements of Visual Function 76
        Visual Acuity Testing 76
        Refraction 76
        Glare Testing 76
        Contrast Sensitivity 76
    External Examination 77
        Motility 77
        Pupils 77
    Slit-Lamp Examination 78
        Conjunctiva 78
        Cornea 78
        Anterior Chamber and Iris 79
        Crystalline Lens 79
        Limitations of Slit-Lamp Examination 80
    Fundus Evaluation 80
        Ophthalmoscopy 80
        Optic Nerve 80
        Fundus Evaluation With Opaque Media 80
    Special Tests 81
        Potential Acuity Estimation 81
        Visual Field Testing 81
        Objective Tests of Macular Function 82
    Preoperative Measurements 82
        Biometry 82
        Corneal Topography 83
        Additional Evaluation of the Cornea 84
    IOL Power Determination 84
        Preventing Errors in IOL Calculation, Selection, and Insertion 84
        IOL Calculation 85
        Improving Outcomes 86
        IOL Calculation Following Refractive Surgery 86
    Patient Preparation and Informed Consent 88

7 Surgery for Cataract ... 89

- The Remote Past ... 89
  - Ancient and Medieval Techniques ... 89
  - Early Extracapsular Cataract Extraction ... 90
  - Early Intracapsular Cataract Extraction ... 92
- The Recent Past ... 93
  - Modern Advances in Intracapsular Surgery ... 93
  - The Renaissance of Extracapsular Extraction ... 94
  - The Modern ECCE Procedure ... 94
- Ophthalmic Viscosurgical Devices ... 96
  - Physical Properties ... 97
  - Characteristics of OVDs ... 98
- Anesthesia for Cataract Surgery ... 98
- Phacoemulsification ... 102
  - Ultrasonics Terminology ... 102
  - Vacuum Terminology ... 104
  - Phaco Instrumentation ... 104
  - Phaco Power Delivery ... 106
  - Irrigation ... 108
  - Aspiration ... 108
- A Basic Outline of the Phaco Procedure ... 110
  - Exposure of the Globe ... 110
  - Paracentesis ... 110
  - Scleral Tunnel Incisions ... 111
  - Clear Corneal Incision ... 113
  - Continuous Curvilinear Capsulorrhexis ... 115
  - Hydrodissection ... 117
  - Hydrodelineation ... 118
  - Nuclear Rotation ... 118
  - Instrument Settings for Phacoemulsification ... 118
  - Location of Emulsification ... 119
  - Techniques of Nucleus Disassembly ... 121
  - Strategies for Irrigation and Aspiration ... 125
- Advances in Energy Delivery ... 126
- Alternative Technologies for Nucleus Removal ... 127
  - Laser Photolysis ... 127
  - Fluid-Based Phacolysis ... 127
  - Femtosecond Laser Cataract Extraction ... 127
- Antimicrobial Prophylaxis ... 127
  - Before Surgery ... 127
  - In Surgery ... 128
  - After Surgery ... 129
- Modification of Preexisting Astigmatism ... 130
  - Incision Size and Location ... 130
  - Astigmatic Keratotomy ... 130

    Limbal Relaxing Incisions 130
    Toric IOLs 131
Pars Plana Lensectomy 132
    Indications 132
    Contraindications 132
Intraocular Lens Implantation 132
    Historical Perspectives 132
    Posterior Chamber IOLs 133
    Multifocal Lenses 136
    Pseudoaccommodative Lenses 137
    Other Designs 137
    IOL Power Determination 138
    Techniques of Lens Implantation 138
    Procedure 138
    Relative Contraindications to Lens Implantation 140
Outcomes of Cataract Surgery 141

8 Complications of Cataract Surgery 143
Corneal Complications 146
    Corneal Edema 146
    Incision and Wound Complications 148
    Detachment of Descemet Membrane 149
    Induced Astigmatism 150
    Corneal Melting 150
Other Anterior Segment Complications 151
    Epithelial Downgrowth 151
    Toxic Anterior Segment Syndrome 151
    Shallow or Flat Anterior Chamber 152
    Elevated Intraocular Pressure 154
    Intraoperative Floppy Iris Syndrome 154
    Lens–Iris Diaphragm Retropulsion Syndrome 156
    Iridodialysis and Iris Trauma 157
    Cyclodialysis 157
    Ciliary Block Glaucoma 157
    Chronic Uveitis 158
    Retained Lens Material 159
    Capsular Rupture 160
    Vitreous Prolapse in the Anterior Chamber 162
Complications of IOL Implantation 162
    Decentration and Dislocation 162
    Pupillary Capture 166
    Capsular Block Syndrome 166
    Uveitis-Glaucoma-Hyphema Syndrome 167
    Pseudophakic Bullous Keratopathy 167
    Unexpected Refractive Results 168
    IOL Glare, Dysphotopsia, and Opacification 168

Capsular Opacification and Contraction 169
    Posterior Capsule Opacification 169
    Anterior Capsule Fibrosis and Phimosis 171
    Nd:YAG Laser Capsulotomy 171
Hemorrhage 175
    Systemic Anticoagulation 175
    Retrobulbar Hemorrhage 176
    Hyphema 177
    Suprachoroidal Effusion or Hemorrhage 177
    Expulsive Suprachoroidal Hemorrhage 178
    Delayed Suprachoroidal Hemorrhage 178
Endophthalmitis 179
    Diagnosis 180
    Treatment 180
Retinal Complications 181
    Cystoid Macular Edema 181
    Retinal Light Toxicity 183
    Retinal Detachment 184
Needle Penetration of the Globe 185

9 Preparing for Cataract Surgery in Special Situations 187

Psychosocial Considerations 187
    Claustrophobia 187
    Dementia or Other Mental Disabilities 187
    Patient Communication During Eye Surgery 188
Systemic Considerations 188
    Medical Status 188
    Anticoagulation Therapy or Bleeding Disorders 189
External Ocular Abnormalities 190
    Blepharitis and Acne Rosacea 190
    Keratoconjunctivitis Sicca 190
    Pemphigoid 191
Corneal Conditions 191
    Corneal Disease 191
    Cataract Following Keratoplasty 193
    Cataract Following Refractive Surgery 193
Compromised Visualization of the Lens 194
    Small Pupil 194
    Poor Red Reflex 195
Altered Lens and Zonular Anatomy 195
    Advanced Cataract 195
    Intumescent Cataract 196
    Iris Coloboma and Corectopia 196
    Posterior Polar Cataract 196
    Zonular Dehiscence With Lens Subluxation or Dislocation 197
    Exfoliation Syndrome 199
    Cataract in Aniridia 200

Extremes in Axial Length 200
    High Myopia 200
    High Hyperopia and Nanophthalmos 200
    Hypotony 201
Glaucoma and Cataract 201
    Assessment 201
    Cataract Surgery in the Glaucoma Patient 202
    Cataract Surgery in an Eye With a Functioning Filter. 203
Uveitis 203
Retinal Conditions 204
    Retinal Disease 204
    Cataract Following Pars Plana Vitrectomy 205
    Cataract With Intraocular Silicone Oil 206
Ocular Trauma 206
    Ocular Assessment 206
    Visualization During Surgery 206
    Inflammation 206
    Retained Foreign Matter 207
    Damage to Other Ocular Tissues 207
    Removal of Traumatic Cataract 208
    Vision Rehabilitation 208

Appendix: Surgical Procedures for Extracapsular and Intracapsular
    Cataract Extraction 211
Basic Texts 217
Related Academy Materials 219
Requesting Continuing Medical Education Credit 221
CME Posttest Request Form 223
Study Questions 225
Answer Sheet for Section 11 Study Questions 231
Answers 233
Index 237

General Introduction

The Basic and Clinical Science Course (BCSC) is designed to meet the needs of residents and practitioners for a comprehensive yet concise curriculum of the field of ophthalmology. The BCSC has developed from its original brief outline format, which relied heavily on outside readings, to a more convenient and educationally useful self-contained text. The Academy updates and revises the course annually, with the goals of integrating the basic science and clinical practice of ophthalmology and of keeping ophthalmologists current with new developments in the various subspecialties.

The BCSC incorporates the effort and expertise of more than 80 ophthalmologists, organized into 13 Section faculties, working with Academy editorial staff. In addition, the course continues to benefit from many lasting contributions made by the faculties of previous editions. Members of the Academy's Practicing Ophthalmologists Advisory Committee for Education serve on each faculty and, as a group, review every volume before and after major revisions.

Organization of the Course

The Basic and Clinical Science Course comprises 13 volumes, incorporating fundamental ophthalmic knowledge, subspecialty areas, and special topics:

1. Update on General Medicine
2. Fundamentals and Principles of Ophthalmology
3. Clinical Optics
4. Ophthalmic Pathology and Intraocular Tumors
5. Neuro-Ophthalmology
6. Pediatric Ophthalmology and Strabismus
7. Orbit, Eyelids, and Lacrimal System
8. External Disease and Cornea
9. Intraocular Inflammation and Uveitis
10. Glaucoma
11. Lens and Cataract
12. Retina and Vitreous
13. Refractive Surgery

In addition, a comprehensive Master Index allows the reader to easily locate subjects throughout the entire series.

References

Readers who wish to explore specific topics in greater detail may consult the references cited within each chapter and listed in the Basic Texts section at the back of the book. These references are intended to be selective rather than exhaustive, chosen by the BCSC faculty as being important, current, and readily available to residents and practitioners.

Related Academy educational materials are also listed in the appropriate sections. They include books, online and audiovisual materials, self-assessment programs, clinical modules, and interactive programs.

Study Questions and CME Credit

Each volume of the BCSC is designed as an independent study activity for ophthalmology residents and practitioners. The learning objectives for this volume are given on page 1. The text, illustrations, and references provide the information necessary to achieve the objectives; the study questions allow readers to test their understanding of the material and their mastery of the objectives. Physicians who wish to claim CME credit for this educational activity may do so by following the instructions given at the end of the book.

Conclusion

The Basic and Clinical Science Course has expanded greatly over the years, with the addition of much new text and numerous illustrations. Recent editions have sought to place a greater emphasis on clinical applicability while maintaining a solid foundation in basic science. As with any educational program, it reflects the experience of its authors. As its faculties change and as medicine progresses, new viewpoints are always emerging on controversial subjects and techniques. Not all alternate approaches can be included in this series; as with any educational endeavor, the learner should seek additional sources, including such carefully balanced opinions as the Academy's Preferred Practice Patterns.

The BCSC faculty and staff are continually striving to improve the educational usefulness of the course; you, the reader, can contribute to this ongoing process. If you have any suggestions or questions about the series, please do not hesitate to contact the faculty or the editors.

The authors, editors, and reviewers hope that your study of the BCSC will be of lasting value and that each Section will serve as a practical resource for quality patient care.

Objectives

Upon completion of BCSC Section 11, *Lens and Cataract,* the reader should be able to

- describe the normal anatomy, embryologic development, physiology, and biochemistry of the crystalline lens

- identify congenital anomalies of the lens

- list types of congenital and acquired cataracts

- describe the association of cataracts with aging, trauma, medications, and systemic and ocular diseases

- describe the evaluation and management of patients with cataract and other lens abnormalities

- state the principles of cataract surgery techniques and associated surgical technology

- design an appropriate differential diagnosis and management plan for intraoperative and postoperative complications of cataract surgery

- identify special circumstances in which cataract surgery techniques should be modified and develop appropriate treatment plans

Introduction

The ancient Greeks and Romans believed that the lens was the part of the eye responsible for the faculty of seeing. They theorized that the optic nerves were hollow channels through which "visual spirits" traveled from the brain to meet visual rays from the outside world at the lens, which they thought was located in the center of the globe. The visual information would then flow back to the brain. This concept was known as the *emanation theory of vision*. Celsus (25 BC–AD 50) drew the lens in the center of the globe, with an empty space called the *locus vacuus* anterior to it, in AD 30 (Fig I-1).

These erroneous ideas about lens position and function persisted through the Middle Ages and into the Renaissance, as shown by the drawings of the Belgian anatomist Andreas Vesalius in 1543 (Fig I-2). However, the true position of the crystalline lens was illustrated by the Italian anatomist Fabricius ab Aquapendente in 1600 (Fig I-3); and the Swiss physician Felix Plater (1536–1614) first postulated that the retina, and not the lens, was the part of the eye responsible for sight.

Today, many areas of lens physiology and biochemistry are still subjects of active research. No medical treatment, for example, can yet prevent the formation or progression of cataract in the lens of the otherwise healthy adult eye, and theories about cataract formation and innovative forms of management continue to be controversial. Although various risk factors for cataract development (UV-B radiation, diabetes mellitus, drug use, smoking, alcohol use, severe malnutrition, and oxidative damage) have been identified, data to develop guidelines for reducing the risk of cataract remain inconclusive.

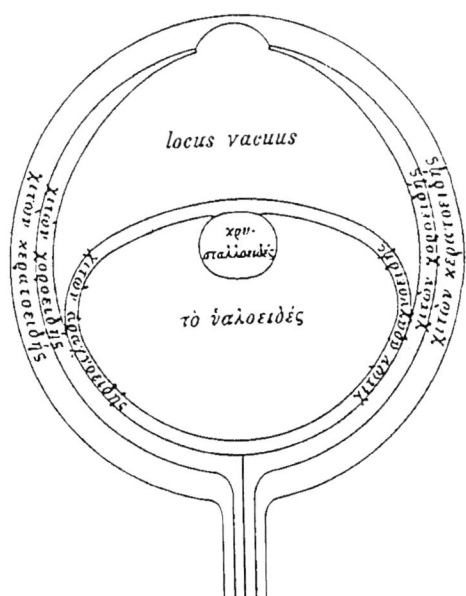

Figure I-1 The eye, after Celsus. *(From Gorin G. History of Ophthalmology. Wilmington: Publish or Perish, Inc; 1982.)*

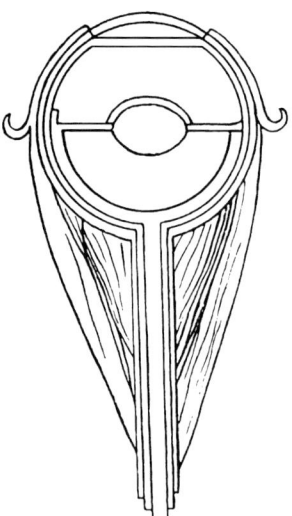

Figure I-2 Schematic eye from *De fabrica corporis humani* of Andreas Vesalius (1514–1564). *(Reproduced by permission from the Ophthalmic Publishing Company. Feigenbaum A. Early history of cataract and the ancient operation for cataract. Am J Ophthalmol. 1960;49:307.)*

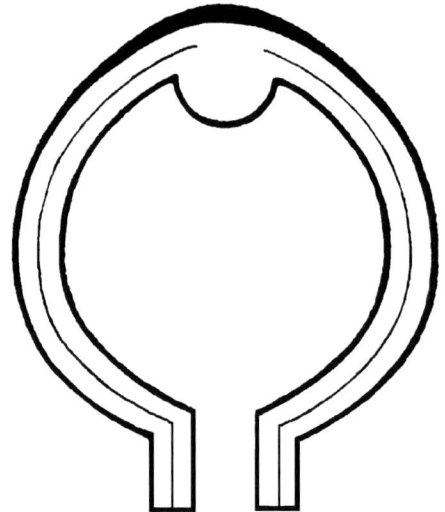

Figure I-3 Sketch from *De oculo* of Fabricius ab Aquapendente (1537–1619), showing correct position of the lens within the eyeball. *(Reproduced by permission from the Ophthalmic Publishing Company. Feigenbaum A. Early history of cataract and the ancient operation for cataract. Am J Ophthalmol. 1960;49:307.)*

Cataract is the leading cause of preventable blindness in the world, whereas cataract extraction with intraocular lens (IOL) implantation is perhaps the most effective surgical procedure in all of medicine. More than 2.4 million cataract procedures are performed on the population older than age 65 in the United States each year, and the visual disability associated with cataract formation accounts for more than 8 million physician office visits each year.

The prevalence of lens disorders and continuing developments in their management make the basic and clinical science of the lens an important subject in ophthalmology training. The goal of Section 11 is to provide a curriculum for the study of all aspects of the lens, including the structure and function of the normal lens, the features of diseases involving the lens, and the surgical management of cataract.

CHAPTER 1
Anatomy

Normal Crystalline Lens

The crystalline lens is a transparent, biconvex structure whose functions are

- to maintain its own clarity
- to refract light
- to provide accommodation

The lens has no blood supply or innervation after fetal development, and it depends entirely on the aqueous humor to meet its metabolic requirements and to carry off its wastes. It lies posterior to the iris and anterior to the vitreous body (Fig 1-1). The lens is suspended in position by the zonules of Zinn, which consist of delicate yet strong fibers that support and attach it to the ciliary body. The lens is composed of the capsule, lens epithelium, cortex, and nucleus (Fig 1-2).

The anterior and posterior poles of the lens are joined by an imaginary line called the *optic axis,* which passes through them. Lines on the surface passing from one pole to the other are referred to as *meridians.* The *equator* of the lens is its greatest circumference.

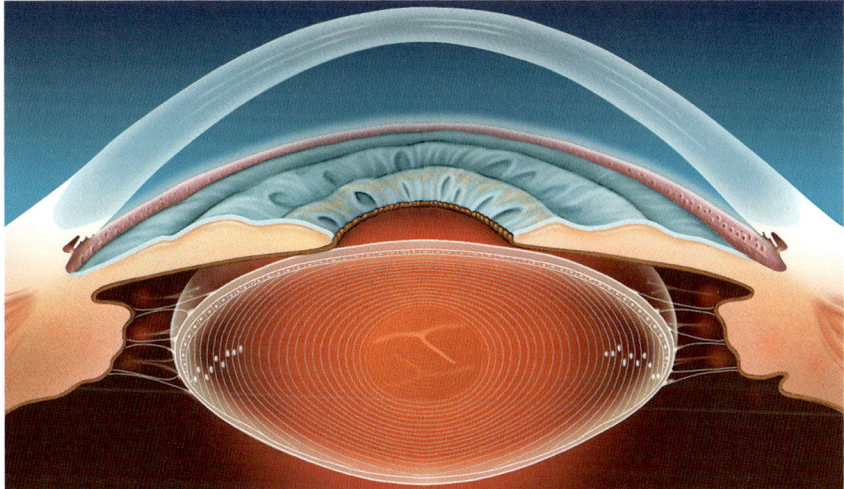

Figure 1-1 Cross section of the human crystalline lens, showing the relationship of the lens to surrounding ocular structures. *(Illustration by Christine Gralapp.)*

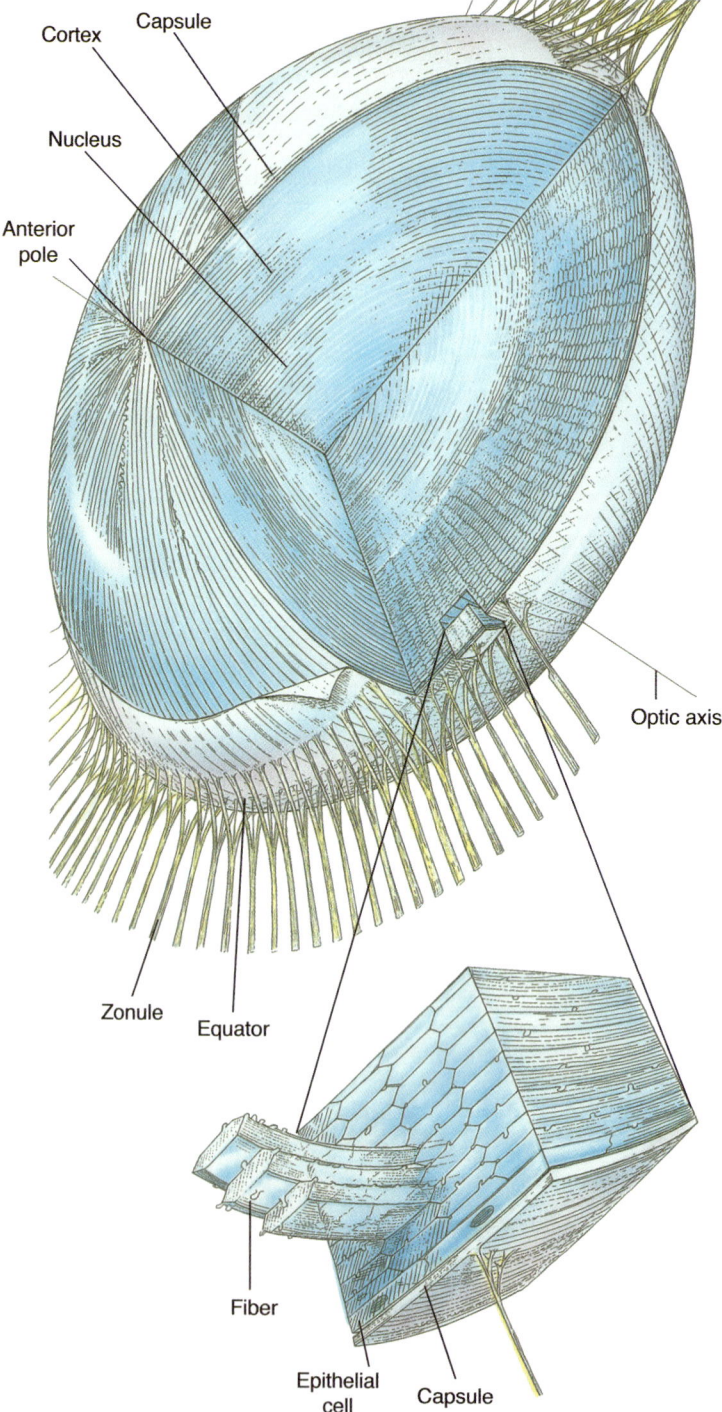

Figure 1-2 Structure of the normal human lens. *(Illustration by Carol Donner. Reproduced with permission from Koretz JF, Handelman GH. How the human eye focuses.* Scientific American. *July 1988:94.)*

The lens is able to refract light because its index of refraction—normally about 1.4 centrally and 1.36 peripherally—is different from that of the aqueous and vitreous that surround it. In its nonaccommodative state, the lens contributes about 15–20 diopters (D) of the approximately 60 D of convergent refractive power of the average human eye; the air–cornea interface provides the rest, or 40–45 D.

The lens continues to grow throughout life. At birth, it measures about 6.4 mm equatorially and 3.5 mm anteroposteriorly and weighs approximately 90 mg. The adult lens typically measures 9 mm equatorially and 5 mm anteroposteriorly and weighs approximately 255 mg. With age, the relative thickness of the cortex increases; the lens also adopts an increasingly curved shape so that older lenses have more refractive power. However, the index of refraction decreases with age, probably as a result of the increasing presence of insoluble protein particles. Thus, the eye may become either more hyperopic or more myopic with age, depending on the balance of these opposing changes.

Capsule

The lens capsule is an elastic, transparent basement membrane composed of type IV collagen laid down by the epithelial cells. The capsule contains the lens substance and is capable of molding it during accommodative changes. The outer layer of the lens capsule, the *zonular lamella,* also serves as the point of attachment for the zonular fibers. The lens capsule is thickest in the anterior and posterior preequatorial zones and thinnest in the region of the central posterior pole, where it may be as thin as 2–4 μm. The anterior lens capsule is considerably thicker than the posterior capsule at birth, and it increases in thickness throughout life (Fig 1-3).

Zonular Fibers

The lens is supported by zonular fibers (also referred to as the *zonules of Zinn*) that consist of microfibrils composed of elastic tissue. These fibers originate from basal laminae of the nonpigmented epithelium of the pars plana and pars plicata of the ciliary body. The zonular fibers insert, in a continuous fashion, on the lens capsule in the equatorial region, anteriorly 1.5 mm onto the anterior lens capsule and posteriorly 1.25 mm onto the posterior lens capsule. With age, the equatorial zonular fibers regress, leaving separate anterior and

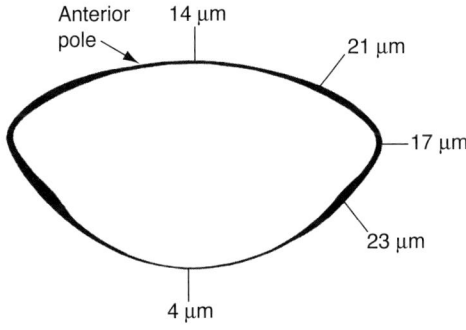

Figure 1-3 Schematic of adult human lens capsule showing relative thickness of capsule in different zones. *(Illustration by Christine Gralapp.)*

posterior layers that appear in a triangular shape on cross section of the zonular ring. The fibers are 5–30 μm in diameter; light microscopy shows them to be eosinophilic structures that have a positive periodic acid–Schiff (PAS) reaction. Ultrastructurally, the strands, or fibrils, composing the fibers are 8–10 nm in diameter, with 12–14 nm of banding.

Lens Epithelium

Immediately behind the anterior lens capsule is a single layer of epithelial cells. These cells are metabolically active and carry out all normal cell activities, including the biosynthesis of DNA, RNA, protein, and lipid. They also generate adenosine triphosphate to meet the energy demands of the lens. The epithelial cells are mitotic, with the greatest activity of premitotic (replicative, or S-phase) DNA synthesis occurring in a ring around the anterior lens known as the *germinative zone*. These newly formed cells migrate toward the equator, where they differentiate into fibers. As the epithelial cells migrate toward the bow region of the lens, they begin the process of terminal differentiation into lens fibers (Fig 1-4).

Perhaps the most dramatic morphologic change occurs when the epithelial cells elongate to form lens fiber cells. This change is associated with a tremendous increase in the mass of cellular proteins in the fiber cell membranes. At the same time, the cells lose organelles, including cell nuclei, mitochondria, and ribosomes. The loss of these organelles is optically advantageous, because light passing through the lens is no longer absorbed or scattered by these structures. However, because these new lens fiber cells lack the metabolic functions previously carried out by the organelles, they are now dependent on glycolysis for energy production (see Chapter 2).

Nucleus and Cortex

No cells are lost from the lens; as new fibers are laid down, they crowd and compact the previously formed fibers, with the older layers located toward the center. The oldest of

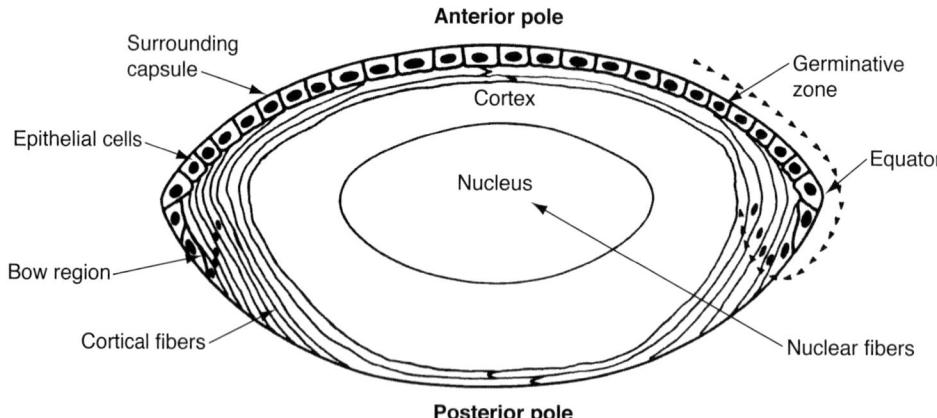

Figure 1-4 Schematic of the mammalian lens in cross section. *Arrowheads* indicate direction of cell migration from the epithelium to the cortex. *(From Anderson RE, ed.* Biochemistry of the Eye. *San Francisco: American Academy of Ophthalmology; 1983;6:112.)*

these, the *embryonic and fetal lens nuclei,* were produced in embryonic life and persist in the center of the lens (see Chapter 3, Fig 3-1). The outermost fibers are the most recently formed and make up the cortex of the lens.

Lens sutures (see Chapter 3, Fig 3-1) are formed by the arrangement of interdigitations of apical cell processes (anterior sutures) and basal cell processes (posterior sutures). Multiple optical zones, as well as the Y-sutures located within the lens nucleus, are visible by slit-lamp biomicroscopy. (See Chapter 3 for further discussion of the embryonic nucleus and lens sutures.) These zones of demarcation occur because strata of epithelial cells with differing optical densities are laid down throughout life. There is no morphologic distinction between the cortex and the nucleus; rather, the transition between these regions is gradual. Although some surgical texts make distinctions between the nucleus, epinucleus, and cortex, these terms relate only to potential differences in the behavior and appearance of the material during surgical procedures.

> Kuszak JR, Clark JI, Cooper KE, et al. Biology of the lens: lens transparency as a function of embryology, anatomy and physiology. In: Albert DM, Jakobiec FA, eds. *Principles and Practice of Ophthalmology.* 2nd ed. Philadelphia: Saunders; 2000:1355–1408.
> Snell RS, Lemp MA. *Clinical Anatomy of the Eye.* 2nd ed. Boston: Blackwell; 1998:197–204.

CHAPTER 2

Biochemistry and Physiology

See BCSC Section 2, *Fundamentals and Principles of Ophthalmology,* for additional discussion of several of the topics discussed in this chapter.

Molecular Biology

Crystallin Proteins

The human lens has a protein concentration of 33% of its wet weight, which is at least twice that of most other tissues. Lens proteins are often divided into 2 groups based on water solubility (Fig 2-1). The water-soluble fraction of the young lens accounts for approximately 80% of lens proteins and consists mainly of a group of proteins called *crystallins*. The crystallins can be subdivided into 2 major groups, α- and β,γ-crystallins.

α-Crystallins represent about one-third of the lens proteins by mass. In their native state, they are the largest of the crystallins, with a molecular mass in the 600–800 range. However, they may associate with other crystallins, yielding complexes greater than 2×10^6. There are 2 α-crystallin subunits, αA and αB, each with a molecular mass of approximately 20, which form heteromeric complexes containing about 30 subunits. The

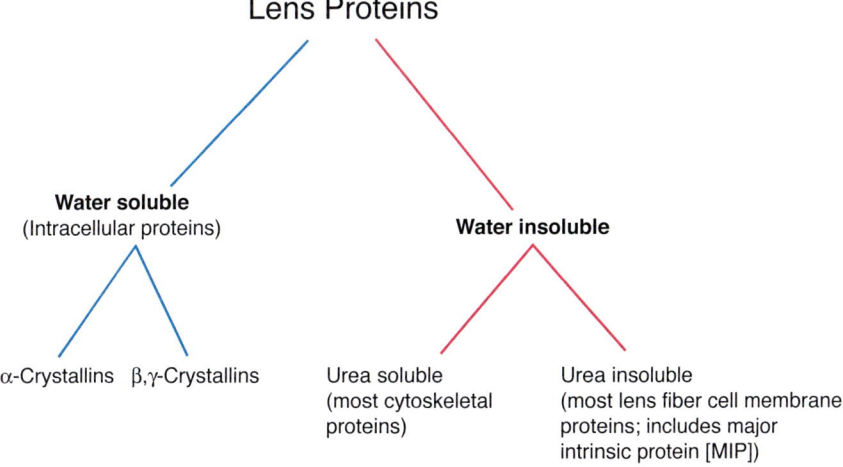

Figure 2-1 Overview of lens proteins.

sequence of the α-crystallins identifies them as members of the family of small "heat-shock proteins." α-Crystallin complexes bind to partially denatured proteins and prevent them from aggregating. Their primary function in lens fiber cells appears to be to inhibit the complete denaturation and insolubilization of the other crystallins.

β,γ-Crystallins are subdivided into 2 groups, based on molecular mass and isoelectric points. The *β-crystallins,* a complex group of oligomers composed of polypeptides, account for 55% (by weight) of the water-soluble proteins in the lens, and they are encoded by 7 genes. β-Crystallins have molecular masses ranging from 23 to 32. The individual polypeptides associate with each other, forming dimers and higher-order complexes in their native state. By gel chromatography, the β-crystallins can be separated into βH (β high molecular mass) and βL (β low molecular mass) fractions.

The *γ-crystallins* are the smallest of the crystallins, with a molecular mass in the range of 20 or less. The native γ-crystallins do not associate with each other or with other proteins and, therefore, have the lowest molecular mass of the crystallin fractions. They make up approximately 15% of adult mammal lens protein. In humans, the gamma family is encoded by 4 genes. X-ray crystallographic studies have determined the 3-dimensional structure of the γ-crystallins to high resolution. Fourfold repetition of a core 3-dimensional structural motif suggests that the β,γ-crystallins might have arisen from double duplication and fusion of a gene for a 40-residue polypeptide. The basic structure of the β-crystallins and γ-crystallins has been maintained through hundreds of millions of years of vertebrate evolution.

Membrane Structural Proteins and Cytoskeletal Proteins

The water-insoluble fraction of lens proteins can be further separated into 2 fractions, 1 soluble and 1 insoluble in 8 M urea. The *urea-soluble fraction* of the young lens contains cytoskeletal proteins that provide the structural framework of the lens cells. Microfilaments and microtubules found in lens cells are similar to those found in other cell types. However, the lens contains 2 types of intermediate filaments that are unusual: one class is made from the protein *vimentin,* which is not usually found in epithelial cells; the other class, the *beaded filaments,* is composed of the proteins phakinin and filensin, which are specific to the lens. Genetic disruption of the structure of the beaded filaments leads to disruption of the structure of the lens fiber cells and formation of a cataract.

The *urea-insoluble fraction* of the young lens contains the plasma membranes of the lens fiber cells. Several proteins are associated with these fiber cell plasma membranes. One makes up nearly 50% of the membrane proteins and is known as the *major intrinsic protein (MIP;* also known as *aquaporin 0),* a member of a class of proteins called *aquaporins.* Other members of the aquaporin family are found throughout the body, where they serve predominantly as water channels. MIP first appears in the lens just as the fibers begin to elongate. With age, this protein, which has a molecular mass of 28, undergoes proteolytic cleavage, forming a protein fragment with a molecular mass of 22. The relative proportions of these 2 proteins become about equal at 20–30 years of age. As expected, the protein with molecular mass of 22 predominates in the nucleus.

Increase of Water-Insoluble Proteins With Age

Over time, lens proteins aggregate to form very large particles that become water insoluble and that scatter light, thus increasing the opacity of the lens. However, it should be noted that the water-insoluble protein fraction increases with age even if the lens remains relatively transparent. Conversion of the water-soluble proteins into water-insoluble proteins appears to be a natural process in lens fiber maturation, but it may occur to excess in cataractous lenses.

In cataracts with significant browning of the lens nucleus *(brunescent cataracts),* the increase in the amount of water-insoluble protein correlates well with the degree of opacification. In markedly brunescent cataracts, as much as 90% of the nuclear proteins may be in the insoluble fraction. Associated oxidative changes occur, including protein-to-protein and protein-to-glutathione disulfide bond formation. These changes result in decreased levels of the reduced form of glutathione and increased levels of glutathione disulfide (oxidized glutathione) in the cytoplasm of the nuclear fiber cells. It is the general view that glutathione is essential to maintain a reducing environment in the lens cytoplasm. Depletion of the reduced form of glutathione accelerates protein cross-linking, protein aggregation, and light scattering. In addition to the increased formation of disulfide bonds, nuclear proteins are highly cross-linked by nondisulfide bonds. This insoluble protein fraction contains yellow-to-brown pigments that are found in higher concentration in nuclear cataracts. Increased fluorescence is generated by the nondisulfide cross-links that form in brunescent nuclear cataracts.

> Hejtmancik JF, Piatigorsky J. Lens proteins and their molecular biology. In: Albert DM, Jakobiec FA, eds. *Principles and Practice of Ophthalmology.* 2nd ed. Philadelphia: Saunders; 2000:1409–1428.

Carbohydrate Metabolism

The goal of lens metabolism is the maintenance of lens transparency. In the lens, energy production largely depends on glucose metabolism. Glucose enters the lens from the aqueous both by *simple diffusion* and by a mediated transfer process called *facilitated diffusion.* Most of the glucose transported into the lens is phosphorylated to glucose-6-phosphate (G6P) by the enzyme hexokinase. This reaction is 70–100 times slower than that of other enzymes involved in lens glycolysis and is, therefore, rate-limited in the lens. Once formed, G6P enters 1 of 2 metabolic pathways: anaerobic glycolysis or the hexose monophosphate (HMP) shunt (Fig 2-2).

The more active of these 2 pathways is anaerobic glycolysis, which provides most of the high-energy phosphate bonds required for lens metabolism. Substrate-linked phosphorylation of adenosine diphosphate (ADP) to adenosine triphosphate (ATP) occurs at 2 steps along the pathway from glucose metabolism to lactate. The rate-limiting step in the glycolytic pathway itself is at the level of the enzyme phosphofructokinase, which is regulated through feedback control by metabolic products of the glycolytic pathway. This pathway is much less efficient than aerobic glycolysis, because only 2 net molecules of

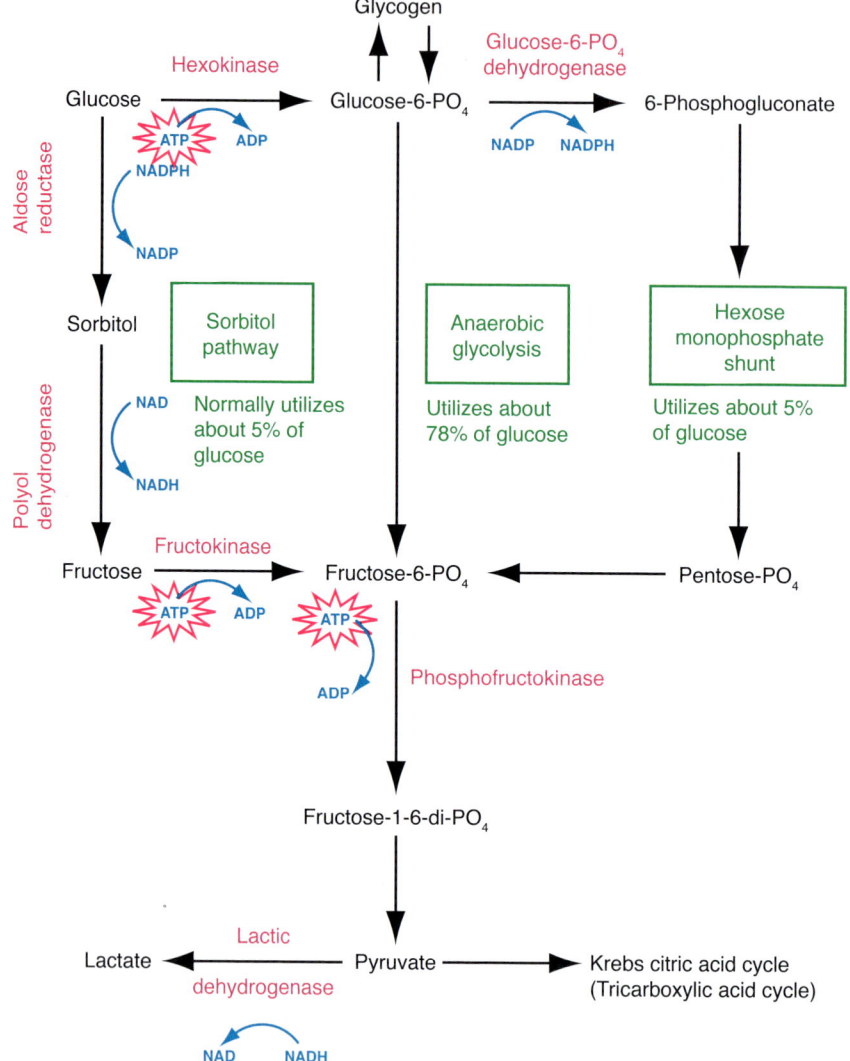

Figure 2-2 Simplified scheme of glucose metabolism in the lens. *(Adapted with permission from Hart WM Jr, ed.* Adler's Physiology of the Eye: Clinical Application. *9th ed. St Louis: Mosby; 1992:362.)*

ATP are produced for each glucose molecule utilized, whereas aerobic glycolysis produces an additional 36 molecules of ATP from each glucose molecule metabolized in the citric acid cycle (oxidative metabolism). Because of the low oxygen tension in the lens, only about 3% of the lens glucose passes through the Krebs citric acid cycle (tricarboxylic acid cycle) to produce ATP; however, even this low level of aerobic metabolism produces approximately 25% of the lens ATP.

That the lens is not dependent on oxygen is demonstrated by its ability to sustain normal metabolism in a nitrogen environment. Provided with ample glucose, the anoxic in vitro lens remains completely transparent, has normal levels of ATP, and maintains its ion and amino acid pump activities. However, when deprived of glucose, the lens cannot maintain these functions and becomes hazy after several hours, even in the presence of oxygen.

The less active pathway for utilization of G6P in the lens is the HMP shunt, also known as the *pentose phosphate pathway*. Approximately 5% of lens glucose is metabolized by this route, although the pathway is stimulated in the presence of elevated levels of glucose. HMP shunt activity is higher in the lens than in most tissues, but the role of the HMP shunt is far from established. As in other tissues, the HMP shunt may provide NADPH (the reduced form of nicotinamide adenine dinucleotide phosphate [NADP]) for fatty acid biosynthesis and ribose for nucleotide biosynthesis. It does provide the NADPH necessary for glutathione reductase and aldose reductase activities in the lens. The carbohydrate products of the HMP shunt enter the glycolytic pathway and are metabolized to lactate.

The glucose that is not phosphorylated to G6P enters the sorbitol pathway, which is yet another pathway for lens glucose metabolism, or it is converted into gluconic acid. Aldose reductase is the key enzyme in this pathway and has been found to play a pivotal role in the development of "sugar" cataracts. The Michaelis constant (K_m) of aldose reductase for glucose is approximately 700 times that for hexokinase. Because the affinity is actually the inverse of K_m, aldose reductase has a very low affinity for glucose compared to hexokinase. Less than 4% of lens glucose is normally converted to sorbitol.

As previously noted, the hexokinase reaction is rate-limited in phosphorylating glucose in the lens and is inhibited by the feedback mechanisms of the products of glycolysis. Therefore, when glucose increases in the lens, as occurs in hyperglycemic states, the sorbitol pathway is activated relatively more than the glycolytic pathway; and sorbitol accumulates. Sorbitol is metabolized to fructose by the enzyme polyol dehydrogenase. Unfortunately, this enzyme has a relatively low affinity (high K_m), meaning that considerable sorbitol will accumulate before being further metabolized. This characteristic, combined with the poor permeability of the lens to sorbitol, results in retention of sorbitol in the lens.

A high NADPH:NADH ratio drives the reaction in the direction of sorbitol accumulation. The accumulation of NADP that occurs as a consequence of activation of the sorbitol pathway may cause the HMP shunt stimulation that is observed in the presence of an elevated lens glucose level. In addition to sorbitol, fructose levels increase in a lens incubated in a high-glucose environment. Together, the 2 sugars increase the osmotic pressure within the lens, drawing in water. At first, the energy-dependent pumps of the lens are able to compensate, but ultimately they are overwhelmed. The result is swelling of the fibers, disruption of the normal cytoskeletal architecture, and opacification of the lens.

The pivotal role of aldose reductase in cataractogenesis in animals is apparent from studies of the development of cataract in various hyperglycemic animal species. Those species that have high aldose reductase activities develop lens opacities, whereas those lacking aldose reductase do not. In addition, specific inhibitors of this enzymatic activity, applied either systemically or topically to 1 eye, decrease the rate of onset and the severity of glucose cataracts in experimental studies.

Oxidative Damage and Protective Mechanisms

Free radicals are generated in the course of normal cellular metabolic activities and may also be produced by external agents such as radiant energy. These free radicals are highly reactive and can damage lens fibers. Peroxidation of lens fiber plasma or plasma membrane lipids has been suggested as a factor contributing to lens opacification. In the process of lipid peroxidation, the oxidizing agent removes a hydrogen atom from the polyunsaturated fatty acid, forming a fatty acid radical, which, in turn, attacks molecular oxygen, forming a lipid peroxy radical. This reaction may propagate the chain leading to the formation of lipid peroxide (LOOH), which, in turn, may eventually react to yield malondialdehyde (MDA), a potent cross-linking agent. It has been hypothesized that MDA cross-reacts with membrane lipids and proteins, rendering them incapable of performing their normal functions.

Because oxygen tension in and around the lens is normally low, free radical reactions may not involve molecular oxygen; instead, the free radicals may react directly with molecules. DNA is easily damaged by free radicals. Although some of the damage to the lens is reparable, some of it may be permanent. Free radicals can also attack the proteins or membrane lipids in the lens cortex. No repair mechanisms are known to ameliorate such damage. In lens fibers, where protein synthesis no longer takes place, free radical damage may lead to polymerization and cross-linking of lipids and proteins, resulting in an increase in the water-insoluble protein content.

The lens is equipped with several enzymes that protect against free radical or oxidative damage. These include glutathione peroxidase, catalase, and superoxide dismutase. Superoxide dismutase catalyzes the destruction of the superoxide anion, O_2^-, and produces hydrogen peroxide: $2O_2^- + 2H^+ \rightarrow H_2O_2 + O_2$. Catalase breaks down the peroxide by the reaction: $2H_2O_2 \rightarrow 2H_2O + O_2$. Glutathione peroxidase catalyzes the reaction: $2GSH + LOOH \rightarrow GSSG + LOH + H_2O$. The glutathione disulfide (GSSG) is then reconverted to glutathione (GSH) by glutathione reductase, using the pyridine nucleotide NADPH provided by the HMP shunt as the reducing agent: $GSSG + NADPH + H^+ \rightarrow 2GSH + NADP^+$. Thus, glutathione acts indirectly as a major free radical scavenger in the lens. In addition, both vitamin E and ascorbic acid are present in the lens. Each of these substances can act as a free radical scavenger and thus protect against oxidative damage.

Increasing oxygen levels within the eye may have a role in cataract formation. Exposure of the lens to an increased level of oxygen during long-term hyperbaric oxygen therapy leads to a myopic shift, increased opacification of the lens nucleus, and, in many cases, the formation of nuclear cataracts. The lens is also exposed to increased levels of oxygen acutely during retinal surgery and chronically following vitrectomy. Because vitrectomy is associated with very high rates of nuclear cataract formation, it has been suggested that the low oxygen level existing around the lens protects it from oxidative damage and that loss of the gel structure of the vitreous body increases exposure of the lens to oxygen and the risk of nuclear cataracts.

> Andley UP, Liang JJN, Lou MF. Biochemical mechanisms of age-related cataract. In: Albert DM, Jakobiec FA, eds. *Principles and Practice of Ophthalmology*. 2nd ed. Philadelphia: Saunders; 2000:1428–1449.

Beebe DC. Lens. In: Kaufman PL, Alm A, eds. *Adler's Physiology of the Eye: Clinical Application*. 10th ed. St Louis: Mosby; 2003:117–158.

Bloemendal H, de Jong W, Jaenicke R, Lubsen NH, Slingsby C, Tardieu A. Aging and vision: structure, stability and function of lens crystallins. *Prog Biophys Mol Biol*. 2004;86(3):407–485.

Jaffe NS, Horwitz J. Evolution and molecular biology of lens proteins. In: Podos SM, Yanoff M, eds. *Textbook of Ophthalmology, Vol 3: Lens and Cataract*. New York: Gower Medical Publishing; 1992.

Lens Physiology

Throughout life, lens epithelial cells at the equator divide and develop into lens fibers, resulting in continual growth of the lens (see Chapter 1, Figs 1-2 and 1-4). The lens cells with the highest metabolic rate are found in the epithelium and the outer cortex. These superficial cells utilize oxygen and glucose for the active transport of electrolytes, carbohydrates, and amino acids into the lens. Because the lens is avascular, the task of maintaining transparency poses several challenges. The older cells, found toward the center of the lens, must be able to communicate with the superficial cells and the environment outside the lens. This communication is accomplished through low-resistance gap junctions that facilitate the exchange of small molecules from cell to cell. Lens fiber cells also have abundant water channels in their membranes, made from MIP. It is not yet certain whether MIP serves primarily as a water channel, as an adhesion molecule that minimizes the extracellular space between fiber cells, or as both in the lens. Minimizing the extracellular space between fiber cells is important to reduce the scattering of light as it passes through the lens.

Maintenance of Lens Water and Cation Balance

Perhaps the most important aspect of lens physiology is the mechanism that controls water and electrolyte balance, which is critical to lens transparency. Because transparency is highly dependent on the structural and macromolecular components of the lens, perturbation of cellular hydration can readily lead to opacification. It is noteworthy that disruption of water and electrolyte balance is not a feature of nuclear cataracts. In cortical cataracts, however, the water content rises significantly.

The normal human lens contains approximately 66% water and 33% protein, and this amount changes very little with aging. The lens cortex is more hydrated than the lens nucleus. About 5% of the lens volume is the water found between the lens fibers in the extracellular spaces. Within the lens, sodium and potassium concentrations are maintained at 20 millimolar (mM) and 120 mM, respectively.

Lens epithelium: site of active transport

The lens is dehydrated and has higher levels of potassium ions (K^+) and amino acids than the surrounding aqueous and vitreous. Conversely, the lens contains lower levels of sodium ions (Na^+), chloride ions (Cl^-), and water than the surrounding environment. The cation balance between the inside and outside of the lens is the result both of the permeability properties of the lens cell membranes and of the activity of the sodium pumps that reside within the cell membranes of the lens epithelium and each lens fiber. The sodium pumps function by pumping sodium ions out while taking potassium ions in. This mechanism depends on the breakdown of adenosine triphosphate (ATP) and is regulated by the enzyme Na^+,K^+-ATPase. This balance is easily disrupted by the specific ATPase inhibitor ouabain. Inhibition of Na^+,K^+-ATPase leads to loss of cation balance and elevated water content in the lens.

Pump–leak theory

The combination of active transport and membrane permeability is often referred to as the pump–leak system of the lens (Fig 2-3). According to the *pump–leak theory*, potassium and various other molecules, such as amino acids, are actively transported into the lens via the epithelium anteriorly. They then diffuse out with the concentration gradient through the back of the lens, where there are no active-transport mechanisms. Conversely, sodium flows in through the back of the lens with the concentration gradient and then is actively exchanged for potassium by the epithelium. In support of this theory, an anteroposterior gradient was found for both ions: potassium was concentrated in the anterior lens; sodium, in the posterior lens. Most of the Na^+,K^+-ATPase activity is found in the lens epithelium and the superficial cortical fiber cells. The active-transport mechanisms are lost if the capsule and attached epithelium are removed from the lens but not if the capsule

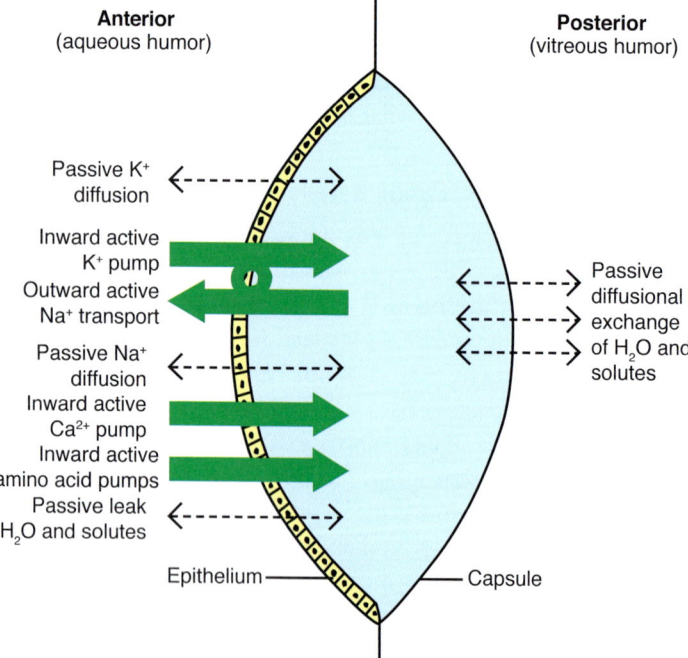

Figure 2-3 The pump–leak hypothesis of pathways of solute movement in the lens. The major site of active-transport mechanisms is the anterior epithelium, whereas passive diffusion occurs over both surfaces of the lens. *(Modified with permission from Paterson CA, Delamere NA. The lens. In: Hart WM Jr, ed. Adler's Physiology of the Eye. 9th ed. St Louis: Mosby; 1992:365.)*

alone is removed by enzymatic degradation with collagenase. These findings support the hypothesis that the epithelium is the primary site for active transport in the lens.

Accommodation and Presbyopia

Accommodation, the mechanism by which the eye changes focus from distant to near images, is produced by a change in lens shape resulting from the action of the ciliary muscle on the zonular fibers. The lens substance is most malleable during childhood and the young-adult years, progressively losing its ability to change shape with age.

According to the Helmholtz theory of accommodation, most of the accommodative change in lens shape occurs at the central anterior lens surface. The central anterior capsule is thinner than the peripheral capsule (see Chapter 1, Fig 1-3), and the anterior zonular fibers insert slightly closer to the visual axis than do the posterior zonular fibers, resulting in a central anterior bulge with accommodation. The curvature of the posterior lens surface changes minimally with accommodation. The central posterior capsule, which is the thinnest area of the capsule, maintains the same curvature regardless of zonular tension.

The ciliary muscle is a ring-shaped muscle that, on contraction, has the opposite effect from that intuitively expected of a sphincter. When a sphincter muscle contracts, it usually tightens its grip. However, when the ciliary muscle contracts, the diameter of the muscle ring is reduced, thereby relaxing the tension on the zonular fibers and allowing the lens to become more spherical. Thus, when the ciliary muscle contracts, the axial thickness of the lens increases, the diameter of the lens decreases, and the dioptric power of the eye increases, producing accommodation. When the ciliary muscle relaxes, the zonular tension increases, the lens flattens, and the dioptric power of the eye decreases (Table 2-1).

The accommodative response may be stimulated by the known or apparent size and distance of an object or by blur, chromatic aberration, or a continual oscillation of ciliary tone. Accommodation is mediated by the parasympathetic fibers of cranial nerve III (oculomotor). Parasympathomimetic drugs (eg, pilocarpine) induce accommodation, whereas parasympatholytic medications (eg, atropine) block accommodation. Drugs that relax the ciliary muscle are called *cycloplegics*.

The *amplitude of accommodation* is the amount of change in the eye's refractive power that is produced by accommodation. It diminishes with age and may be affected

Table 2-1 Changes With Accommodation

	With Accommodation	Without Accommodation
Ciliary muscle action	Contraction	Relaxation
Ciliary ring diameter	Decreases	Increases
Zonular tension	Decreases	Increases
Lens shape	More spherical	Flatter
Lens equatorial diameter	Decreases	Increases
Axial lens thickness	Increases	Decreases
Central anterior lens capsule curvature	Steepens	Flattens
Central posterior lens capsule curvature	Minimal change	Minimal change
Lens dioptric power	Increases	Decreases

by some medications and diseases. Adolescents generally have 12–16 D of accommodation, whereas adults at age 40 have 4–8 D. After age 50, accommodation decreases to less than 2 D.

Hardening of the lens with age is the principal cause of this loss of accommodation, which is called *presbyopia*. Once an individual is about 40 years of age or older, the rigidity of the lens nucleus reduces accommodation, as contraction of the ciliary muscle no longer results in increased convexity and dioptric power of the anterior surface of the lens. This decreased accommodation then becomes clinically significant. Studies have shown that, throughout life, the hardness or stiffness of the human lens increases more than 1000-fold. (See also BCSC Section 3, *Clinical Optics*.) Researchers continue to explore other factors that may contribute to presbyopia, such as changes in lens dimensions, in the elasticity of the lens capsule, and in the geometry of zonular attachments with age.

> Glasser A, Kaufman PL. Accommodation and presbyopia. In: Kaufman PL, Alm A, eds. *Adler's Physiology of the Eye: Clinical Application*. 10th ed. St Louis: Mosby; 2003:197–233.
>
> Heys KR, Cram SL, Truscott RJ. Massive increase in the stiffness of the human lens nucleus with age: the basis for presbyopia? *Mol Vis*. 2004;10:956–963.
>
> Winkler J, Wirbelauer C, Frank V, Laqua H. Quantitative distribution of glycosaminoglycans in young and senile (cataractous) anterior lens capsules. *Exp Eye Res*. 2001;72(3):311–318.

This chapter was prepared with the assistance of David Beebe, PhD.

CHAPTER 3

Embryology and Developmental Defects

Normal Development

The formation of the human crystalline lens begins very early in embryogenesis (Fig 3-1). At approximately 25 days of gestation, 2 lateral evaginations, called the *optic vesicles,* form from the forebrain, or diencephalon. As the optic vesicles enlarge and extend laterally, they become closely apposed and adherent to the *surface ectoderm,* a single layer of cuboidal cells, in 2 patches on either side of the head.

Lens Placode

The ectoderm cells that overlie the optic vesicles become columnar at approximately 27 days of gestation. This area of thickened cells is called the *lens placode*. Growth factors of the *bone morphogenetic protein (BMP)* family are required for the formation of the lens placode and for subsequent lens formation.

Lens Pit

The lens pit appears at 29 days of gestation as an indentation (infolding) of the lens placode. The lens pit deepens and invaginates to form the lens vesicle.

Lens Vesicle

As the lens pit continues to invaginate, the stalk of cells connecting it to the surface ectoderm degenerates by programmed cell death (apoptosis), thereby separating the lens cells from the surface ectoderm. The resultant sphere, a single layer of cuboidal cells encased in a basement membrane (the *lens capsule*), is called the *lens vesicle*. At the time of its formation at 30 days' gestation, the lens vesicle is approximately 0.2 mm in diameter.

Because the lens vesicle was formed through a process of invagination of the surface ectoderm, the apices of the cuboidal cells are oriented toward the lumen of the lens vesicle, with the base of each cell attached to the capsule around the periphery of the vesicle. At the same time that the lens vesicle is forming, the optic vesicle is invaginating to form the 2-layered *optic cup*.

22 • Lens and Cataract

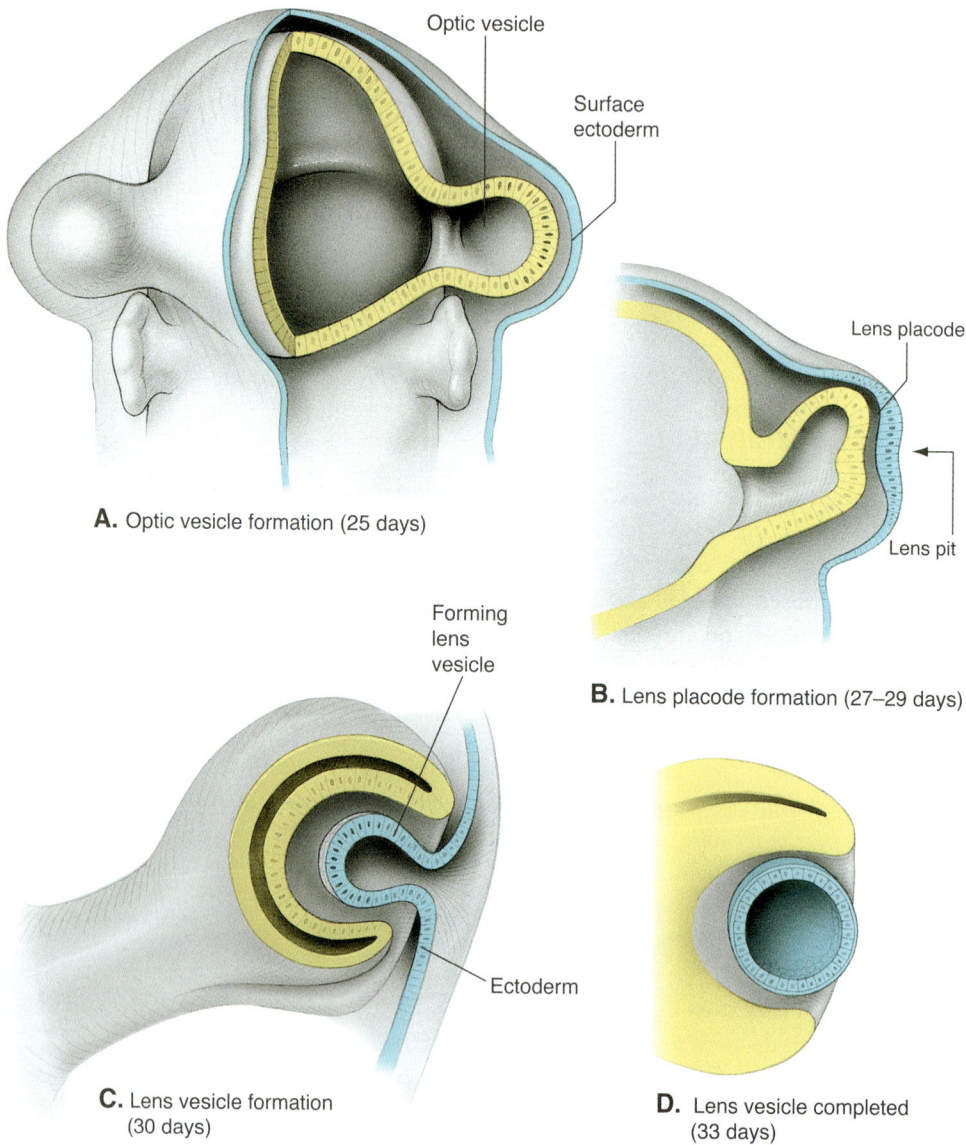

Figure 3-1 Embryologic development of the lens. See text for detailed description of artwork. *(Illustration by Christine Gralapp.)* *(Continued on next page)*

Primary Lens Fibers and the Embryonic Nucleus

The cells in the posterior layer of the lens vesicle stop dividing and begin to elongate. As they elongate, they begin to fill the lumen of the lens vesicle. At approximately 40 days of gestation, the lumen of the lens vesicle is obliterated. The elongated cells are called the *primary lens fibers*. As the fiber cells mature, their nuclei and other membrane-bound organelles undergo degradation, a process that reduces light scattering. The primary lens fibers make up the embryonic nucleus that will ultimately occupy the central area of the lens in adult life.

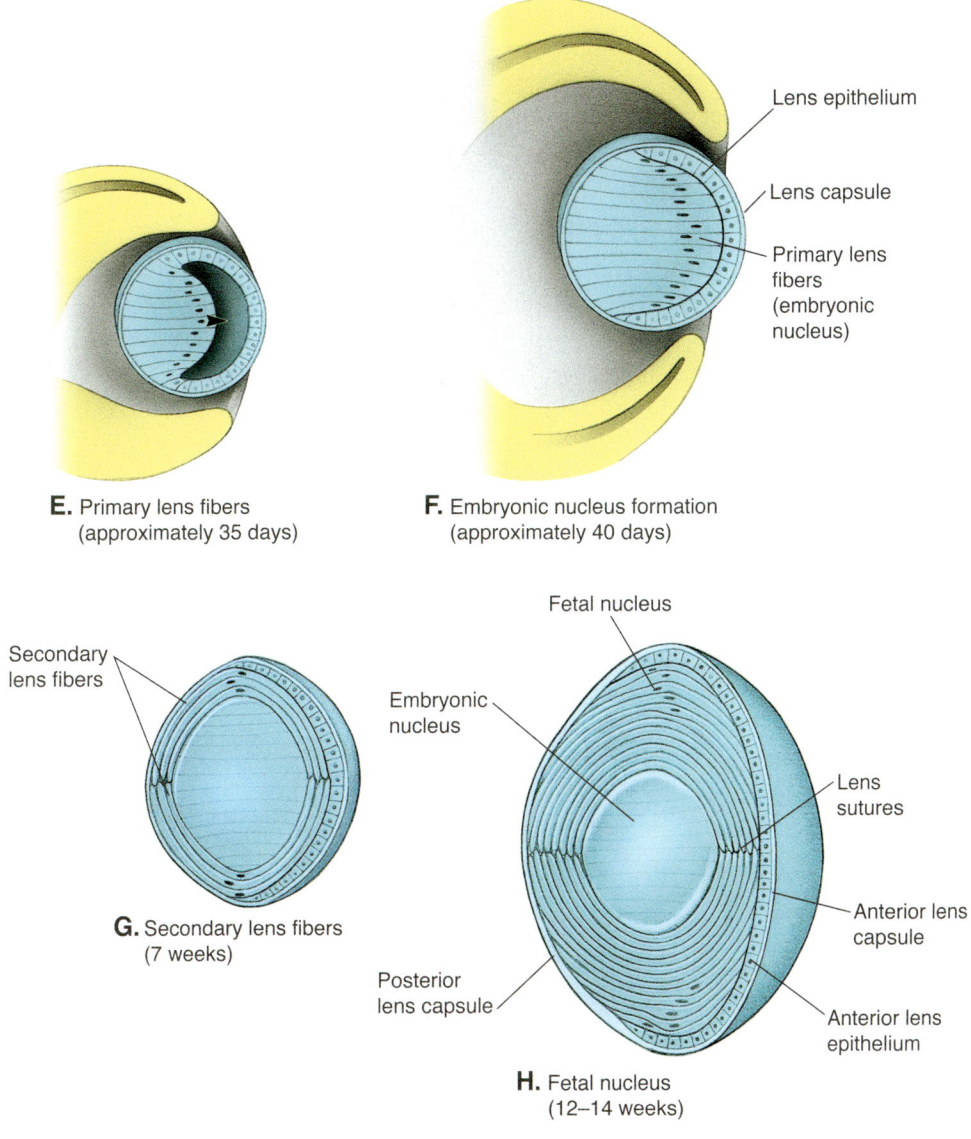

Figure 3-1 *(continued)*

The cells of the anterior lens vesicle remain as a monolayer of cuboidal cells, the *lens epithelium*. Subsequent growth of the lens is due to proliferation within the epithelium. The *lens capsule* develops as a basement membrane elaborated by the lens epithelium anteriorly and by lens fibers posteriorly.

Secondary Lens Fibers

After they proliferate, the epithelial cells near the lens equator elongate to form secondary lens fibers. The anterior aspect of each developing lens fiber extends anteriorly beneath the lens epithelium, toward the anterior pole of the lens. The posterior aspect of each developing lens fiber extends posteriorly along the capsule, toward the posterior pole of the lens. In this manner, new lens fibers are continually formed, layer upon layer. As each secondary fiber cell detaches from the capsule, it loses its nucleus and membrane-bound organelles. The secondary lens fibers formed between 2 and 8 months of gestation make up the *fetal nucleus.*

Lens Sutures and the Fetal Nucleus

As lens fibers grow anteriorly and posteriorly, a pattern emerges where the ends of the fibers meet and interdigitate with the ends of fibers arising on the opposite side of the lens, near the anterior and posterior poles. These patterns of cell association are known as *sutures*. Y-shaped sutures are recognizable at about 8 weeks of gestation, with an erect Y-suture appearing anteriorly and an inverted Y-suture posteriorly (Fig 3-2). As the lens fibers continue to form and the lens continues to grow, the pattern of lens sutures becomes increasingly complex, resulting in 12 or more suture branches in the adult eye. The influences responsible for the precise formation and changing organization of the suture pattern remain a mystery.

The human lens weighs approximately 90 mg at birth, and it increases in mass at the rate of about 2 mg per year as new fibers form throughout life. The central, or oldest, lens

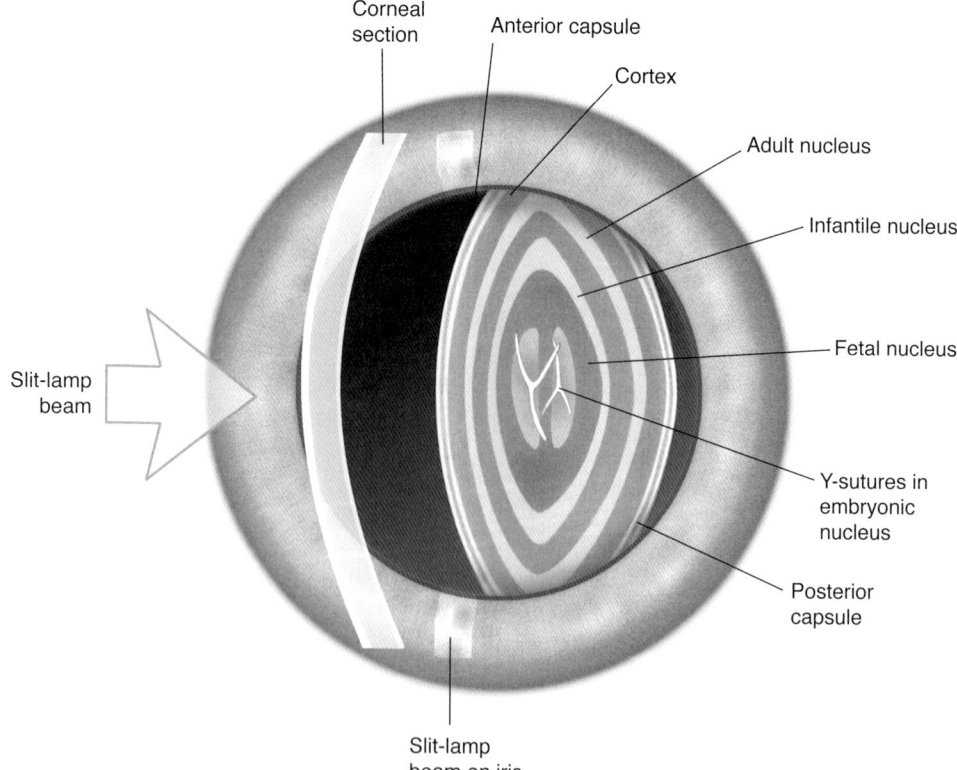

Figure 3-2 Y-shaped sutures, formed during embryogenesis, are visible within the adult lens with the use of the slit lamp. *(Illustration by Christine Gralapp.)*

fibers gradually become less malleable, and the lens nucleus becomes more rigid. This process progressively reduces the amplitude of accommodation.

Tunica Vasculosa Lentis

At about 1 month of gestation, the hyaloid artery, which enters the eye at the optic disc, branches to form a network of capillaries, the tunica vasculosa lentis, on the posterior surface of the lens capsule (Fig 3-3). These capillaries grow toward the equator of the lens, where they anastomose with a second network of capillaries, called the *anterior pupillary membrane*, which derives from the ciliary veins and which covers the anterior surface of the lens. At approximately 9 weeks' gestation, the capillary network surrounding the lens is fully developed; it disappears by an orderly process of programmed cell death shortly before birth. Sometimes a remnant of the tunica vasculosa lentis persists as a small opacity or strand, called a *Mittendorf dot* (discussed later), on the posterior aspect of the lens. In other eyes, remnants of the pupillary membrane are often visible as pupillary strands.

Zonules of Zinn

Experimental evidence suggests that the zonular fibers are secreted by the ciliary epithelium, although how these fibers insert into the lens capsule is not known. The zonular fibers begin to develop at the end of the third month of gestation.

Duke-Elder S, ed. *System of Ophthalmology*. St Louis: Mosby; 1973:127–137.

Kuszak JR, Clark JI, Cooper KE, et al. Biology of the lens: lens transparency as a function of embryology, anatomy, and physiology. In: Albert DM, Jakobiec FA, eds. *Principles and Practice of Ophthalmology*. 2nd ed. Philadelphia: Saunders; 2000:1355–1408.

Kuszak JR, Costello MJ. Embryology and anatomy of human lenses. In: Tasman W, Jaeger EA, eds. *Duane's Clinical Ophthalmology*. Vol 1. Philadelphia: Lippincott; 2002:1–20.

Streeten BW. Zonular apparatus; Worgul BV. The lens. In: Jakobiec FA, ed. *Ocular Anatomy, Embryology, and Teratology*. Philadelphia: Harper & Row; 1982:331–353.

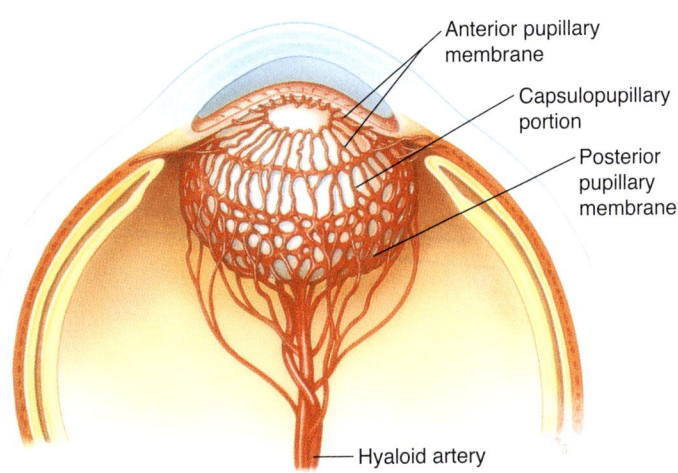

Figure 3-3 Components of the tunica vasculosa lentis. *(Illustration by Christine Gralapp.)*

Congenital Anomalies and Abnormalities

Congenital Aphakia

The lens is absent in congenital aphakia, a very rare anomaly. Two forms of congenital aphakia have been described. In *primary aphakia*, the lens placode fails to form from the surface ectoderm in the developing embryo. In *secondary aphakia*, the more common type, the developing lens is spontaneously absorbed. Both forms of aphakia are usually associated with other malformations of the eye.

Lenticonus and Lentiglobus

Lenticonus is a localized, cone-shaped deformation of the anterior or posterior lens surface (Fig 3-4). Posterior lenticonus is more common than anterior lenticonus and is usually unilateral and axial in location. Anterior lenticonus is often bilateral and may be associated with Alport syndrome.

In lentiglobus, the localized deformation of the lens surface is spherical. Posterior lentiglobus is more common than anterior lentiglobus and is often associated with posterior pole opacities that vary in density.

Retinoscopy through the center of the lens reveals a distorted and myopic reflex in both lenticonus and lentiglobus. These deformations can also be seen in the red reflex, where, by retroillumination, they appear as an "oil droplet." (This condition should not be confused with the "oil droplet" cataract of galactosemia, which is discussed in Chapter 4.) The posterior bulging may progress with initial worsening of the myopia, followed by opacification of the defect. Surrounding cortical lamellae may also opacify.

Lens Coloboma

A lens coloboma is an anomaly of lens shape (Fig 3-5). Lens colobomas can be classified into 2 types: *primary coloboma*, a wedge-shaped defect or indentation of the lens periphery that occurs as an isolated anomaly; and *secondary coloboma*, a flattening or indentation of the lens periphery caused by the lack of ciliary body or zonular development. Lens colobomas are typically located inferiorly and may be associated with colobomas of the

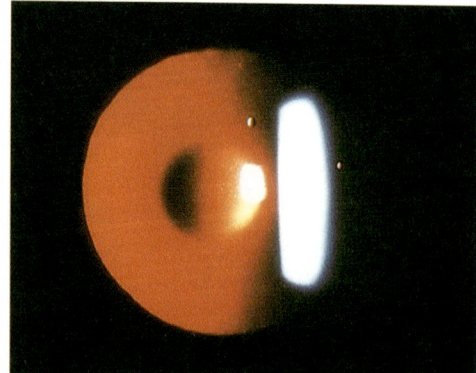

Figure 3-4 Posterior lenticonus as viewed by retroillumination.

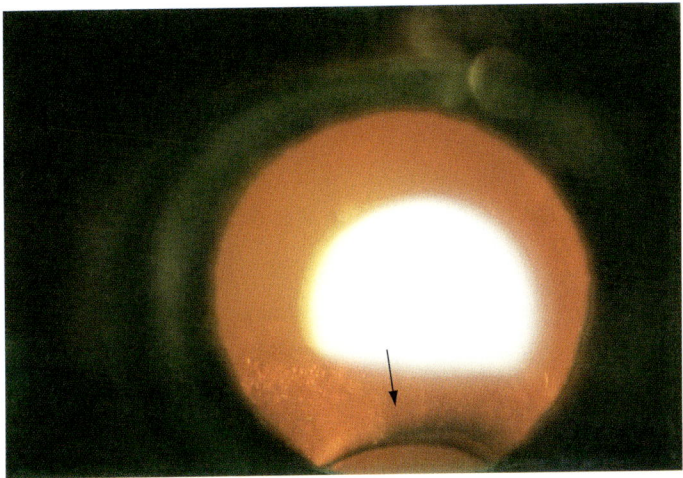

Figure 3-5 Coloboma of the lens *(arrow)* as viewed by retroillumination.

uvea. Cortical lens opacification or thickening of the lens capsule may appear adjacent to the coloboma. The zonular attachments in the region of the coloboma usually are weakened or absent.

Mittendorf Dot

Mittendorf dot, mentioned earlier in this chapter, is a common anomaly observed in many healthy eyes. A small, dense white spot generally located inferonasal to the posterior pole of the lens, a Mittendorf dot is a remnant of the posterior pupillary membrane of the tunica vasculosa lentis. It marks the place where the hyaloid artery came into contact with the posterior surface of the lens in utero. Sometimes a Mittendorf dot is associated with a fibrous tail or remnant of the hyaloid artery projecting into the vitreous body.

Epicapsular Star

Another very common remnant of the tunica vasculosa lentis is an epicapsular star (Fig 3-6). As its name suggests, this anomaly is a star-shaped distribution of tiny brown or golden flecks on the central anterior lens capsule. It may be unilateral or bilateral.

Peters Anomaly

Peters anomaly is part of a spectrum of disorders known as *anterior segment dysgenesis syndrome,* also referred to as *neurocristopathy* or *mesodermal dysgenesis.* (See also BCSC Section 6, *Pediatric Ophthalmology and Strabismus.*) Peters anomaly is characterized by a central or paracentral corneal opacity (leukoma) associated with thinning or absence of adjacent endothelium and Descemet membrane. In normal ocular development, the lens vesicle separates from the surface ectoderm (the future corneal epithelium) at about 33 days' gestation. Peters anomaly is typically linked with the absence of this separation. It is often associated with mutations in or deletion of 1 allele of the genes normally involved

28 • Lens and Cataract

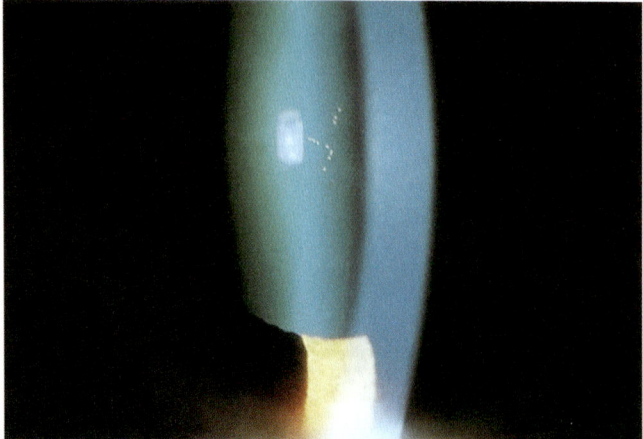

Figure 3-6 Epicapsular star.

in anterior segment development, including the transcription factors *PAX6*, *PITX2*, and *FOXC1*. Patients with Peters anomaly may also display the following lens anomalies:

- adhesions between lens and cornea
- anterior cortical or polar cataract
- a misshapen lens displaced anteriorly into the pupillary space and the anterior chamber
- microspherophakia

Microspherophakia

Microspherophakia is a developmental abnormality in which the lens is small in diameter and spherical. The entire lens equator can be visualized at the slit lamp when the pupil is widely dilated (Fig 3-7). The spherical shape of the lens results in increased refractive power, which causes the eye to be highly myopic.

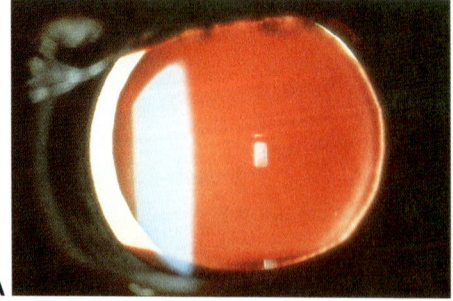
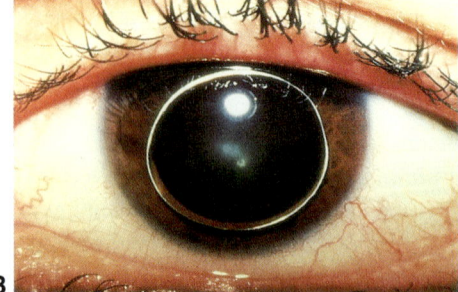

Figure 3-7 Microspherophakia. **A,** When the pupil is dilated, the entire lens equator can be seen at the slit lamp. **B,** Anterior dislocation of a microspherophakic lens. *(Part A courtesy of Karla J. Johns, MD.)*

Faulty development of the secondary lens fibers during embryogenesis is believed to be the cause of microspherophakia. Microspherophakia is most often seen as a part of Weill-Marchesani syndrome, but it may also occur as an isolated hereditary abnormality or, occasionally, in association with Peters anomaly, Marfan syndrome, Alport syndrome, Lowe syndrome, or congenital rubella. Individuals with Weill-Marchesani syndrome commonly have small stature, short and stubby fingers, and broad hands with reduced joint mobility. Weill-Marchesani syndrome is usually inherited as an autosomal recessive trait.

The spherical lens can block the pupil, causing secondary angle-closure glaucoma. Use of miotics aggravates this condition by increasing pupillary block and allowing additional forward lens displacement. Cycloplegics are the medical treatment of choice to break an attack of angle-closure glaucoma in patients with microspherophakia, because they decrease pupillary block by tightening the zonular fibers, decreasing the anteroposterior lens diameter, and pulling the lens posteriorly. A laser iridotomy may also be useful in relieving angle closure in patients with microspherophakia. (See also BCSC Section 10, *Glaucoma*.)

Aniridia

Aniridia is an uncommon panocular syndrome in which the most dramatic manifestation is partial or nearly complete absence of the iris (Fig 3-8). Aniridia has been linked to the loss of 1 allele of the *PAX6* gene, a transcription factor that is important for the development and function of the cornea, lens, and retina. Associated findings include corneal pannus and epitheliopathy, glaucoma, foveal and optic nerve hypoplasia, and nystagmus. Aniridia is almost always bilateral. Two-thirds of cases are familial; one-third of cases are sporadic. Sporadic cases of aniridia are associated with a high incidence of Wilms tumor and the WAGR complex (Wilms tumor, aniridia, genitourinary malformations, and mental retardation).

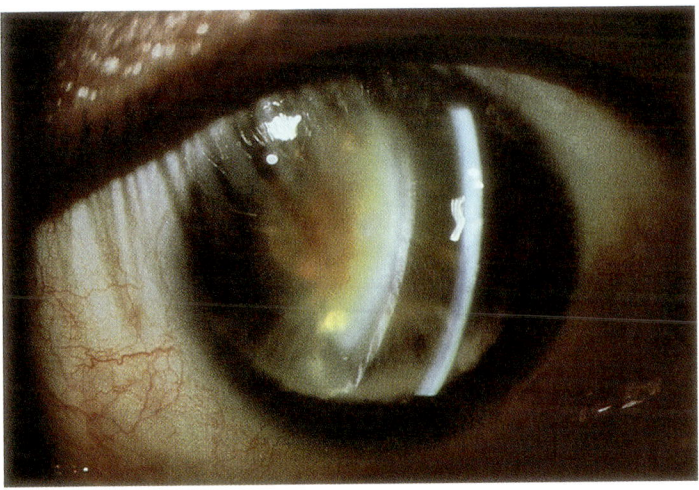

Figure 3-8 Cataract in aniridic patient.

Anterior and posterior polar lens opacities may be present at birth in patients with aniridia. Cortical, subcapsular, and lamellar opacities develop in 50%–85% of patients within the first 2 decades of life. The lens opacities may progress and further impair vision. Poor zonular integrity and ectopia lentis have also been reported in patients with aniridia.

Congenital Cataract

Cataracts that are present at birth or that develop within the first year of life are called *congenital* or *infantile* cataracts. Because some lens opacities escape detection at birth and are noted only on later examination, these terms are used interchangeably by many physicians. In this book, we will use the term *congenital cataract* for both categories of lens opacities. These cataracts are fairly common, occurring in 1 of every 2000 live births, and cover a broad spectrum of severity. Whereas some lens opacities do not progress and are visually insignificant, others can produce profound visual impairment.

Congenital cataracts may be unilateral or bilateral. They can be classified by morphology, presumed or defined genetic etiology, presence of specific metabolic disorders, or associated ocular anomalies or systemic findings (Table 3-1). In general, approximately one-third of congenital cataracts are a component of a more extensive syndrome or disease (eg, cataract resulting from congenital rubella syndrome), one-third occur as an isolated inherited trait, and one-third result from undetermined causes. Metabolic diseases tend to be more commonly associated with bilateral cataracts. (For a discussion of the systemic evaluation of patients with congenital cataracts, see BCSC Section 6, *Pediatric Ophthalmology and Strabismus*.) Congenital cataracts occur in a variety of morphologic configurations, including lamellar, polar, sutural, coronary, cerulean, nuclear, capsular, complete, and membranous.

Lamellar

Of the congenital cataracts, lamellar, or zonular, cataracts are the most common type (Fig 3-9). They are characteristically bilateral and symmetric, and their effect on visual acuity varies with the size and density of the opacity. Lamellar cataracts may be inherited as an autosomal dominant trait. In some cases, they may occur as a result of a transient toxic influence during embryonic lens development. The earlier this toxic influence occurs, the smaller and deeper is the resulting lamellar cataract.

Lamellar cataracts are opacifications of specific layers or zones of the lens. Clinically, the cataract is visible as an opacified layer that surrounds a clearer center and is itself surrounded by a layer of clear cortex. Viewed from the front, the lamellar cataract has a disc-shaped configuration. Often, additional arcuate opacities within the cortex straddle the equator of the lamellar cataract; these horseshoe-shaped opacities are called *riders*.

Polar

Polar cataracts are lens opacities that involve the subcapsular cortex and capsule of the anterior or posterior pole of the lens. *Anterior polar cataracts* are usually small, bilateral, symmetric, nonprogressive opacities that do not impair vision (Fig 3-10). They are frequently inherited in an autosomal dominant pattern. Anterior polar cataracts are sometimes seen

Table 3-1 Etiology of Pediatric Cataracts

Bilateral cataracts
Idiopathic
Hereditary cataracts (autosomal dominant most common; also autosomal recessive or X-linked)
Genetic and metabolic diseases
    Down syndrome
    Hallermann-Streiff syndrome
    Lowe syndrome
    Galactosemia
    Marfan syndrome
    Trisomy 13–15
    Hypoglycemia
    Alport syndrome
    Myotonic dystrophy
    Fabry disease
    Hypoparathyroidism
    Conradi syndrome
Maternal infection
    Rubella
    Cytomegalovirus
    Varicella
    Syphilis
    Toxoplasmosis
Ocular anomalies
    Aniridia
    Anterior segment dysgenesis syndrome
Toxic
    Corticosteroids
    Radiation (may also be unilateral)

Unilateral cataracts
Idiopathic
Ocular anomalies
    Persistent fetal vasculature (PFV)
    Anterior segment dysgenesis
    Posterior lenticonus
    Posterior pole tumors
Traumatic (rule out child abuse)
Rubella
Masked bilateral cataract

in association with other ocular abnormalities, including microphthalmos, persistent pupillary membrane, and anterior lenticonus. They do not require treatment but often cause anisometropia.

Posterior polar cataracts generally produce more visual impairment than do anterior polar cataracts because they tend to be larger and are positioned closer to the nodal point of the eye. Capsular fragility has been reported. Posterior polar cataracts are usually stable but occasionally progress. They may be familial or sporadic. Familial posterior polar cataracts are usually bilateral and inherited in an autosomal dominant pattern. Sporadic posterior polar cataracts are often unilateral and may be associated with remnants of the tunica vasculosa lentis or with an abnormality of the posterior capsule such as lenticonus or lentiglobus.

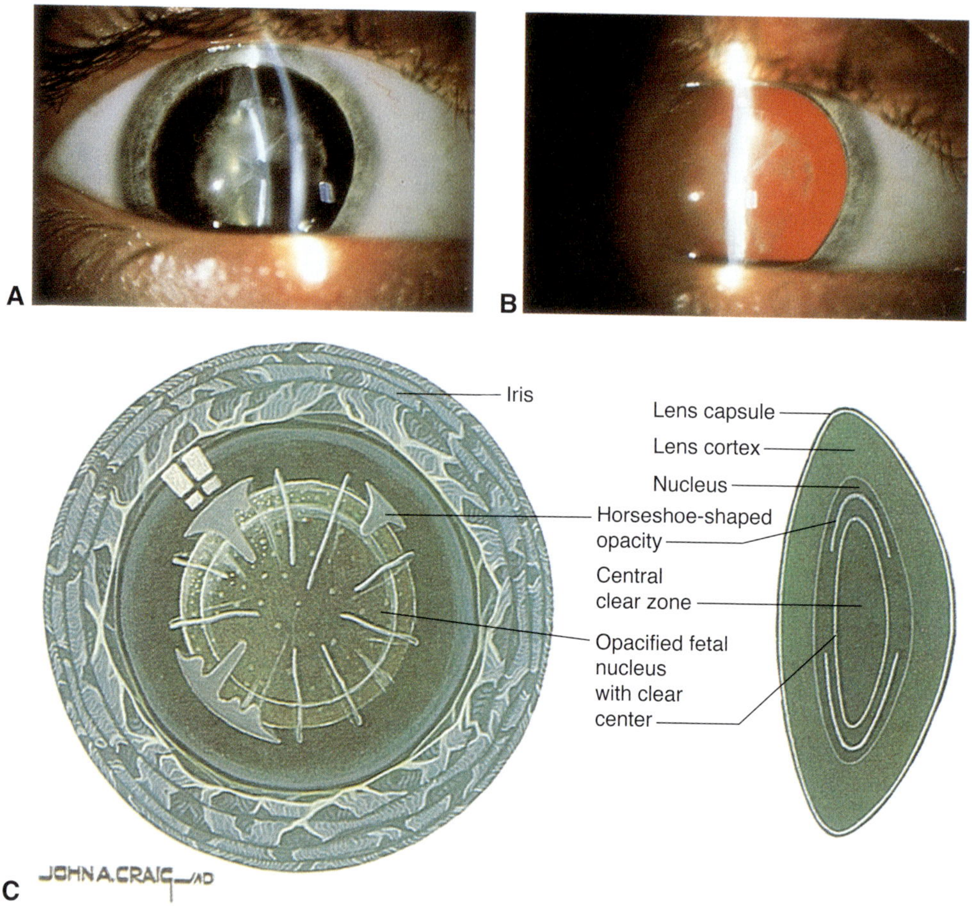

32 • Lens and Cataract

Figure 3-9 **A,** Lamellar cataract. **B,** Lamellar cataract viewed by retroillumination. **C,** Schematic of lamellar cataract. *(Courtesy of CIBA Pharmaceutical Co., division of CIBA-GEIGY Corp. Reproduced with permission from* Clinical Symposia. *Illustration by John A. Craig.)*

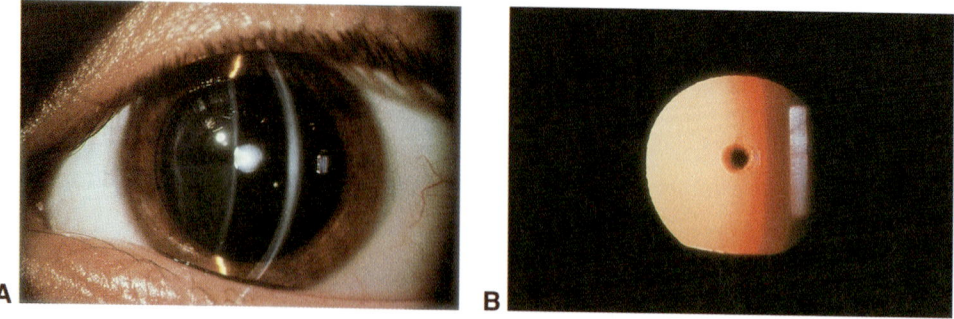

Figure 3-10 **A,** Anterior polar cataract. **B,** Anterior polar cataract viewed by retroillumination.

Sutural

The sutural, or stellate, cataract is an opacification of the Y-sutures of the fetal nucleus. It usually does not impair vision (Fig 3-11). These opacities often have branches or knobs projecting from them. Sutural cataracts are bilateral and symmetric and are frequently inherited in an autosomal dominant pattern.

Coronary

Coronary cataracts are so named because they consist of a group of club-shaped cortical opacities that are arranged around the equator of the lens like a crown, or corona. They cannot be seen unless the pupil is dilated, and they usually do not affect visual acuity. Coronary cataracts are often inherited in an autosomal dominant pattern.

Cerulean

Cerulean cataracts are small bluish opacities located in the lens cortex (Fig 3-12); hence, they are also known as *blue-dot cataracts*. They are nonprogressive and usually do not cause visual symptoms.

Nuclear

Congenital nuclear cataracts are opacities of the embryonic nucleus alone or of both embryonic and fetal nuclei (Fig 3-13). They are usually bilateral, with a wide spectrum of severity. Lens opacification may involve the complete nucleus or be limited to discrete layers within the nucleus. Eyes with congenital nuclear cataracts tend to be microphthalmic, and they are at increased risk of developing aphakic glaucoma.

Capsular

Capsular cataracts are small opacifications of the lens epithelium and anterior lens capsule that spare the cortex. They are differentiated from anterior polar cataracts by their

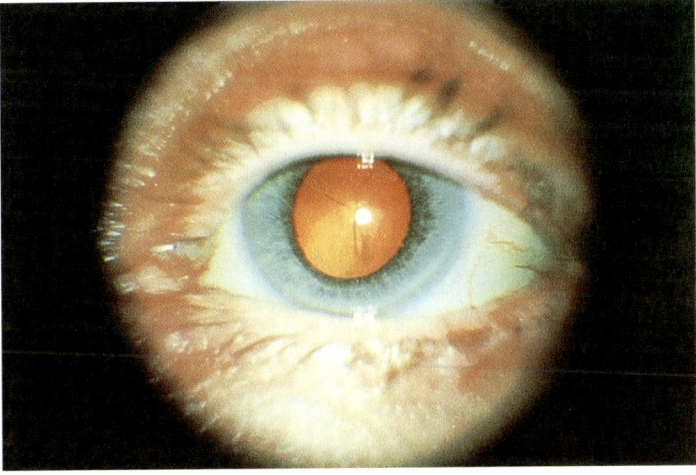

Figure 3-11 Sutural cataract.

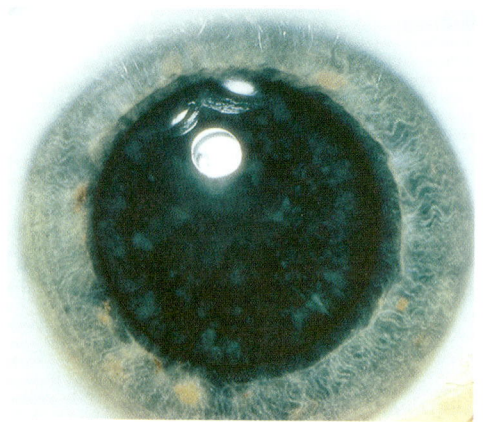

Figure 3-12 A cerulean cataract consists of small bluish opacities in the cortex. *(Courtesy of Karla J. Johns, MD.)*

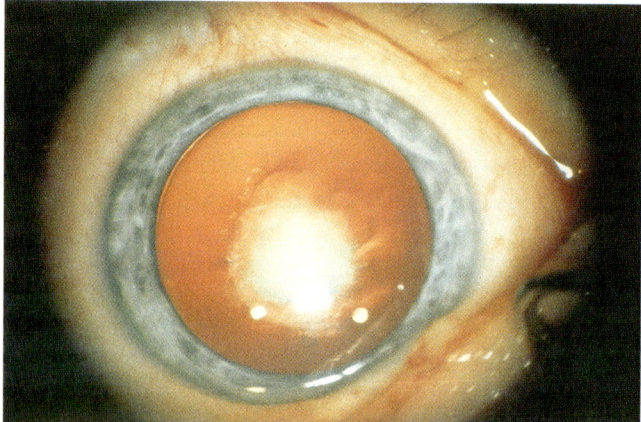

Figure 3-13 Congenital nuclear cataract. *(Reproduced from Day SH.* Understanding and Preventing Amblyopia. Eye Care Skills for the Primary Care Physician Series *[slidescript]. San Francisco: American Academy of Ophthalmology; 1987.)*

protrusion into the anterior chamber. Capsular cataracts generally do not adversely affect vision.

Complete

With complete, or total, cataract, all of the lens fibers are opacified. The red reflex is completely obscured, and the retina cannot be seen with either direct or indirect ophthalmoscopy. Some cataracts may be subtotal at birth and progress rapidly to become complete cataracts. Complete cataracts may be unilateral or bilateral, and they produce profound visual impairment.

Membranous

Membranous cataracts occur when lens proteins are resorbed from either an intact or a traumatized lens, allowing the anterior and posterior lens capsules to fuse into a dense white membrane (Fig 3-14). The resulting opacity and lens distortion generally cause significant visual disability.

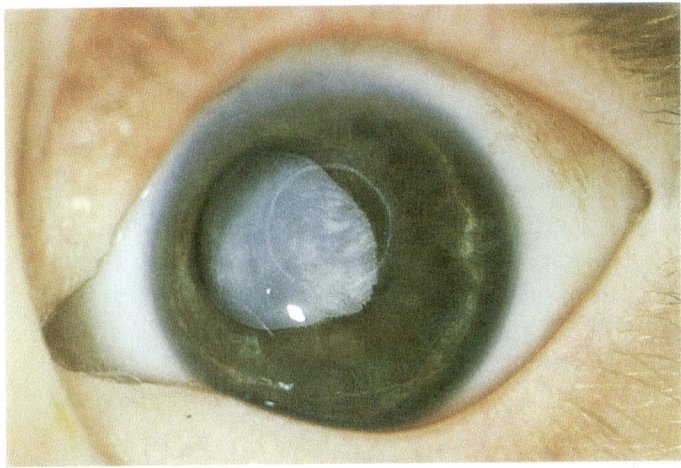

Figure 3-14 Membranous cataract.

Rubella

Maternal infection with the rubella virus, an RNA togavirus, can cause fetal damage, especially if the infection occurs during the first trimester of pregnancy. Systemic manifestations of congenital rubella infection include cardiac defects, deafness, and mental disability.

Cataracts resulting from *congenital rubella syndrome* are characterized by pearly white nuclear opacifications. Sometimes the entire lens is opacified (complete cataract), and the cortex may liquefy. Histologically, lens-fiber nuclei are retained deep within the lens substance. Live virus particles may be recovered from the lens as late as 3 years after the patient's birth. Cataract removal may be complicated by excessive postoperative inflammation caused by release of these live virus particles. (See also BCSC Section 6, *Pediatric Ophthalmology and Strabismus*.)

Other ocular manifestations of congenital rubella syndrome include diffuse pigmentary retinopathy, microphthalmos, glaucoma, and transient or permanent corneal clouding. Although congenital rubella syndrome may cause cataract or glaucoma, both conditions are usually not present simultaneously in the same eye.

Developmental Defects

Ectopia Lentis

Ectopia lentis is a displacement of the lens that may be congenital, developmental, or acquired. A *subluxated* lens is partially displaced from its normal position but remains in the pupillary area. A *luxated,* or *dislocated,* lens is completely displaced from the pupil, implying separation of all zonular attachments. Findings associated with lens subluxation include decreased vision, marked astigmatism, monocular diplopia, and iridodonesis (tremulous iris). Potential complications of ectopia lentis include cataract and displacement of the lens into the anterior chamber or into the vitreous. Dislocation into the anterior chamber or pupil may cause pupillary block and angle-closure glaucoma. Dislocation of the lens posteriorly into the vitreous cavity often has no adverse sequelae aside from a profound change in refractive error.

Trauma is the most common cause of acquired lens displacement. Nontraumatic ectopia lentis is commonly associated with Marfan syndrome, homocystinuria, aniridia, and congenital glaucoma. Less frequently, it appears with Ehlers-Danlos syndrome, hyperlysinemia, and sulfite oxidase deficiency. Ectopia lentis may occur as an isolated anomaly (simple ectopia lentis), usually inherited as an autosomal dominant trait. Ectopia lentis can also be associated with pupillary abnormalities in the ocular syndrome ectopia lentis et pupillae (discussed later in this chapter).

Marfan syndrome

Marfan syndrome is a heritable disorder with ocular, cardiac, and skeletal manifestations. Though usually inherited as an autosomal dominant trait, the disorder appears with no family history in approximately 15% of cases. Marfan syndrome is caused by mutations in the fibrillin gene on chromosome 15. Affected individuals are tall, with arachnodactyly (Fig 3-15A) and chest wall deformities. Associated cardiac abnormalities include dilated aortic root and mitral valve prolapse.

From 50% to 80% of patients with Marfan syndrome exhibit ectopia lentis (Fig 3-15B). The lens subluxation tends to be bilateral and symmetric (usually superior and temporal), but variations do occur. The zonular attachments commonly remain intact but become stretched and elongated. Ectopia lentis in Marfan syndrome is probably congenital in most cases. Progression of lens subluxation is observed in some patients over time, but in many patients the lens position remains stable.

Ocular abnormalities associated with Marfan syndrome include axial myopia and an increased risk of retinal detachment. Patients with Marfan syndrome may develop pupillary block glaucoma if the lens dislocates into the pupil or anterior chamber. Open-angle glaucoma may also occur. In addition, children with lens subluxation may develop amblyopia if their refractive error shows significant asymmetry or remains uncorrected in early childhood.

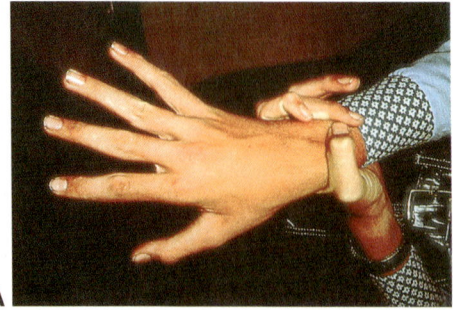
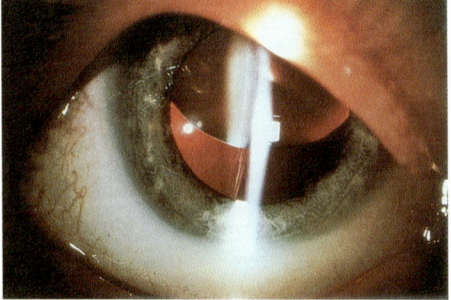

Figure 3-15 Marfan syndrome. **A,** Arachnodactyly in a patient with Marfan syndrome. **B,** Subluxated lens in Marfan syndrome. *(Part A courtesy of Karla J. Johns, MD.)*

Spectacle or contact lens correction of the refractive error provides satisfactory visual acuity in most cases. Pupillary dilation is sometimes helpful. The clinician may refract both the phakic and the aphakic portions of the pupil to determine the optimum visual acuity. A reading add is often necessary because the subluxated lens lacks sufficient accommodation.

In some cases, adequate visual acuity cannot be obtained with spectacle or contact lens correction, and removal of the lens may be indicated. Lens extraction—either extracapsular or intracapsular—in patients with Marfan syndrome is associated with a high rate of complications such as vitreous loss and complex retinal detachment. (Intracapsular and extracapsular cataract extraction are discussed in detail in Chapter 7.) Improved results have been reported with lensectomy using vitrectomy instrumentation, although the long-term results are not yet known.

Homocystinuria

Homocystinuria is an autosomal recessive disorder, an inborn error of methionine metabolism. Serum levels of homocystine and methionine are elevated. Affected individuals are healthy at birth but develop seizures and osteoporosis and soon display mental disability. They are usually tall and have light-colored hair. Patients with homocystinuria are also prone to thromboembolic episodes, and surgery and general anesthesia are thought to increase the risk of thromboembolism.

Lens dislocation in homocystinuria tends to be bilateral and symmetric. The dislocation appears in infancy in approximately 30% of affected individuals, and by the age of 15 years, it appears in 80% of those affected. The lenses are usually subluxated inferiorly and nasally, but variations have been reported. Because zonular fibers of the lens are known to have a high concentration of cysteine, deficiency of cysteine is thought to disturb normal zonular development; affected fibers tend to be brittle and easily disrupted. Studies of infants with homocystinuria treated with a low-methionine, high-cysteine diet and vitamin supplementation with the coenzyme pyridoxine (vitamin B_6) have shown that this therapy holds promise in reducing the incidence of ectopia lentis. (See also BCSC Section 6, *Pediatric Ophthalmology and Strabismus*.)

Hyperlysinemia

Hyperlysinemia, an inborn error of metabolism of the amino acid lysine, is associated with ectopia lentis. Affected individuals also show mental disability and muscular hypotony.

Genetic Contributions to Age-Related Cataracts

Studies of identical and fraternal twins and of familial associations suggest that a large proportion of the risk of age-related cataracts is inherited. It is estimated that inheritance accounts for more than 50% of the risk of cortical cataracts. Recent studies identified mutations in the gene associated with congenital and age-related cortical cataracts, *EPHA2*, which has been mapped to 1p36. This is the first gene known to cause hereditary, nonsyndromic age-related cortical cataracts, although mutations at this locus account for only a small fraction of cortical opacities. Similarly, 35%–50% of the risk of nuclear cataracts can be traced to inheritance. Identification of the genes associated with increased risk of cortical and nuclear cataracts is important, because understanding the biochemical pathways in which they function may suggest ways to slow the progression or prevent the development of age-related cataracts in a large number of cases.

> Jun G, Guo H, Klein BE, et al. EPHA2 is associated with age-related cortical cataract in mice and humans. *PLoS Genet.* 2009;5(7):e1000584.
>
> Shiels A, Bennett TM, Knopf HL, et al. The EPHA2 gene is associated with cataracts linked to chromosome 1p. *Mol Vis.* 2008;14:2042–2055.

Ectopia Lentis et Pupillae

In the autosomal recessive disorder ectopia lentis et pupillae, the lens and the pupil are displaced in opposite directions. The pupil is irregular, usually slit shaped, and displaced from the normal position. The dislocated lens may bisect the pupil or may be completely luxated from the pupillary space. This disorder is usually bilateral but not symmetric. Characteristically, the iris dilates poorly. Associated ocular anomalies include severe axial myopia, retinal detachment, enlarged corneal diameter, cataract, and abnormal iris transillumination.

Persistent Fetal Vasculature

Persistent fetal vasculature (PFV), also known as *persistent hyperplastic primary vitreous (PHPV)*, is a congenital, nonhereditary ocular malformation that frequently involves the lens. In 90% of patients, it is unilateral. A white, fibrous retrolental tissue is present, often in association with posterior cortical opacification. Progressive cataract formation often occurs, sometimes leading to a complete cataract. Other abnormalities associated with PFV include elongated ciliary processes, prominent radial iris vessels, and persistent hyaloid artery. (See also BCSC Section 6, *Pediatric Ophthalmology and Strabismus,* and Section 12, *Retina and Vitreous.*)

> Beebe DC. The lens. In: Kaufman PL, Alm A, eds. *Adler's Physiology of the Eye: Clinical Application.* 10th ed. St Louis: Mosby; 2003:117–158.
>
> Goldberg MF. Persistent fetal vasculature (PFV): an integrated interpretation of signs and symptoms associated with persistent hyperplastic primary vitreous (PHPV). LIV Edward Jackson Memorial Lecture. *Am J Ophthalmol.* 1997;124(5):587–626.
>
> Hiles DA, Kilty LA. Disorders of the lens. In: Isenberg SJ, ed. *The Eye in Infancy.* 2nd ed. St Louis: Mosby; 1994:336–373.
>
> Lambert S. Lens. In: Taylor D, ed. *Paediatric Ophthalmology.* 2nd ed. Boston: Blackwell Science; 1997:445–476.
>
> Shortt AJ, Lanigan B, O'Keefe M. Pars plana lensectomy for the management of ectopia lentis in children. *J Pediatr Ophthalmol Strabismus.* 2004;41(5):289–294.
>
> Streeten BW. Pathology of the lens. In: Albert DM, Jakobiec FA, eds. *Principles and Practice of Ophthalmology.* 2nd ed. Philadelphia: Saunders; 2000:3685–3749.

CHAPTER 4

Pathology

Age-Related Lens Changes

As the lens ages, it increases in mass and thickness and decreases in accommodative power. As new layers of cortical fibers form concentrically, the lens nucleus undergoes compression and hardening (nuclear sclerosis). Chemical modification and proteolytic cleavage of crystallins (lens proteins) result in the formation of high-molecular-mass protein aggregates. These aggregates may become large enough to cause abrupt fluctuations in the local refractive index of the lens, thereby scattering light and reducing transparency. Chemical modification of lens nuclear proteins also increases pigmentation, such that the lens becomes increasingly yellow or brown with advancing age (Fig 4-1). Other age-related changes include decreased concentrations of glutathione and potassium and increased concentrations of sodium and calcium in the lens cell cytoplasm.

A very common cause of visual impairment in older adults is *age-related cataract*, the pathogenesis of which is multifactorial and not completely understood. There are 3 main types of age-related cataracts: nuclear, cortical, and posterior subcapsular. In many patients, components of more than one type are present. (See also BCSC Section 4, *Ophthalmic Pathology and Intraocular Tumors*.)

Nuclear Cataracts

Some degree of nuclear sclerosis and yellowing is normal in adult patients after the age of 50. In general, this condition interferes only minimally with visual function. An excessive amount of light scattering and yellowing is called a *nuclear cataract*, which causes a central opacity (Fig 4-2). The ophthalmologist can evaluate the degree of increased color and of opacification by using a slit-lamp biomicroscope and by examining the red reflex with the pupil dilated.

Nuclear cataracts tend to progress slowly. Although they are usually bilateral, they may be asymmetric. Nuclear cataracts typically cause greater impairment of distance vision than of near vision. In the early stages, the progressive hardening of the lens nucleus frequently causes an increase in the refractive index of the lens and thus a myopic shift in refraction *(lenticular myopia)*. In hyperopic eyes, the myopic shift enables otherwise presbyopic individuals to read without spectacles, a condition referred to as *second sight*. Occasionally, the abrupt change in refractive index between the sclerotic nucleus (or other

40 • Lens and Cataract

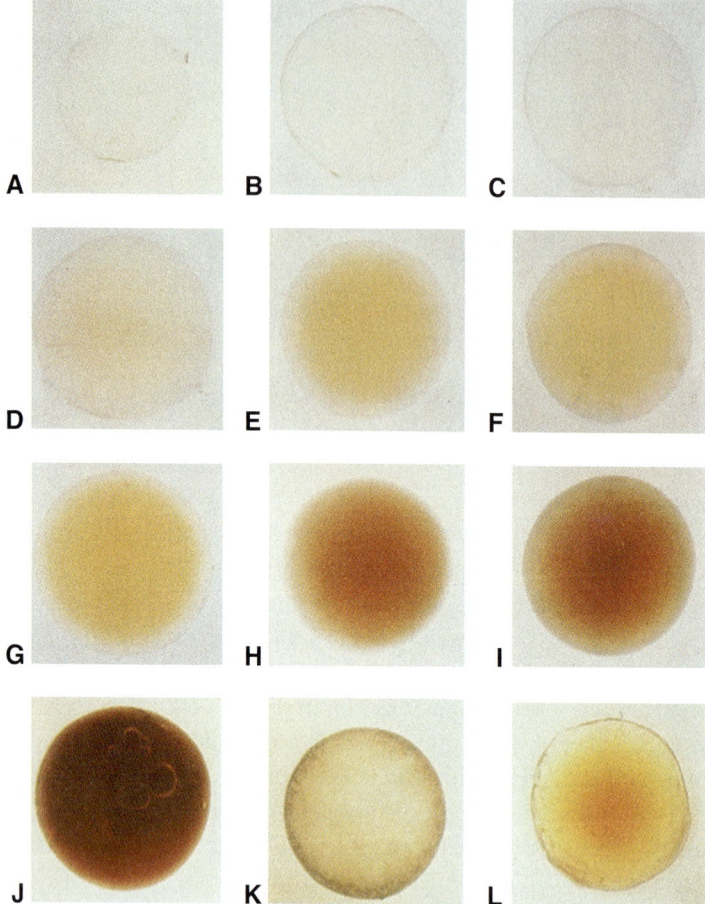

Figure 4-1 Increasing yellow-to-brown coloration of the human lens from 6 months *(A)* through 8 years *(B)*, 12 years *(C)*, 25 years *(D)*, 47 years *(E)*, 60 years *(F)*, 70 years *(G)*, 82 years *(H)*, and 91 years *(I)*. Brown nuclear cataract in 70-year-old patient *(J)*, cortical cataract in 68-year-old *(K)*, and mixed nuclear and cortical cataract in 74-year-old *(L)*. *(Reproduced with permission from Lerman S. Phototoxicity: clinical considerations.* Focal Points: Clinical Modules for Ophthalmologists. *San Francisco: American Academy of Ophthalmology; 1987, module 8.)*

lens opacities) and the lens cortex can cause monocular diplopia. Progressive yellowing or browning of the lens causes patients to have poor color discrimination, especially at the blue end of the visible light spectrum. Photopic retinal function may decrease with advanced nuclear cataract. In very advanced cases, the lens nucleus becomes opaque and brown and is called a *brunescent* nuclear cataract.

Histologically, the nucleus in nuclear cataract is difficult to distinguish from the nucleus of normal, aged lenses. Investigations by electron microscopy have identified an increased number of lamellar membrane whorls in some nuclear cataracts. The degree to which protein aggregates or these membrane modifications contribute to the increased light scattering of nuclear cataracts is unclear.

CHAPTER 4: Pathology • 41

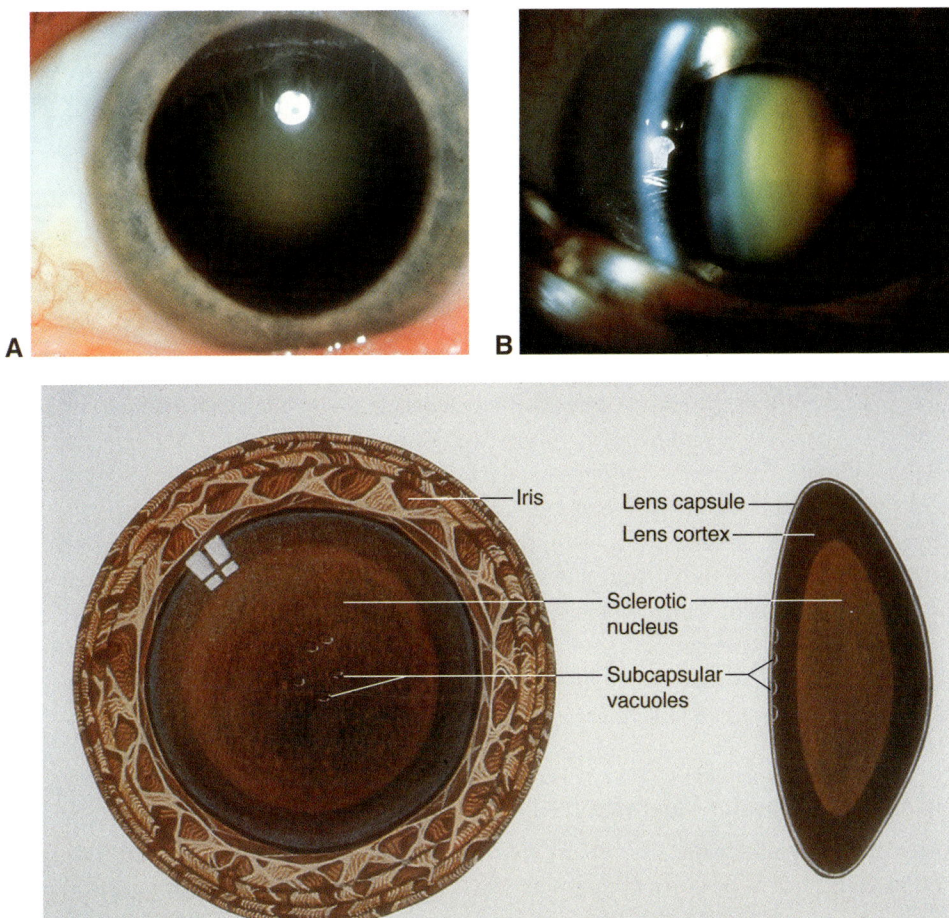

Figure 4-2 Nuclear cataract viewed with diffuse illumination **(A)** and with a slit beam **(B)**. **C,** Schematic of nuclear cataract. *(Courtesy of CIBA Pharmaceutical Co., division of CIBA-GEIGY Corp. Modified with permission from* Clinical Symposia. *Illustration by John A. Craig.)*

Cortical Cataracts

In contrast to nuclear cataracts, cortical cataracts are associated with the local disruption of the structure of mature lens fiber cells. Once membrane integrity is compromised, essential metabolites are lost from the affected cells. This loss leads to extensive protein oxidation and precipitation. Cortical cataracts are usually bilateral but are often asymmetric. Their effect on visual function varies greatly, depending on the location of the opacification relative to the visual axis. A common symptom of cortical cataracts is glare from intense focal light sources, such as car headlights. Monocular diplopia may also result. Cortical cataracts vary greatly in their rate of progression, with some cortical opacities remaining unchanged for prolonged periods and others progressing rapidly.

The first signs of cortical cataract formation visible with the slit-lamp biomicroscope are vacuoles (Fig 4-3) and water clefts in the anterior or posterior cortex. The cortical lamellae may be separated by fluid. Wedge-shaped opacities (often called *cortical spokes* or *cuneiform opacities*) form near the periphery of the lens, with the pointed end of the opacities oriented toward the center (Fig 4-4). Since these peripheral opacities occur in fiber cells that extend from the posterior to the anterior sutures, they affect only the equatorial regions of the fiber cells. In the initial stages of the cataract, affected fiber cells remain clear at their anterior and posterior ends. The cortical spokes appear as white opacities when viewed with the slit-lamp biomicroscope and as dark shadows when viewed on retroillumination. The wedge-shaped opacities may spread to adjacent fiber cells and along the length of affected fibers, causing the degree of opacity to increase and extend toward the visual axis. When the entire cortex from the capsule to the nucleus becomes white and opaque, the cataract is said to be *mature* (Fig 4-5). In mature opacities, the lens takes up water, swelling to become an *intumescent* cortical cataract.

When degenerated cortical material leaks through the lens capsule, leaving the capsule wrinkled and shrunken (Fig 4-6), the cataract is referred to as *hypermature*. When further liquefaction of the cortex allows free movement of the nucleus within the capsular bag (Fig 4-7), the term *morgagnian* cataract is used.

Histologically, cortical cataracts are characterized by local swelling and disruption of the lens fiber cells. Globules of eosinophilic material (morgagnian globules) are observed in slitlike spaces between lens fibers.

Posterior Subcapsular Cataracts

Posterior subcapsular cataracts (PSCs) are often seen in patients younger than those presenting with nuclear or cortical cataracts. PSCs are located in the posterior cortical layer

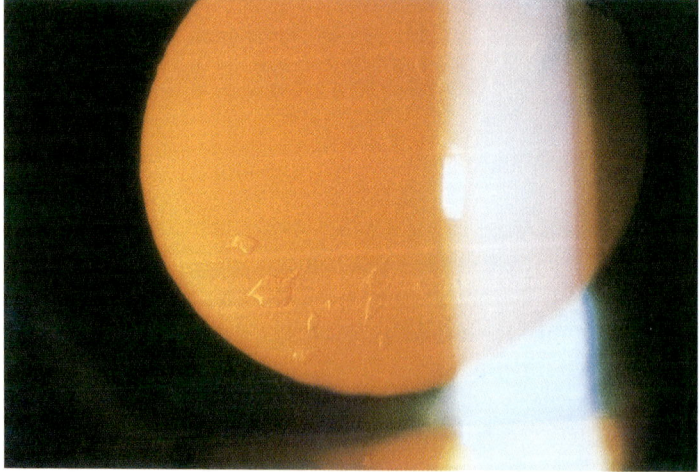

Figure 4-3 Vacuoles in early cortical cataract development.

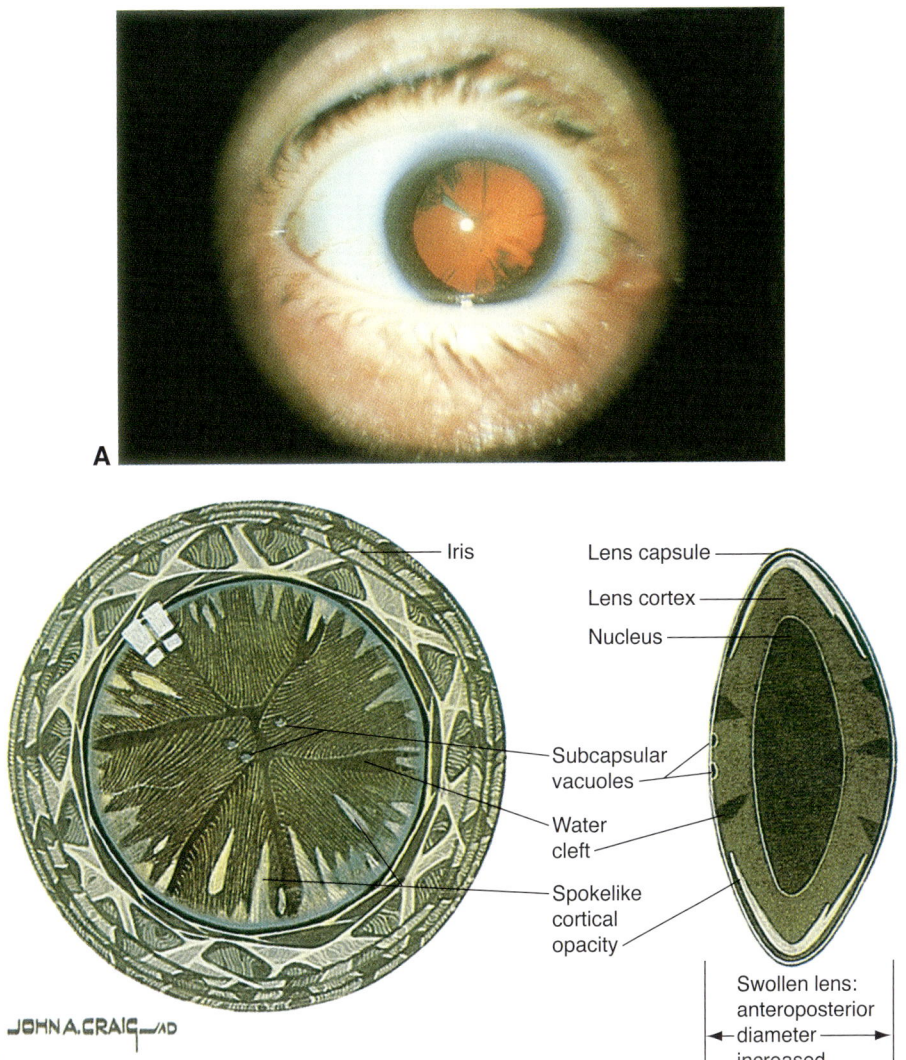

Figure 4-4 **A,** Cortical cataract viewed by retroillumination. **B,** Schematic of immature cortical cataract. *(Courtesy of CIBA Pharmaceutical Co., division of CIBA-GEIGY Corp. Reproduced with permission from Clinical Symposia. Illustration by John A. Craig.)*

and are usually axial (Fig 4-8). The first indication of PSC formation is a subtle iridescent sheen in the posterior cortical layers visible with the slit lamp. In later stages, granular opacities and a plaquelike opacity of the posterior subcapsular cortex appear.

The patient often complains of glare and poor vision under bright lighting conditions because the PSC obscures more of the pupillary aperture when miosis is induced by bright lights, accommodation, or miotics. Near vision tends to be reduced more than distance vision. Some patients experience monocular diplopia. Slit-lamp detection of PSCs can best be accomplished through a dilated pupil. Retroillumination is also helpful.

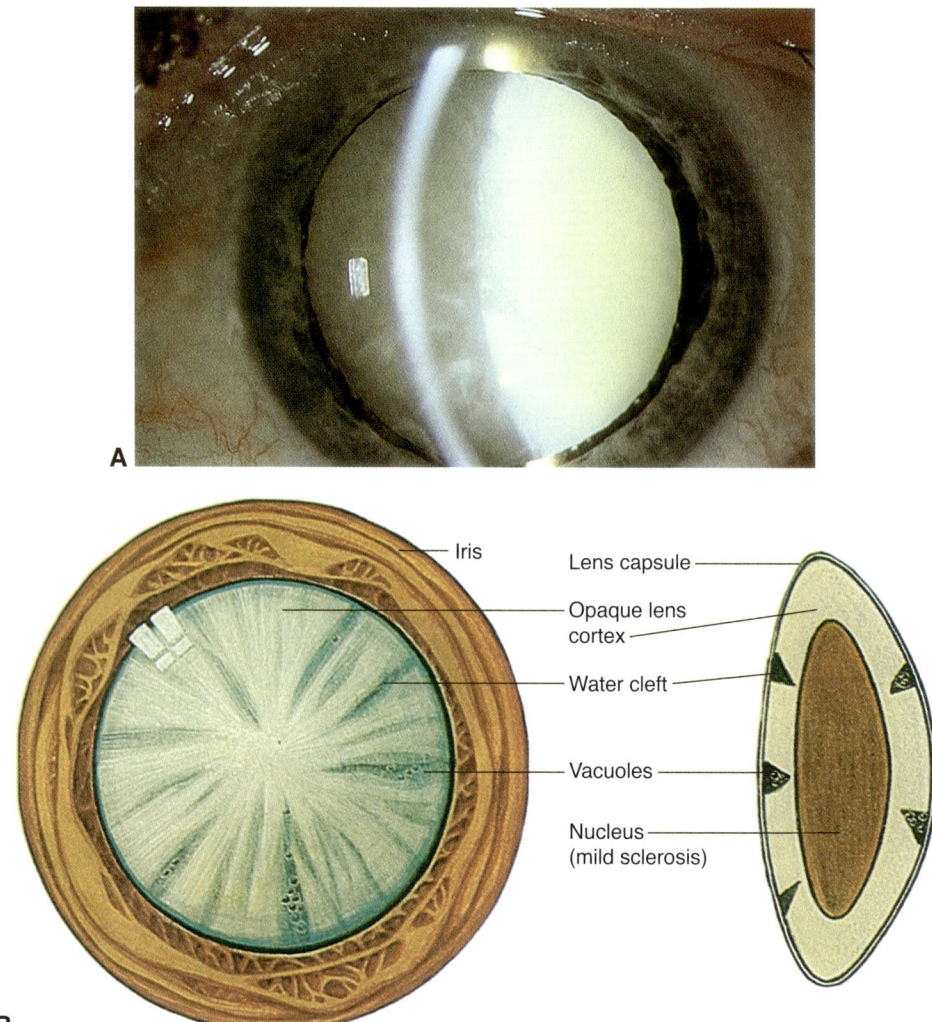

Figure 4-5 A, Mature cortical cataract. **B,** Schematic of mature cortical cataract. *(Courtesy of CIBA Pharmaceutical Co., division of CIBA-GEIGY Corp. Reproduced with permission from* Clinical Symposia. *Illustration by John A. Craig.)*

As stated earlier, PSCs are one of the main types of cataract related to aging. However, they can also occur as a result of trauma; systemic, topical, or intraocular corticosteroid use; inflammation; exposure to ionizing radiation; and alcoholism.

Histologically, PSC is associated with posterior migration of the lens epithelial cells from the lens equator to the visual axis on the inner surface of the posterior capsule. During their migration to or after their arrival at the posterior axis, the cells undergo aberrant enlargement. These swollen cells are called *Wedl,* or *bladder,* cells.

Hammond CJ, Duncan DD, Snieder H, et al. The heritability of age-related cortical cataract: the twin eye study. *Invest Ophthalmol Vis Sci.* 2001;42(3):601–605.

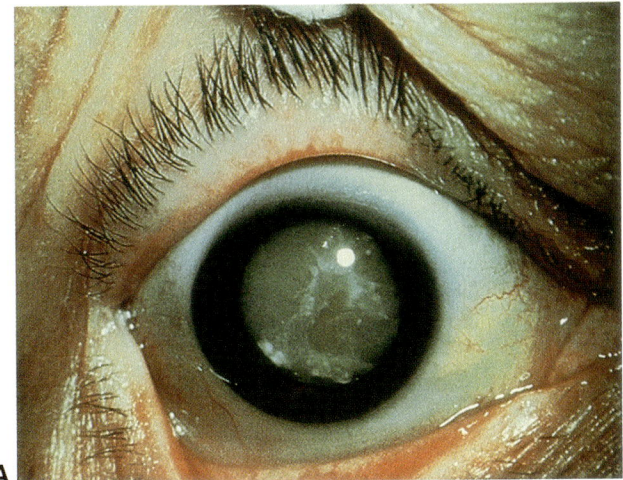

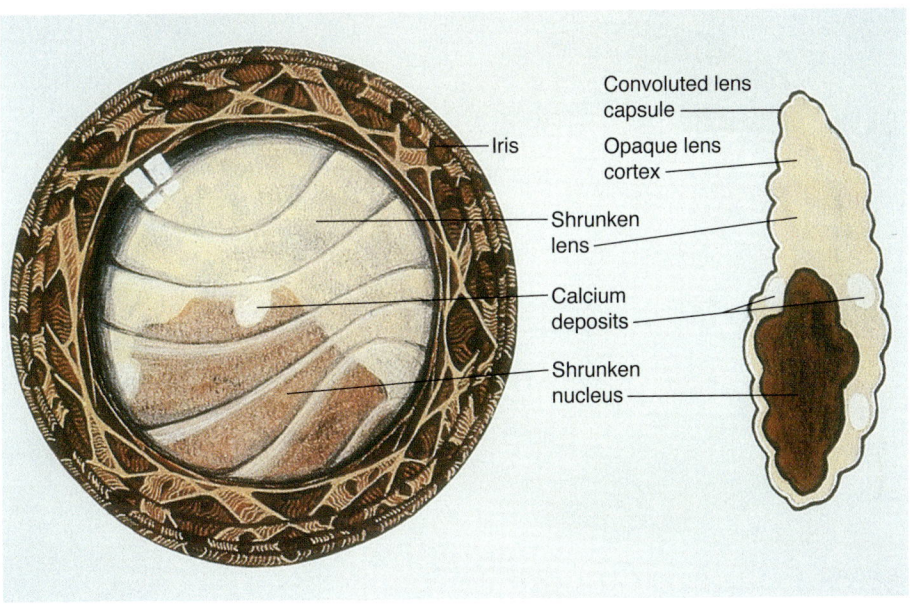

Figure 4-6 A, Hypermature cortical cataract. **B,** Schematic of hypermature cortical cataract. *(Courtesy of CIBA Pharmaceutical Co., division of CIBA-GEIGY Corp. Reproduced with permission from* Clinical Symposia. *Illustration by John A. Craig.)*

Hammond CJ, Snieder H, Spector TD, Gilbert CE. Genetic and environmental factors in age-related nuclear cataracts in monozygotic and dizygotic twins. *N Engl J Med.* 2000; 342(24):1786–1790.

Heiba IM, Elston RC, Klein BE, Klein R. Genetic etiology of nuclear cataract: evidence for a major gene. *Am J Med Genet.* 1993;47(8):1208–1214.

Iyengar SK, Klein BE, Klein R, et al. Identification of a major locus for age-related cortical cataract on chromosome 6p12-q12 in the Beaver Dam Eye Study. *Proc Natl Acad Sci USA.* 2004;101(40):14485–14490.

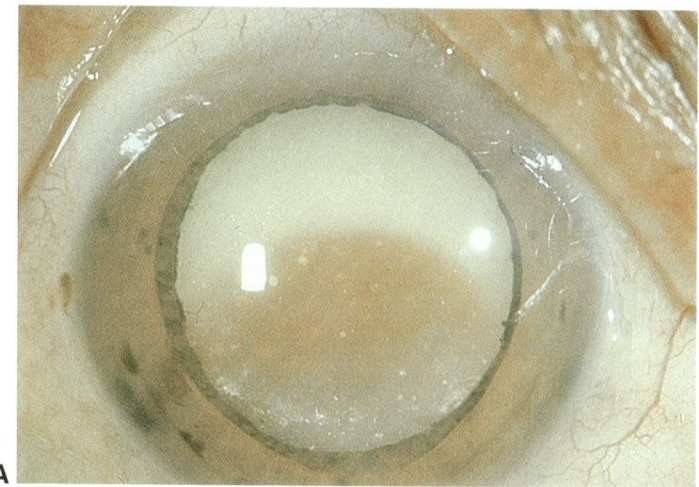
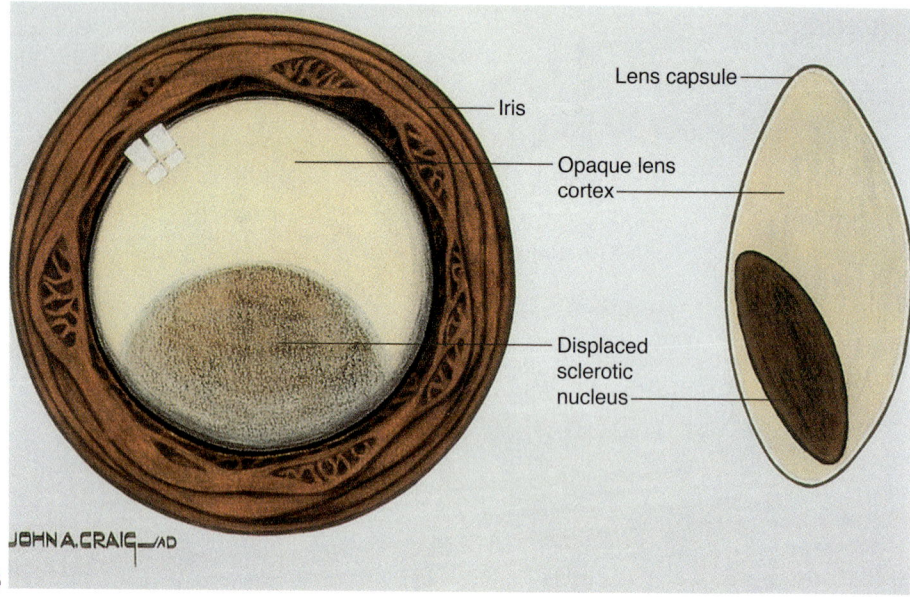

Figure 4-7 **A,** Morgagnian cataract. **B,** Schematic of morgagnian cataract. *(Courtesy of CIBA Pharmaceutical Co., division of CIBA-GEIGY Corp. Modified with permission from* Clinical Symposia. *Illustration by John A. Craig.)*

Klein BE, Klein R, Lee KE. Incidence of age-related cataract: the Beaver Dam Eye Study. *Arch Ophthalmol.* 1998;116(2):219–225.

Kuszak JR, Deutsch TA, Brown HG. Anatomy of aged and senile cataractous lenses. In: Albert DM, Jakobiec FA, eds. *Principles and Practice of Ophthalmology.* Philadelphia: Saunders; 1994: 564–575.

West SK, Duncan DD, Muñoz B, et al. Sunlight exposure and risk of lens opacities in a population-based study: the Salisbury Eye Evaluation Project. *JAMA.* 1998;280(8):714–718.

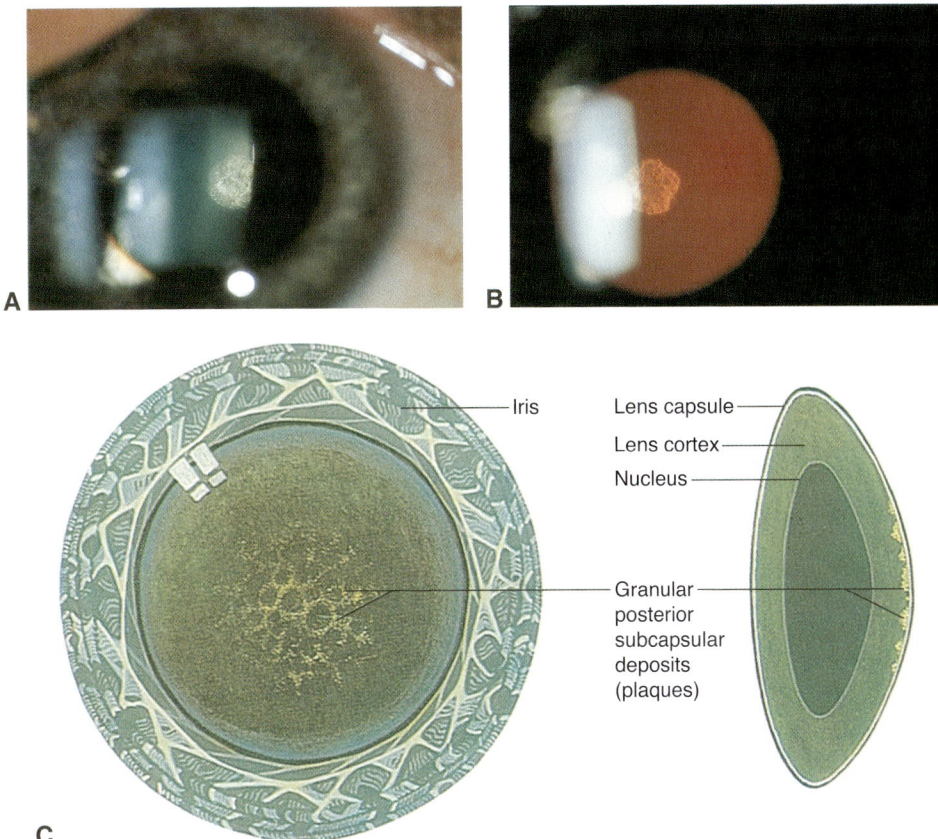

Figure 4-8 Posterior subcapsular cataract (PSC) viewed at the slit lamp **(A)** and with indirect illumination **(B). C,** Schematic of PSC. *(Courtesy of CIBA Pharmaceutical Co., division of CIBA-GEIGY Corp. Reproduced with permission from* Clinical Symposia. *Illustration by John A. Craig.)*

West SK, Valmadrid CT. Epidemiology of risk factors for age-related cataract. *Surv Ophthalmol.* 1995;39(4):323–334.

Young RW. *Age-Related Cataract.* New York: Oxford University Press; 1991.

Drug-Induced Lens Changes

Corticosteroids

Long-term use of corticosteroids may cause PSCs. The incidence of corticosteroid-induced PSCs is related to dose and duration of treatment. Cataract formation has been reported following administration of corticosteroids by several routes: systemic, topical, subconjunctival, and inhaled. The increasing use of high-dose intraocular steroids to treat retinal neovascularization and inflammation has resulted in a substantial rise in the incidence of

PSCs and of steroid-induced ocular hypertension. Coincidentally, the patients who are susceptible to steroid-induced increases in intraocular pressure (IOP) are frequently those who develop PSCs after intravitreal injection of triamcinolone acetonide. The advent of slow-release steroid repositories such as fluocinolone acetonide 0.59 mg and dexamethasone intravitreal implant 0.7 mg has not altered the IOP-elevating and PSC-producing effects of these medications on the eye.

Histologically and clinically, PSC formation occurring subsequent to corticosteroid use cannot be distinguished from senescent PSC formation. Some steroid-induced PSCs in children may resolve with cessation of the drug.

> Fraunfelder FT, Fraunfelder FW. *Drug-Induced Ocular Side Effects*. 5th ed. Boston: Butterworth-Heinemann; 2001.
>
> Gillies MC, Kuzniarz M, Craig J, Ball M, Luo W, Simpson JM. Intravitreal triamcinolone-induced elevated intraocular pressure is associated with the development of posterior subcapsular cataract. *Ophthalmology*. 2005;112(1):139–143.
>
> Jaffe GJ, Martin D, Callanan D, et al. Fluocinolone acetonide implant (Retisert) for noninfectious posterior uveitis: thirty-four-week results of a multicenter randomized clinical study. *Ophthalmology*. 2006;113(6):1020–1027.
>
> Kiernan DF, Mieler WF. The use of intraocular corticosteroids. *Expert Opin Pharmacother*. 2009;10(15):2511–2525.
>
> Urban RC Jr, Cotlier E. Corticosteroid-induced cataracts. *Surv Ophthalmol*. 1986;31(2): 102–110.

Phenothiazines

Phenothiazines, a major group of psychotropic medications, can cause pigmented deposits in the anterior lens epithelium in an axial configuration (Fig 4-9). The occurrence of these deposits appears to be dependent on both drug dose and treatment duration. In addition, they are more likely to be seen with the use of some phenothiazines, notably

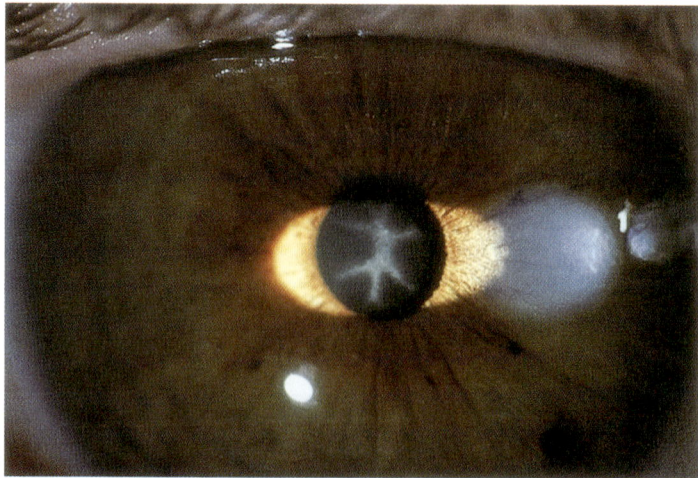

Figure 4-9 Pigmented deposits on anterior lens capsule in patient treated with phenothiazines.

chlorpromazine and thioridazine, than with others. The visual changes associated with phenothiazine use are generally insignificant.

Miotics

The use of anticholinesterases can cause cataracts. The incidence of cataracts has been reported as high as 20% in patients after 55 months of pilocarpine use and 60% in patients after echothiophate iodide use. Usually, this type of cataract first appears as small vacuoles within and posterior to the anterior lens capsule and epithelium. These vacuoles are best appreciated on retroillumination. The cataract may progress to posterior cortical and nuclear lens changes. Cataract formation is more likely in patients receiving anticholinesterase therapy over a long period and in those receiving more frequent dosing. Although visually significant cataracts are common in elderly patients using topical anticholinesterases, progressive cataract formation has not been reported in children given echothiophate for the treatment of accommodative esotropia. The use of these medications has declined with the advent of other classes of medications for the treatment of glaucoma, and indirect-acting anticholinesterase agents are irritating, cataractogenic, and difficult to obtain.

Amiodarone

The use of amiodarone, an antiarrhythmia medication, has been reported to cause stellate pigment deposition in the anterior cortical axis. Only very rarely is this condition visually significant. Amiodarone is also deposited in the corneal epithelium and can cause a rare optic neuropathy.

Statins

Studies in dogs showed that some 3-hydroxy-3-methylglutaryl coenzyme A (HMG-CoA) reductase inhibitors (statins) are associated with cataract when given in excessive doses. Long-term use of statins in humans has been shown not to be associated with an increased cataract risk; moreover, a longitudinal study reported a 50% reduction in the 5-year incidence of nuclear cataracts in patients treated with statins. However, concomitant use of simvastatin and erythromycin, which increases circulating statin levels, may be associated with approximately a twofold increased risk of cataract.

> Klein BE, Klein R, Lee KE, Grady LM. Statin use and incident nuclear cataract. *JAMA*. 2006; 295(23):2752–2758.
> Schlienger RG, Haefeli WE, Jick H, Meier CR. Risk of cataract in patients treated with statins. *Arch Intern Med*. 2001;161(16):2021–2026.

Tamoxifen

In a recent study, the association previously suggested between cataract development and tamoxifen use was not substantiated. Research on and discussion of this subject continue.

> Bradbury BD, Lash TL, Kaye JA, Jick SS. Tamoxifen and cataracts: a null association. *Breast Cancer Res Treat*. 2004;87(2):189–196.

Trauma

Traumatic lens damage may be caused by mechanical injury and by physical forces (radiation, chemicals, electrical current).

Contusion

Vossius ring

Blunt injury to the eye can sometimes cause a ring of pigment from the pupillary ruff to be imprinted on the anterior surface of the lens; this is referred to as a *Vossius ring*. Although a Vossius ring is visually insignificant and gradually resolves with time, it serves as an indicator of prior blunt trauma.

Traumatic cataract

A blunt, nonperforating injury may cause lens opacification either as an acute event or as a late sequela. A contusion cataract may involve only a portion of the lens or the entire lens. Often, the initial manifestation of a contusion cataract is a stellate or rosette-shaped opacification *(rosette cataract)*, usually axial in location, that involves the posterior lens capsule (Fig 4-10). In some cases, blunt trauma causes both dislocation and cataract formation (Fig 4-11). Mild contusion cataracts can improve spontaneously in rare cases.

Dislocation and subluxation

During a blunt injury to the eye, rapid expansion of the globe in an equatorial plane immediately follows compression. This rapid equatorial expansion can disrupt the zonular fibers, causing dislocation or subluxation of the lens. The lens may be dislocated in any direction, including posteriorly into the vitreous cavity or anteriorly into the anterior chamber.

Symptoms and signs of traumatic lens subluxation include fluctuation of vision, impaired accommodation, monocular diplopia, and high astigmatism. Often, iridodonesis

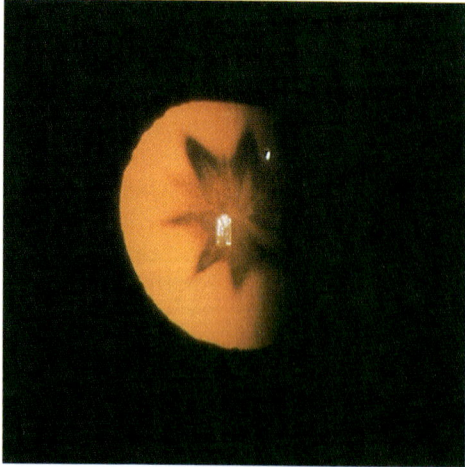

Figure 4-10 Stellate lens opacity following contusion.

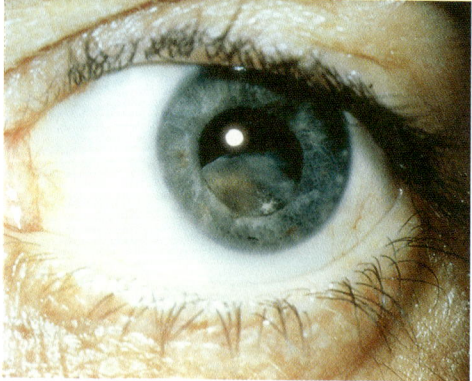

Figure 4-11 Dislocated cataractous lens following blunt trauma. *(Courtesy of Karla J. Johns, MD.)*

or phacodonesis is present. Retroillumination of the lens at the slit lamp through a dilated pupil may reveal the zonular disruption. In some cases, blunt trauma causes both dislocation and cataract formation.

> Irvine JA, Smith RE. Lens injuries. In: Shingleton BJ, Hersh PS, Kenyon KR, eds. *Eye Trauma.* St Louis: Mosby; 1991:126–135.

Perforating and Penetrating Injury

A perforating or penetrating injury of the lens often results in opacification of the cortex at the site of the rupture, usually progressing rapidly to complete opacification (Fig 4-12). Occasionally, a small perforating injury of the lens capsule heals, resulting in a stationary focal cortical cataract (Fig 4-13).

Intralenticular Foreign Bodies

In rare instances, a small foreign body can perforate the cornea and the anterior lens capsule and become lodged within the lens. If the foreign body is not composed of a ferric or cupric material and the anterior lens capsule seals the perforation site, the foreign body may be retained within the lens without significant complication. Intralenticular foreign bodies may cause cataract formation in some cases but do not always lead to lens opacification.

Radiation

Ionizing radiation

The lens is extremely sensitive to ionizing radiation; however, as much as 20 years may pass after exposure before a cataract becomes clinically apparent. This period of latency

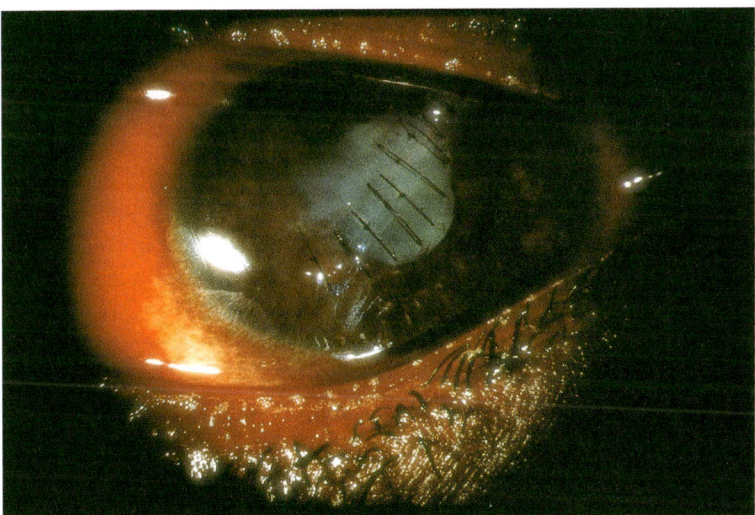

Figure 4-12 Complete cortical opacification after perforating injury, with disruption of the lens capsule.

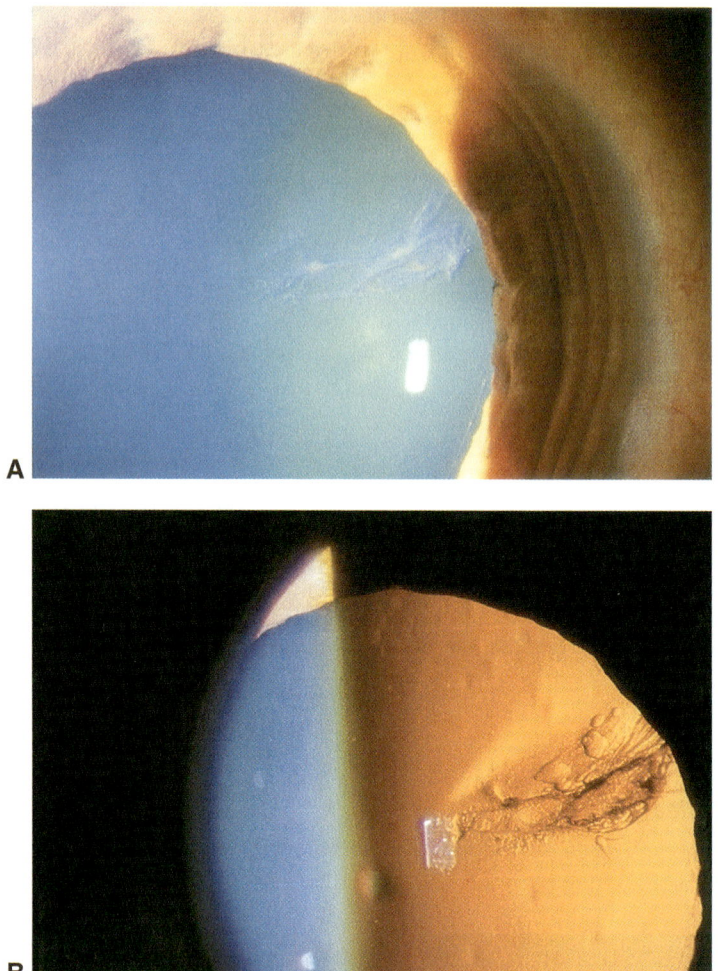

Figure 4-13 A, Focal cortical cataract from a small perforating injury to the lens capsule. **B,** Focal cortical cataract viewed by retroillumination.

is related to the dose of radiation and to the patient's age; younger patients are more susceptible because they have more actively growing lens cells. Ionizing radiation in the x-ray range (0.001–10.0 nm wavelength) can cause cataracts in some individuals in doses as low as 2 Gy in one fraction. (A routine chest x-ray equals 0.01 Gy exposure to the thorax.)

The first clinical signs of radiation-induced cataract are often punctate opacities within the posterior capsule and feathery anterior subcapsular opacities that radiate toward the equator of the lens. These opacities may progress to complete opacification of the lens.

Infrared radiation (glassblowers' cataract)

Exposure of the eye to infrared radiation and intense heat over time can cause the outer layers of the anterior lens capsule to peel off as a single layer. Such true exfoliation of the lens capsule, in which the exfoliated outer lamella tends to scroll up on itself, is rarely seen today. Cortical cataract may be associated. (See the section Exfoliation Syndrome.)

Ultraviolet radiation

Experimental evidence suggests that the lens is susceptible to damage from ultraviolet (UV) radiation. Epidemiologic evidence indicates that long-term exposure to sunlight is associated with increased risk of cortical cataracts. Although sunlight exposure accounts for only about 10% of the total risk of cortical cataract in the general population in temperate climates, this risk is avoidable. Since exposure to UV radiation can produce other morbidity, clinicians should encourage their patients to avoid excessive sunlight exposure. Lenses sold in the United States must conform to the American National Standards Institute (ANSI) requirements aimed at reducing UV transmission. Prescription corrective lenses and nonprescription sunglasses decrease UV transmission by more than 80%, and wearing a hat with a brim decreases ocular sun exposure by 30%–50%.

> Cruickshanks KF, Klein BE, Klein R. Ultraviolet light exposure and lens opacities: the Beaver Dam Eye Study. *Am J Public Health*. 1992;82(12):1658–1662.

Microwave radiation

Microwave radiation has been shown to cause cataracts in laboratory animals. Human case reports and epidemiologic studies are more controversial and less conclusive than experimental studies. Cataracts caused by microwave radiation are likely to be anterior and/or posterior subcapsular opacities.

> Lipman RM, Tripathi BJ, Tripathi RC. Cataracts induced by microwave and ionizing radiation. *Surv Ophthalmol*. 1988;33(3):200–210.

Chemical Injuries

Alkali injuries to the ocular surface often result in cataract, in addition to damaging the cornea, conjunctiva, and iris. Alkali compounds penetrate the eye readily, causing an increase in aqueous pH and a decrease in the level of aqueous glucose and ascorbate. Cortical cataract formation may occur acutely or as a delayed effect of chemical injury. Because acid tends to penetrate the eye less easily than does alkali, acid injuries are less likely to result in cataract formation.

Metallosis

Siderosis bulbi

Iron intraocular foreign bodies can result in siderosis bulbi, a condition characterized by deposition of iron molecules in the trabecular meshwork, lens epithelium, iris, and retina (Fig 4-14A). The epithelium and cortical fibers of the affected lens at first show a yellowish tinge, followed later by a rusty brown discoloration (Fig 4-14B). Lens involvement occurs more rapidly if the retained foreign body is embedded close to the lens. Later manifestations of siderosis bulbi are complete cortical cataract formation and retinal dysfunction. (See also BCSC Section 12, *Retina and Vitreous*.)

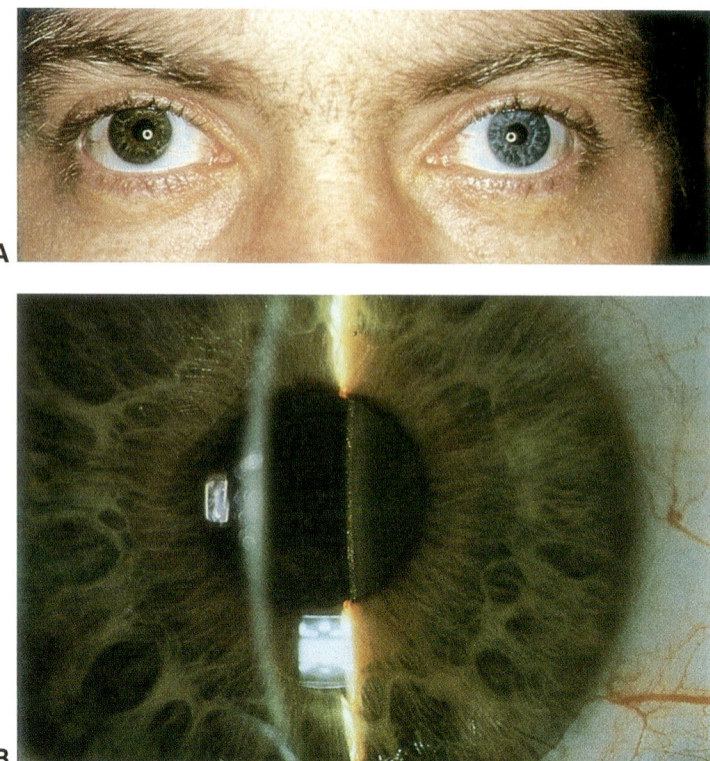

Figure 4-14 Siderosis bulbi. **A,** Heterochromia iridis caused by siderosis bulbi. **B,** Discoloration of lens capsule and cortex.

Chalcosis

Chalcosis occurs when an intraocular copper-containing foreign body deposits copper in the Descemet membrane, anterior lens capsule, or other intraocular basement membranes. A resulting "sunflower" cataract is a petal-shaped deposition of yellow or brown pigment in the lens capsule that radiates from the anterior axial pole of the lens to the equator. Usually, this cataract causes no significant loss of vision. However, intraocular foreign bodies containing almost pure copper (more than 90%) can cause a severe inflammatory reaction and intraocular necrosis.

Electrical Injury

Electrical shock can cause protein coagulation and cataract formation. Lens manifestations are more likely when the transmission of current involves the patient's head. Initially, lens vacuoles appear in the anterior midperiphery of the lens, followed by linear opacities in the anterior subcapsular cortex. A cataract induced by an electrical injury may regress, remain stationary, or mature to complete cataract over months or years (Fig 4-15).

Portellos M, Orlin SE, Kozart DM. Electric cataracts [photo essay]. *Arch Ophthalmol.* 1996; 114(8):1022–1023.

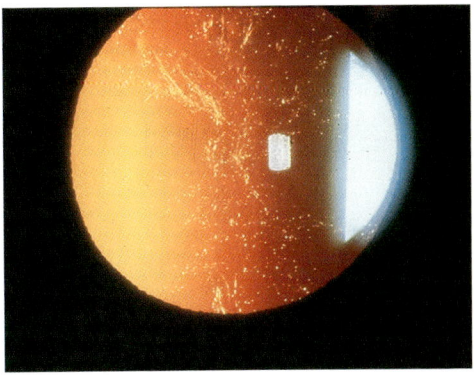

Figure 4-15 Electrical injury. *(Courtesy of Karla J. Johns, MD.)*

Metabolic Cataract

Diabetes Mellitus

Diabetes mellitus can affect lens clarity as well as the refractive index and accommodative amplitude of the lens. As the blood glucose level increases, so, also, does the glucose content in the aqueous humor. (See Chapter 2 for discussion of glucose-induced lens changes.) Acute myopic shifts may indicate undiagnosed or poorly controlled diabetes. Patients with type 1 diabetes have a decreased amplitude of accommodation compared to age-matched controls, and presbyopia may present at a younger age in patients with diabetes. (See also Chapter 9.)

Cataract is a common cause of visual impairment in patients with diabetes. Acute *diabetic cataract,* or *"snowflake" cataract,* consists of bilateral, widespread subcapsular lens changes of abrupt onset, typically in young people with uncontrolled diabetes mellitus (Fig 4-16). Multiple gray-white subcapsular opacities that have a snowflake appearance are seen initially in the superficial anterior and posterior lens cortex. Vacuoles and clefts form in the underlying cortex. Intumescence and maturity of the cortical cataract follow shortly thereafter. Although acute diabetic cataracts are rarely encountered in clinical practice today, rapidly maturing bilateral cortical cataracts in a child or young adult should alert the clinician to the possibility of diabetes mellitus.

Diabetic patients develop age-related lens changes that are indistinguishable from nondiabetic age-related cataracts, except that these lens changes tend to occur at a younger age in patients with diabetes than in those without the disease. The increased risk or earlier onset of age-related cataracts in diabetic patients may be a result of the accumulation of sorbitol within the lens and accompanying changes in hydration, increased nonenzymatic glycosylation (glycation) of lens proteins, or greater oxidative stress from alterations in lens metabolism.

> Flynn HW Jr, Smiddy WE, eds. *Diabetes and Ocular Disease: Past, Present, and Future Therapies.* Ophthalmology Monograph 14. San Francisco: American Academy of Ophthalmology; 2000:49–53, 226.
>
> Gold DH, Weingeist TA, eds. *The Eye in Systemic Disease.* Philadelphia: Lippincott; 1990:90, 330–331, 390, 434.

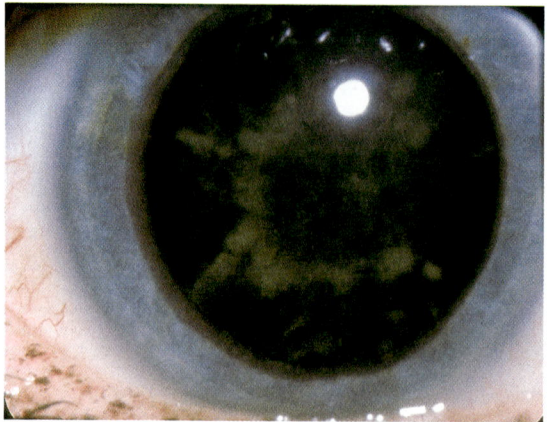

Figure 4-16 Diabetic cataract, or "snowflake" cataract, consists of gray-white subcapsular opacities. This type of cataract is seen, in rare cases, in patients with uncontrolled diabetes mellitus. *(Courtesy of Karla J. Johns, MD.)*

Johns KJ. Diabetes and the lens. In: Feman SS, ed. *Ocular Problems in Diabetes Mellitus.* Boston: Blackwell; 1992:221–244.

Galactosemia

Galactosemia is an inherited autosomal recessive inability to convert galactose to glucose. As a consequence of this inability, excessive galactose accumulates in body tissues, with further metabolic conversion of galactose to galactitol (dulcitol), the sugar alcohol of galactose. Galactosemia can result from defects in 1 of 3 enzymes involved in the metabolism of galactose: galactose 1-phosphate uridyltransferase (Gal-1-PUT), galactokinase, or UDPgalactose 4-epimerase. The most common and the severest form, known as *classic galactosemia,* is caused by a defect in Gal-1-PUT.

In classic galactosemia, symptoms of malnutrition, hepatomegaly, jaundice, and mental deficiency present within the first few weeks of life. The disease is fatal if undiagnosed and untreated. The diagnosis of classic galactosemia can be confirmed by demonstration of galactose in the urine.

Typically, the nucleus and deep cortex become increasingly opacified, causing an "oil droplet" appearance on retroillumination (Fig 4-17). If the disease remains untreated, the cataracts progress to total opacification. Treatment of galactosemia includes elimination of milk and milk products from the diet. In some cases, early cataract formation can be reversed by timely diagnosis and dietary intervention.

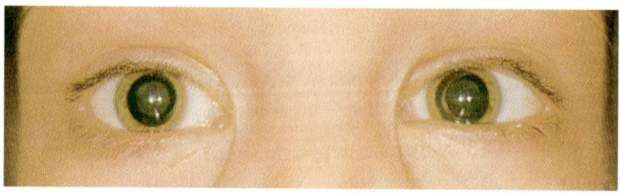

Figure 4-17 "Oil droplet" bilateral cataracts in patient with galactosemia.

Deficiencies of the 2 other enzymes, galactokinase and epimerase, can also cause galactosemia. These deficiencies are less common, however, and cause less severe systemic abnormalities. Cataracts caused by deficiencies in these enzymes tend to present later in life than those seen in classic galactosemia.

> Burke JP, O'Keefe M, Bowell R, Naughten ER. Ophthalmic findings in classical galactosemia: a screened population. *J Pediatr Ophthalmol Strabismus.* 1989;26(4):165–168.

Hypocalcemia

Cataracts may occur in association with any condition that results in hypocalcemia. Hypocalcemia may be idiopathic, or it may appear as a result of unintended destruction of the parathyroid glands during thyroid surgery. Usually bilateral, hypocalcemic (tetanic) cataracts are punctate iridescent opacities in the anterior and posterior cortex. They lie beneath the lens capsule and are usually separated from it by a zone of clear lens. These discrete opacities may remain stable or may mature into complete cortical cataracts.

Wilson Disease

Wilson disease (hepatolenticular degeneration) is an inherited autosomal recessive disorder of copper metabolism. The characteristic ocular manifestation of Wilson disease is the Kayser-Fleischer ring, a golden brown discoloration of the Descemet membrane around the periphery of the cornea. In addition, a characteristic "sunflower" cataract often develops. Reddish brown pigment (cuprous oxide) is deposited in the anterior lens capsule and subcapsular cortex in a stellate shape that resembles the petals of a sunflower. In most cases, the sunflower cataract does not produce serious visual impairment.

Myotonic Dystrophy

Myotonic dystrophy is an inherited autosomal dominant condition characterized by delayed relaxation of contracted muscles, ptosis, weakness of the facial musculature, cardiac conduction defects, and prominent frontal balding in affected male patients. Patients with this disorder typically develop polychromatic iridescent crystals in the lens cortex (Fig 4-18), with sequential PSC progressing to complete cortical opacification. These crystals are also noted unilaterally in patients without myotonic dystrophy. Ultrastructurally, polychromatic iridescent crystals are composed of whorls of plasmalemma from the lens fibers. The crystals are occasionally seen in the lens cortex of patients who do not have myotonic dystrophy; these crystals are thought to be caused by cholesterol crystal deposition in the lens.

Effects of Nutrition, Alcohol, and Smoking

Although nutritional deficiencies have been demonstrated to cause cataracts in animal models, this etiology has been difficult to confirm in humans. Numerous population-based studies have found that lower socioeconomic status, lower education level, and poorer overall nutrition are associated with increased prevalence of age-related cataracts. The identification of specific dietary deficiencies that lead to cataract formation and of

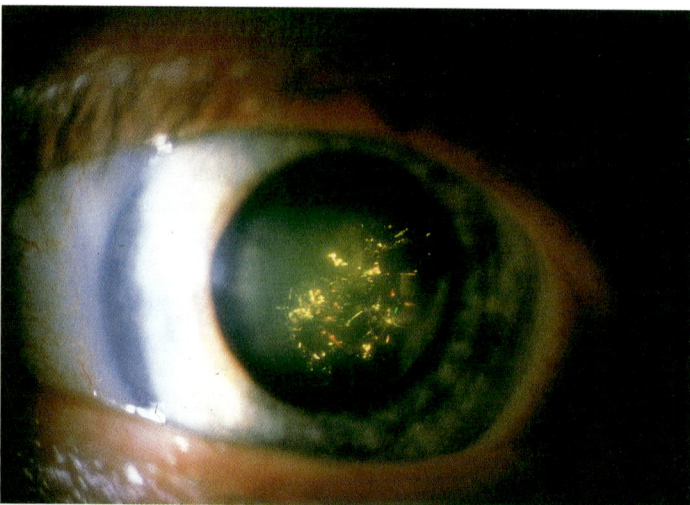

Figure 4-18 Polychromatic iridescent crystals in a patient with myotonic dystrophy. *(Courtesy of Karla J. Johns, MD.)*

supplements that protect against it has been more difficult. Some studies have suggested that taking multivitamin supplements, vitamin A, vitamin C, vitamin E, niacin, thiamine, riboflavin, beta carotene, or increased protein may have a protective effect on cataract development. Other studies have found that vitamins C and E have little or no effect on cataract development. Most recently, the Age-Related Eye Disease Study (AREDS) showed that, over 7 years, increased intake of vitamins C and E and beta carotene did not decrease the development or progression of cataract. Use of the multivitamin supplement offered to all AREDS participants was moderately protective against the development of nuclear opacities. It is important to remember that high-dose vitamin use may pose risks. Smokers taking high doses of beta carotene have been shown to have an increased risk of lung cancer, of death from lung cancer, and of death from cardiovascular disease. In addition, women taking supplemental doses of vitamin A have been shown to be at increased risk of hip fracture.

Lutein and zeaxanthin are the only carotenoids found in human lenses, and recent studies have shown a moderate decrease in cataract risk with the increased frequency of intake of food high in lutein (eg, spinach, kale, and broccoli). Eating cooked spinach more than twice a week decreased the risk of cataract. This decreased risk was unrelated to a healthful lifestyle. In contrast to the effects of such dietary supplements, severe episodes of diarrhea associated with severe dehydration may be linked to an increased risk of cataract formation.

Smoking, the use of smokeless tobacco products, and excessive alcohol consumption are significant, avoidable risk factors for cataracts. In numerous studies worldwide, these practices have consistently been associated with an increase in the frequency of nuclear opacities. Although patients may know the general health risks of smoking and excessive alcohol consumption, they may not know about the risks of ocular conditions such as macular degeneration and cataract that are related to these practices. Ophthalmologists can inform their patients about these risks, and they are in a strong position to encourage individuals to stop smoking and reduce alcohol consumption.

> Age-Related Eye Disease Study Research Group. A randomized, placebo-controlled, clinical trial of high-dose supplementation with vitamins C and E and beta carotene for age-related cataract and vision loss: AREDS report no. 9. *Arch Ophthalmol.* 2001;119(10):1439–1452.
>
> Berendschot TT, Broekmans WM, Klöpping-Ketelaars IA, Kardinaal AF, Van Poppel G, Van Norren D. Lens aging in relation to nutritional determinants and possible risk factors for age-related cataract. *Arch Ophthalmol.* 2002;120(12):1732–1737.
>
> Christen WG, Manson JE, Seddon JM, et al. A prospective study of cigarette smoking and risk of cataract in men. *JAMA.* 1992;268(8):989–993.
>
> Cumming RG, Mitchell P, Smith W. Diet and cataract: the Blue Mountains Eye Study. *Ophthalmology.* 2000;107(3):450–456.
>
> Goodman GE, Thornquist MD, Balmes J, et al. The Beta-Carotene and Retinol Efficacy Trial: incidence of lung cancer and cardiovascular disease mortality during 6-year follow-up after stopping beta-carotene and retinol supplements. *J Natl Cancer Inst.* 2004;96(23):1743–1750.
>
> Kanthan GL, Mitchell P, Burlutsky G, Wang JJ. Alcohol consumption and the long-term incidence of cataract and cataract surgery: the Blue Mountains Eye Study. *Am J Ophthalmol.* 2010;150(3):434–440.
>
> Lyle BJ, Mares-Perlman JA, Klein BE, Klein R, Greger JL. Antioxidant intake and risk of incident age-related nuclear cataracts in the Beaver Dam Eye Study. *Am J Epidemiol.* 1999;149:801–809.
>
> Milton RC, Sperduto RD, Clemons TE, Ferris FL III; Age-Related Eye Disease Study Research Group. Centrum use and progression of age-related cataract in the Age-Related Eye Disease Study: a propensity score approach. AREDS report no. 21. *Ophthalmology.* 2006;113(8):1264–1270.
>
> Opotowsky AR, Bilezikian JP. Serum vitamin A concentration and the risk of hip fracture among women 50 to 74 years old in the United States: a prospective analysis of the NHANES I follow-up study. *Am J Med.* 2004;117(3):169–174.
>
> Raju P, George R, Ve Ramesh S, Arvind H, Baskaran M, Vijaya L. Influence of tobacco use on cataract development. *Br J Ophthalmol.* 2006;90(11):1374–1377. Epub 2006 Jul 12.

Cataract Associated With Uveitis

Lens changes often occur as a result of chronic uveitis or associated corticosteroid therapy. Typically, a PSC appears; anterior lens changes may also occur. The formation of posterior synechiae is common in uveitis, often with thickening of the anterior lens capsule, which may have an associated fibrous pupillary membrane. Lens changes in cataract secondary to uveitis may progress to a mature cataract. Calcium deposits may be observed on the anterior capsule or within the lens substance.

Cortical cataract formation occurs in up to 70% of cases of Fuchs heterochromic uveitis (Fig 4-19). Because posterior synechiae do not commonly occur in this syndrome, formation of pupillary membranes is unlikely, and long-term corticosteroid therapy is not indicated. Cataract extraction in patients with Fuchs heterochromic uveitis generally has a favorable prognosis. Intraoperative anterior chamber hemorrhages have been reported in approximately 25% of cases.

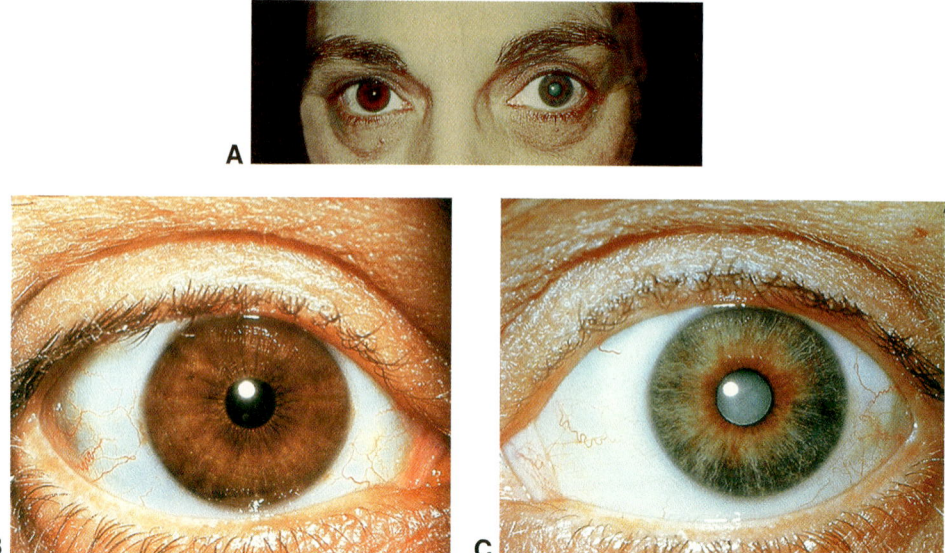

Figure 4-19 Fuchs heterochromic uveitis. **A,** Patient with Fuchs heterochromic uveitis. In this case, the affected eye is lighter. **B,** Normal right eye. **C,** Cataract formation in affected left eye. *(Courtesy of Karla J. Johns, MD.)*

Cataracts Associated With Ocular Treatments

Posterior subcapsular cataract secondary to corticosteroid treatment is discussed in the previous section. Vitrectomy is another cause of treatment-induced cataract. Transient opacities involving the posterior sutures can occur soon after vitrectomy, but these opacities usually resolve spontaneously. However, more than 60% and up to 95% of patients who undergo vitrectomy during surgical treatment of a variety of retinal problems develop nuclear cataracts within 2 years of the surgery. Postvitrectomy cataracts are less common in patients younger than 50 years. The formation of nuclear cataracts after vitrectomy is associated with increases in oxygen tension in the vitreous intraoperatively and postoperatively. (See Chapter 2 for a discussion of oxygen tension in the lens.) Retinal surgery performed without vitrectomy is not associated with increased lens opacification. In this regard, age-related degeneration of the vitreous body has also been associated with increased risk of nuclear opacification.

Cataracts and Hyperbaric Oxygen Therapy

Lens changes may also occur after hyperbaric oxygen therapy. Several studies found a myopic shift during the course of several weeks of hyperbaric oxygen therapy for different conditions. Since no change in axial length or corneal curvature was detected, the refractive change was presumed to be due to increased nuclear sclerosis. In most cases, the myopic shift resolved after cessation of therapy. In patients exposed to hyperbaric oxygen at least 150 times during a 1-year period, nearly 50% of patients with previously clear lenses developed frank nuclear cataracts, consistent with the increase in oxygenation in the vitreous. (See Chapter 2 for a discussion of oxygen tension in the lens.) An increase in nuclear light scatter was shown in most of the other patients in this treatment group when they were compared with older, sicker patients who were in the same clinic but not eligible for hyperbaric oxygen therapy.

> Harocopos GJ, Shui YB, McKinnon M, Holekamp NM, Gordon MO, Beebe DC. Importance of vitreous liquefaction in age-related cataract. *Invest Ophthalmol Vis Sci.* 2004;45(1):77–85.
> Melberg NS, Thomas MA. Nuclear sclerotic cataract after vitrectomy in patients younger than 50 years of age. *Ophthalmology.* 1995;102(10):1466–1471.
> Palmquist BM, Philipson B, Barr PO. Nuclear cataract and myopia during hyperbaric oxygen therapy. *Br J Ophthalmol.* 1984;68(2):113–117.
> Sawa M, Ohji M, Kusaka S, et al. Nonvitrectomizing vitreous surgery for epiretinal membrane long-term follow-up. *Ophthalmology.* 2005;112(8):1402–1408.

Exfoliation Syndrome

Exfoliation syndrome (pseudoexfoliation) is a systemic disease in which a matrix of fibrotic material is deposited in many bodily organs. In the eye, a basement membrane–like fibrillogranular white material is deposited on the lens, cornea, iris, anterior hyaloid face, ciliary processes, zonular fibers, and trabecular meshwork. These deposits, believed to comprise elastic microfibrils, appear as grayish white flecks that are prominent at the pupillary margin and on the lens capsule (Fig 4-20). Associated with this condition are atrophy of the iris at the pupillary margin, deposition of pigment on the anterior surface of the iris, poorly dilating pupil, increased pigmentation of the trabecular meshwork, capsular fragility, zonular weakness, and open-angle glaucoma. Exfoliation syndrome is a unilateral or bilateral disorder that becomes more apparent with increasing age.

Increased oxidative stress caused by abnormalities in transforming growth factor β (TGF-β) contributes to the formation of cataracts. Patients with this syndrome may also experience weakness of the zonular fibers and spontaneous lens subluxation and

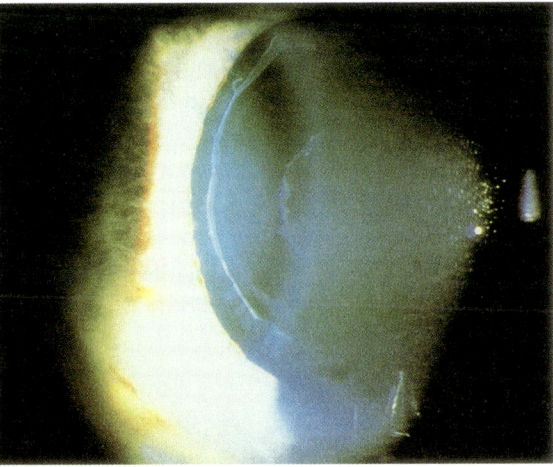

Figure 4-20 In exfoliation syndrome, deposits appear as grayish white flecks that are prominent at the pupillary margin and on the lens capsule.

phacodonesis. Poor zonular integrity may affect cataract surgery technique and intraocular lens implantation. (See Chapter 9 for discussion of cataract surgery in special situations.) The exfoliative material may be elaborated even after the crystalline lens is removed.

> Schlötzer-Schrehardt U, Naumann GO. Ocular and systemic pseudoexfoliation syndrome. *Am J Ophthalmol.* 2006;141(5):921–937.
>
> Zenkel M, Lewczuk P, Jünemann A, Kruse FE, Naumann GO, Schlötzer-Schrehardt U. Proinflammatory cytokines are involved in the initiation of the abnormal matrix process in pseudoexfoliation syndrome/glaucoma. *Am J Pathol.* 2010;176(6):2868–2879. Epub 2010 Apr 15.

Cataract and Atopic Dermatitis

Atopic dermatitis is a chronic, erythematous dermatitis, accompanied by itching and often seen in conjunction with increased levels of immunoglobulin E (IgE) and a history of multiple allergies or asthma. Cataract formation has been reported in up to 25% of patients with atopic dermatitis. The cataracts are usually bilateral, and onset occurs in the second to third decade of life. Typically, these cataracts are anterior subcapsular opacities in the pupillary area that resemble shieldlike plaques.

> Mannis MJ, Macsai MS, Huntley AC, eds. *Eye and Skin Disease*. Philadelphia: Lippincott-Raven; 1996.

Phacoantigenic Uveitis

In the normal eye, minute amounts of lens proteins leak out through the lens capsule. The eye appears to have immunologic tolerance to these small amounts of lens antigens. However, the release of a large amount of lens protein into the anterior chamber disrupts this immunologic tolerance and may trigger a severe inflammatory reaction. Phacoantigenic uveitis, sometimes referred to as *phacoanaphylactic uveitis,* is an immune-mediated granulomatous inflammation initiated by lens proteins released through a ruptured lens capsule. This condition usually occurs following traumatic rupture of the lens capsule or following cataract surgery when cortical material is retained within the eye. Onset occurs days to weeks after the injury or surgery.

The disease is characterized by a red, painful eye with injection, chemosis, and anterior chamber inflammation with cells, flare, and keratic precipitates. Occasionally, glaucoma secondary to blockage of the trabecular meshwork and formation of synechiae may occur. Late complications include cyclitic membrane, hypotony, and phthisis bulbi. In rare instances, phacoantigenic uveitis can give rise to an inflammatory reaction in the fellow eye. Histologic examination shows a zonal granulomatous inflammation surrounding a breach of the lens capsule. Lens extraction is the definitive therapy for the condition. See also BCSC Section 4, *Ophthalmic Pathology and Intraocular Tumors,* and Section 9, *Intraocular Inflammation and Uveitis.*

Lens-Induced Glaucoma

Phacolytic Glaucoma

Phacolytic glaucoma is a complication of a mature or hypermature cataract. Denatured, liquefied high-molecular-mass lens proteins leak through an intact but permeable lens capsule. An immune response is not elicited; rather, macrophages ingest these lens proteins. The trabecular meshwork can become clogged with both the lens proteins and the engorged macrophages. The usual clinical presentation of phacolytic glaucoma consists of abrupt onset of pain and redness in a cataractous eye that has had poor vision for some time. The cornea may be edematous, and significant flare reaction occurs in the anterior chamber. White flocculent material appears in the anterior chamber and often adheres to the lens capsule as well. IOP is markedly elevated; and the anterior chamber angle is open, although the same material may be seen in the trabecular meshwork. Initial treatment of phacolytic glaucoma consists of controlling IOP with antiglaucoma medications and managing inflammation with topical corticosteroids. Surgical removal of the lens is the definitive treatment.

Lens Particle Glaucoma

Following a penetrating lens injury or surgical procedure (ie, extracapsular cataract extraction or phacoemulsification with retained cortical material; or, in rare instances, Nd:YAG laser capsulotomy), particles of lens cortex may migrate into the anterior chamber, where they obstruct aqueous outflow through the trabecular meshwork. In most instances, the onset of glaucoma is delayed by days or weeks after the surgical event or lens injury. Gonioscopy shows that the angle is open, and cortical material can often be seen deposited along the trabecular meshwork. Medical therapy to lower IOP and to reduce intraocular inflammation is indicated. If the IOP and inflammation do not respond quickly to this treatment, surgical removal of the retained lens material may be required.

> Richter C, Epstein DL. Lens-induced open-angle glaucoma. In: Ritch R, Shields MB, Krupin T, eds. *The Glaucomas*. 2nd ed. St Louis: Mosby; 1996.

Phacomorphic Glaucoma

An intumescent cataractous lens can cause pupillary block and induce secondary angle-closure glaucoma, or it can physically push the iris forward and thus cause shallowing of the anterior chamber. Typically, the patient presents with a red, painful eye and a history of decreased vision as a result of cataract formation prior to the acute event (Fig 4-21). The cornea may be edematous, and gonioscopy reveals a closed anterior chamber angle. Initial management includes medical treatment to lower the IOP. The condition responds to laser iridotomy, but definitive treatment consists of cataract extraction.

> Liebman JM, Ritch R. Glaucoma secondary to lens intumescence and dislocation. In: Ritch R, Shields MB, Krupin T, eds. *The Glaucomas*. 2nd ed. St Louis: Mosby; 1996.

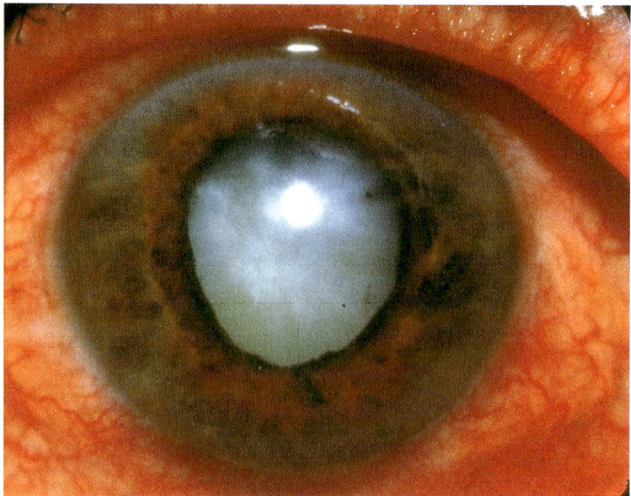

Figure 4-21 Phacomorphic glaucoma.

Glaukomflecken

Glaukomflecken are gray-white epithelial and anterior cortical lens opacities that occur following an episode of markedly elevated IOP, as in acute angle-closure glaucoma. Histologically, glaukomflecken are composed of necrotic lens epithelial cells and degenerated subepithelial cortex.

Ischemia

Ischemic ocular conditions, such as pulseless disease (Takayasu arteritis), thromboangiitis obliterans (Buerger disease), and anterior segment necrosis, can cause PSC. The cataract may progress rapidly to total opacification of the lens.

Cataracts Associated With Degenerative Ocular Disorders

Cataracts can occur secondary to many degenerative ocular diseases, such as retinitis pigmentosa, essential iris atrophy, chronic hypotony, and absolute glaucoma. These secondary cataracts usually begin as PSCs and may progress to total lens opacification. The mechanisms responsible for cataractogenesis in degenerative ocular disorders are not well understood.

CHAPTER 5

Epidemiology of Cataracts

Cataract is the leading cause of blindness and visual impairment throughout the world, according to the World Health Organization (WHO), and it has been shown that visual impairment and age-related cataract may be independent risk factors for increased mortality in older persons. With the general aging of the population, the overall prevalence of vision loss as a result of lenticular opacities increases each year. In 2002, the WHO estimated that cataracts caused reversible blindness in more than 17 million (47.8%) of the 37 million blind individuals worldwide (Table 5-1), and this number is projected to reach 40 million by 2020. The International Agency for the Prevention of Blindness (IAPB) and the WHO collaborated, in 1999, to launch VISION 2020—The Right to Sight, an initiative to develop the infrastructure, personnel, and economic strategy necessary for sustainable provision of high-quality cataract surgical services throughout the underdeveloped world. The WHO has determined that between 2000 and 2020, the number of cataract surgeries performed worldwide will need to triple to keep pace with the needs of the population.

Cataract affects nearly 20.5 million Americans aged 40 years and older, or about 1 in every 6 people in this age range. It is estimated that 2.5 million cataract surgeries were performed in the United States in 2004, of which 2.4 million were performed on Medicare beneficiaries. The rate of cataract surgery in the United States is thus greater than 8000 cataract surgeries per million population, whereas in China the number is fewer than 500 cataract surgeries per million. In parts of the developing world, the number may be as low as 50 surgeries per million.

Because surgery is the only treatment currently available for visually significant lenticular opacity, the growing need for surgical resources compounds the already significant

Table 5-1 Global Estimate of Visual Impairment, by WHO Region (millions), 2002

	Afr	Amr	Emr	Eur	Sear	Wpr
Population	672,238	852,551	502,823	877,886	1,590,832	1,717,536
No. of blind people	6782	2419	4026	2732	11,587	9312
No. with low vision	19,996	13,116	12,444	12,789	33,496	32,481
No. with visual impairment	**26,778**	**15,535**	**16,469**	**15,521**	**45,083**	**41,793**

Afr = WHO African Region; Amr = WHO Region of the Americas; Emr = WHO Eastern Mediterranean Region; Eur = WHO European Region; Sear = WHO South-East Asia Region; Wpr = WHO Western Pacific Region.

Modified with permission from Resnikoff S, Pascolini D, Etya'ale D, et al. Global data on visual impairment in the year 2002. *Bull World Health Organ.* 2004;82(11):849.

socioeconomic impact of cataracts in particular and blindness in general. The problem is especially critical in developing countries, where 1 blind individual takes 2 individuals out of the workforce, if the blind person requires the care of an able adult.

Further complicating the issue of cataract treatment in the developing world is that the monetary resources needed in order to offer expensive, advanced surgical methods to patients are lacking. The emergence of manual small-incision cataract surgery (MSICS) has had a positive impact, however. MSICS evolved after years of innovation and combines modern surgical techniques with methods used in the era of extracapsular cataract surgery. With MSICS, clinicians are able to perform 5-minute cataract operations with sutureless closure for approximately $20 per eye. The effectiveness of this procedure has reduced the backlog of patients needing cataract surgery in Nepal and India, with 98% of these patients receiving high-quality intraocular lenses. The technique used in MSICS is described in the following reference.

> Tabin GC, Feilmeier MR. Cataract surgery in the developing world. *Focal Points: Clinical Modules for Ophthalmologists.* San Francisco: American Academy of Ophthalmology; 2011, module 9.

The economic impact of cataract surgery in the United States alone is enormous. It is estimated that the federal government spends more than $3.4 billion each year treating cataract patients through the Medicare program. In addition to the vast number of cataract operations performed each year in the United States, an even greater number of related office visits and tests contribute to the financial impact of cataracts. Further, patients with vision loss incur significantly higher medical costs, and 90% of these costs are unrelated to the eye.

As discussed in Chapter 4, cataracts may be congenital, metabolic, age-related, or traumatic in origin. Of these, age-related cataracts, because of their prevalence, have the greatest socioeconomic impact. However, the lack of a widely accepted, standardized classification system for lens opacities makes it difficult to evaluate precisely the prevalence and incidence of cataracts. The size, shape, density, and location of age-related lens opacities are variable, and most definitions of cataract require a quantifiable reduction in visual acuity in addition to alterations in lens morphology visible at the slit lamp. Also, examination methods are often subjective and require patient participation. Studies of cataract prevalence and incidence are thus easily biased. Further, most estimates of the frequency of age-related cataract are based on data from select groups rather than from the general population. Finally, in many older patients, eyes may have coexisting pathology, producing vision loss that might have been incorrectly attributed to lens changes.

The Age-Related Eye Disease Study (AREDS), performed during the 1990s, demonstrated, among other findings, a high degree of reliability in grading the severity of lens opacities in a large study cohort with mostly early lens changes. The Beaver Dam Eye Study was a large population-based study that was performed in the late 1980s (data published in the 1990s). It reported that 38.8% of men and 45.9% of women older than 74 years had visually significant cataracts. For this study, "significance" was determined by photographic grading of lens opacities and a specified best-corrected visual acuity (20/32 [logMAR equivalent closest to 20/30 Snellen fraction]), excluding those individuals with severe age-related maculopathy.

A follow-up to the Beaver Dam Eye Study was performed between 1993 and 1995 to estimate the incidence of nuclear, cortical, and posterior subcapsular cataract (PSC) in the study cohort. Incident nuclear cataract occurred in 13.1% of the study cohort, cortical cataract in 8.2%, and PSC in 3.4%. The cumulative incidence of nuclear cataract increased from 2.9% in persons aged 43–54 years at baseline to 40.0% in those aged 75 years or older. For cortical cataract and PSC, the corresponding values were 1.9% and 21.8% and 1.4% and 7.3%, respectively. Women were more likely than men to have nuclear cataracts, even after adjustments for age were made.

Published in 1991, the Baltimore Eye Survey revealed that cataract was the leading cause of blindness (20/200 or worse vision) among persons 40 years and older. Untreated cataract was the source of blindness in 27% of African Americans and 13% of whites.

The Longitudinal Study of Cataract (LSC), published in 1997, was an epidemiologic study of the natural history of and risk factors for lens opacities. In this study, nuclear opacification was linked with increasing age, white race, lower education, gout medication, current smoking, family history of cataract, preexisting PSC, and early use of eyeglasses. The LSC assessed new lens opacities and the progression of lenticular opacities, using a research instrument called the *Lens Opacities Classification System III (LOCS III)*. The median age of study participants was 65 years, and the incidence of new opacities was 6% after 2 years and 8% after 5 years. After 5 years' follow-up, the incidence rates for developing cortical and posterior subcapsular opacities were 7.7% and 4.3%, respectively. The progression of preexisting posterior subcapsular opacities was higher, reaching 55.1% after 5 years of follow-up. Although the incidence rates for both cortical and posterior subcapsular opacities were much higher for those aged 65 years or older than for those younger than 65 years, the progression rates for these two age groups were very similar. The Barbados Eye Study provided prevalence data on lens opacities in a predominantly black population. Cortical opacities were the most frequent type of cataract, and women had a higher frequency of opacification than did men.

In a US-based cohort of 8363 individuals older than 61 years at intake, the cumulative rate of cataract surgery was 7.4% annually over 5 years. A second study indicated that each year, 5.7% of individuals 49 years or older become unilaterally pseudophakic. Applied to data from the most recent US census, these percentages translate to 3.3 million cataract surgeries in patients 62 years or older.

Other studies have linked the risk of developing cortical opacities and PSC with higher body mass index (BMI) at baseline and have shown increased risk with increasing BMI over time. The AREDS found that persons with moderate nuclear opacities were more likely to be female, nonwhite, and smokers and to have large macular drusen. Moderate nuclear opacities were less common in persons with higher educational status, in those with a history of diabetes (only patients with mild background diabetic retinopathy [BDR] were included in the study), and in those taking nonsteroidal anti-inflammatory drugs. Moderate cortical opacities were associated with dark iris color, large macular drusen, weight gain, increased sunlight exposure, and thyroid hormone use; they were less common in persons with higher educational status.

Although reported risk factors for cataract development are not consistent, studies repeatedly show that cataracts are more common in African Americans and that nuclear cataracts are more common in women, smokers, and those with less education. Cigarette smokers of both sexes have repeatedly been shown to have an increased risk of developing nuclear lens opacities. Some smoking-related damage to the lens may be reversible, and smoking cessation reduces the risk of cataract by limiting total dose-related damage to the lens.

Age-Related Eye Disease Study Research Group. The age-related eye disease study (AREDS) system for classifying cataracts from photographs: AREDS report no. 4. *Am J Ophthalmol.* 2001;131(2):167–175.

Age-Related Eye Disease Study Research Group. Risk factors associated with age-related nuclear and cortical cataract: a case-control study in the Age-Related Eye Disease Study. AREDS report no. 5. *Ophthalmology.* 2001;108(8):1400–1408.

Christen WG, Glynn RJ, Ajani UA, et al. Smoking cessation and risk of age-related cataract in men. *JAMA.* 2000;284(6):713–716.

Chylack LT Jr, Wolfe JK, Singer DM, et al. The Lens Opacities Classification System III. The Longitudinal Study of Cataract Study Group. *Arch Ophthalmol.* 1993;111(6):831–836.

Erie JC, Baratz KH, Hodge DO, Schleck CD, Burke JP. Incidence of cataract surgery from 1980 through 2004: 25-year population-based study. *J Cataract Refract Surg.* 2007;33(7):1273–1277.

Hiller R, Podgor MJ, Sperduto RD, et al. A longitudinal study of body mass index and lens opacities. The Framingham Studies. *Ophthalmology.* 1998;105(7):1244–1250.

Hiller R, Sperduto RD, Podgor MJ, et al. Cigarette smoking and the risk of development of lens opacities. The Framingham Studies. *Arch Ophthalmol.* 1997;115(9):1113–1118.

Javitt JC, Zhou Z, Willke RJ. Association between vision loss and higher medical care costs in Medicare beneficiaries: costs are greater for those with progressive vision loss. *Ophthalmology.* 2007;114(2):238–245.

Klein BE, Klein R, Lee KE. Incidence of age-related cataract: the Beaver Dam Eye Study. *Arch Ophthalmol.* 1998;116(2):219–225.

Klein BE, Klein R, Linton KL. Prevalence of age-related lens opacities in a population: the Beaver Dam Eye Study. *Ophthalmology.* 1992;99(4):546–552.

Resnikoff S, Pascolini D, Etya'ale D, et al. Global data on visual impairment in the year 2002. *Bull World Health Organ.* 2004;82(11):844–851.

Sommer A, Tielsch JM, Katz J, et al. Racial differences in the cause-specific prevalence of blindness in east Baltimore. *N Engl J Med.* 1991;325(20):1412–1417.

Williams A, Sloan FA, Lee PP. Longitudinal rates of cataract surgery. *Arch Ophthalmol.* 2006;124(9):1308–1314.

CHAPTER 6

Evaluation and Management of Cataracts in Adults

An ophthalmologist evaluating a patient with cataracts must assess the degree to which the lens opacity affects vision and determine whether surgery will improve the quality of life. The following questions should be considered in the evaluation and management of cataract:

- What is the functional impact of the cataract?
- What are the morphological characteristics of the cataract?
- Is surgery indicated either to improve the patient's quality of life or to aid in the management of other ocular conditions?
- Does the patient have ocular or systemic comorbidities that might affect the decision to proceed with surgery or alter the management plan?
- What are the possible barriers to obtaining informed consent or to ensuring good postoperative care?

In most cases, cataract surgery is an elective procedure. Therefore, the ophthalmologist should not only answer these questions but also inform the patient about the impact of the cataract, the risks and benefits of surgical management, the alternatives to surgery, and any applicable options for the intraocular lens to be used if surgery takes place. Ultimately, it is important that both patient and physician be satisfied that surgery is the appropriate choice for improving vision.

Clinical History: Signs and Symptoms

Decreased Visual Acuity

Often, the clinical history of a patient with decreased vision and function secondary to cataract is straightforward, and the patient tells the ophthalmologist which activities have been curtailed or abandoned. Some patients learn of their decline in visual acuity only after being examined. Others deny that they are having any problems until their limitations are demonstrated or privileges are withdrawn because they are no longer visually competent.

Different types of cataract may have different effects on visual acuity, depending on incident light, pupil size, and degree of myopia (Table 6-1). The presence of even small

Table 6-1 Cataract and Its Effect on Visual Acuity

	Growth Rate	Glare	Effect on Distance	Effect on Near	Induced Myopia
Cortical	Moderate	Moderate	Mild	Mild	None
Nuclear	Slow	Mild	Moderate	None	Moderate
Posterior subcapsular	Rapid	Marked	Mild	Marked	None

posterior subcapsular cataracts (PSCs) can greatly disturb near visual acuity (reading vision) even though distance vision is relatively unaffected. In contrast, the induced myopic shift from "oil droplet" cataracts may worsen distance clarity while preserving reading vision. Color vision disturbances may be noted by the patient, especially when the nucleus of the lens turns yellow or brunescent.

Glare and Altered Contrast Sensitivity

Cataract patients often report an increase in glare, which may vary from increased photosensitivity in brightly lit environments to disabling glare in the daytime or with headlights from oncoming cars. Shorter wavelengths of light cause the most scatter; the color, intensity, and direction of lighting also affect glare. This increased sensitivity is particularly prominent with PSCs and, occasionally, with anterior cortical lens changes.

Contrast sensitivity is the ability to detect subtle variations in shading. Because patients with ocular abnormalities have altered contrast sensitivity in reduced luminance, measurement of contrast sensitivity may provide a more comprehensive estimate of the visual resolution of the eye. A significant loss in contrast sensitivity may occur without a similar loss in Snellen acuity. However, abnormal contrast sensitivity is not a specific indicator of vision loss due to cataract.

Myopic Shift

The development of cataract may increase the dioptric power of the lens, commonly causing a mild to moderate degree of myopic shift. Hyperopic presbyopic patients find that their need for distance spectacles diminishes as they experience this "second sight." This phenomenon is encountered with nuclear sclerotic cataracts and disappears when the optical quality of the crystalline lens further deteriorates. Asymmetric development of lens-induced myopia may produce intolerable anisometropia.

Monocular Diplopia or Polyopia

Occasionally, nuclear changes are localized to the inner layers of the lens nucleus, resulting in multiple refractile areas at the center of the lens. Such areas may best be seen as irregularities in the red reflex on retinoscopy or direct ophthalmoscopy. This type of cataract can result in monocular diplopia or polyopia, including ghost images and occasionally a true second image. Monocular diplopia can also occur with other ocular media opacities or other disorders of the eye (see also BCSC Section 5, *Neuro-Ophthalmology*).

Decreased Visual Function

Assessing the overall effect of the cataract on visual function is almost certainly a more appropriate way to determine visual disability than is acuity testing alone. Patients should be asked whether their vision (at near, at distance, under different lighting conditions) is adequate to perform relevant activities of daily living (ADLs) and any hobbies. While no one test can comprehensively assess the effects of a cataract, questionnaires for measuring functional vision may be useful. These include the Activities of Daily Vision Scale (ADVS), the Visual Function Index (VF-14), the National Eye Institute Visual Function Questionnaire (NEI-VFQ), and the Visual Disability Assessment (VDA).

> Mangione CM, Lee PP, Gutierrez PR, et al. Development of the 25-item National Eye Institute Visual Function Questionnaire. *Arch Ophthalmol.* 2001;119(7):1050–1058.
> Mangione CM, Phillips RS, Seddon JM, et al. Development of the "Activities of Daily Vision Scale": a measure of visual functional status. *Med Care.* 1992;30(12):1111–1126.
> Pesudovs K, Wright TA, Gothwal VK. Visual disability assessment: valid measurement of activity limitation and mobility in cataract patients. *Br J Ophthalmol.* 2010;94(6):777–781.
> Steinberg EP, Tielsch JM, Schein OD, et al. The VF-14: an index of functional impairment in patients with cataract. *Arch Ophthalmol.* 1994;112(5):630–638.

Nonsurgical Management

Nonsurgical approaches may be attempted to improve visual function in cataract patients who do not desire surgery or in those for whom surgical management is not feasible. Careful refraction may improve spectacle correction for distance and near vision. For example, patients who have experienced a myopic shift secondary to cataract may hold reading material closer and may be asymptomatic until a change in their glasses is made; a corresponding increase in the power added for near vision is necessary. Use of specialized tints may reduce glare, and brighter illumination can improve the contrast of reading material. Handheld monoculars may facilitate spotting objects at a distance; high-add spectacles, magnifiers, closed-circuit televisions, and telescopic loupes may be used for reading and close work.

Referral to low vision services may be appropriate. For patients whose visual function could be aided or enhanced by vision rehabilitation, the American Academy of Ophthalmology provides *SmartSight,* which is available at http://one.aao.org/ce/educationalcontent/smartsight.aspx.

In patients with small axial cataracts, pupillary dilation, achieved either pharmacologically or by laser pupilloplasty, may improve visual function by allowing more light to pass through peripheral portions of the lens. However, there is a risk of inducing additional glare with this approach.

Pharmacologic reversal of cataracts is a subject of ongoing research. No commercially available medication has been proven to delay or reverse cataract formation in humans. Aldose reductase inhibitors, which block the conversion of glucose to sorbitol, have been shown to prevent cataracts in animals with experimentally induced diabetes. However, studies in humans show no such effect. Antioxidants such as zinc and beta carotene and vitamins E and C do not slow cataract progression.

> American Academy of Ophthalmology Cataract and Anterior Segment Panel. Preferred Practice Pattern Guidelines. *Cataract in the Adult Eye.* San Francisco: American Academy of Ophthalmology; 2011. Available at: www.aao.org/ppp.
> Ettl A, Daxer A, Göttinger W, Schmid E. Inhibition of experimental diabetic cataract by topical administration of RS-verapamil hydrochloride. *Br J Ophthalmol.* 2004;88(1):44–47.
> Kanthan GL, Wang JJ, Rochtchina E, Mitchell P. Use of antihypertensive medications and topical beta-blockers and the long-term incidence of cataract and cataract surgery. *Br J Ophthalmol.* 2009;93(9):1210–1214.

Indications for Surgery

The most common indication for cataract surgery is the patient's desire for improved vision. The decision to operate is not based solely on a specific level of reduced acuity. Key to the decision is determining whether the patient's reduced visual function would improve sufficiently to warrant cataract surgery. Some governmental agencies and industries have minimum standards of visual function for tasks such as driving, flying, and operating complex equipment. A patient whose best-corrected visual acuity does not meet these visual requisites may need to consider cataract surgery. The ophthalmic surgeon must determine, through discussion with the patient and family, as well as through analysis of the results of subjective and objective testing, whether cataract surgery is advisable. To approve reimbursement for cataract surgery, some third-party payers require that patients have a certain level of vision loss; in such cases, glare testing may be useful for documenting loss of visual function beyond that measured by Snellen acuity.

Medical indications for cataract surgery include phacolytic glaucoma, phacomorphic glaucoma, phacoantigenic uveitis, and dislocation of the lens into the anterior chamber. An additional indication for surgery is the presence of a cataract sufficiently opaque to obscure the view of the fundus and impair the diagnosis or management of other ocular diseases such as diabetic retinopathy, macular degeneration, or glaucoma.

Cataract in elderly persons, especially those with significant deafness or early dementia, may lead to isolation. The quality of life of such patients may be greatly improved with spectacle independence following cataract surgery. Also, cataract extraction has been shown to prevent falls and hip fractures and to reduce morbidity and mortality.

Common indications for surgery in a patient with a monocular cataract include loss of stereopsis, diminished peripheral vision, disabling glare, and symptomatic anisometropia. The presence of cataract in one eye has a negative effect on driving performance and accident avoidance.

When a patient has bilateral visually significant cataracts, surgery is performed first in the eye with the more advanced cataract. In fragile patients with active or severe systemic illness, or in those with other ocular diseases contributing to decreased vision, it may be appropriate to operate first on the eye with better visual potential, should only one surgical procedure be anticipated. Consideration may also be given to operating on the dominant eye first.

After undergoing second-eye cataract surgery, patients have been shown to have significant improvements not only in acuity and satisfaction with their vision but also in measures of bilateral visual function such as stereopsis and contrast sensitivity. But the decision of whether to proceed with cataract surgery on the second eye must be individualized to the patient's needs and visual potential, just as it was for the first eye. Also, before proceeding with the second surgery, the physician and patient should allow sufficient time to confirm the success and safety of the first operation.

Symptomatic anisometropia may occur as a result of the initial cataract surgery. The anisometropia may be unsatisfactorily addressed by nonsurgical treatment and may be disabling enough to the patient to justify surgery on the second eye, even if the cataract is at an early stage of development.

In rare instances, consideration might be given to simultaneous, bilateral surgery. Although most ophthalmologists do not perform this type of procedure because of concern about potential bilateral complications, it may be a viable option for patients who are unable to return for second-eye surgery because of health or travel constraints or for those who have limited access to surgical resources. The surgeon should treat each eye as an entirely separate case by using new gloves, draping, instruments, and equipment.

> Bohigian GM, Kamenetzky SA. Risk management in cataract surgery. *Focal Points: Clinical Modules for Ophthalmologists.* San Francisco: American Academy of Ophthalmology; 2007, module 8.
>
> Castells X, Alonso J, Ribó C, et al. Comparison of the results of first and second cataract eye surgery. *Ophthalmology.* 1999;106(4):676–682.
>
> Castells X, Comas M, Alonso J, et al. In a randomized controlled trial, cataract surgery in both eyes increased benefits compared to surgery in one eye only. *J Clin Epidemiol.* 2006;59(2):201–207.
>
> Ishii K, Kabata T, Oshika T. The impact of cataract surgery on cognitive impairment and depressive mental status in elderly patients. *Am J Ophthalmol.* 2008;146(3): 404–409.
>
> Ivers RQ, Cumming RG, Mitchell P, Attebo K. Visual impairment and falls in older adults: the Blue Mountains Eye Study. *J Am Geriatr Soc.* 1998;46(1):58–64.
>
> Javitt JC, Steinberg EP, Sharkey P, et al. Cataract surgery in one eye or both: a billion dollar per year issue. *Ophthalmology.* 1995;102(11):1583–1592; discussion 1592–1593.
>
> Talbot EM, Perkins A. The benefit of second eye cataract surgery. *Eye.* 1998;12(Pt 6):983–989.

Preoperative Evaluation

The following information should be obtained in order to determine whether cataract surgery is advisable. The parameters suggested should be tailored to the specific patient's situation.

General Health of the Patient

A complete medical history is the starting point for the preoperative evaluation. The ophthalmologist should work with the patient's primary care physician to achieve optimal management of all medical problems, especially diabetes mellitus, ischemic heart disease, chronic obstructive pulmonary disease, bleeding disorders, or adrenal suppression caused by systemic corticosteroid use. The ophthalmologist should be aware of the patient's drug sensitivities and use of medications that might alter the outcome of surgery, such as immunosuppressants and anticoagulants. Given the low risk of hemorrhage with topical anesthesia and clear corneal incisions, anticoagulant medications do not universally need to be discontinued prior to cataract surgery. Any alteration in the patient's use of these medications should ideally be done in consultation with the prescribing physician.

The ophthalmologist should inquire specifically about the use of systemic sympathetic $α_{1a}$-adrenergic antagonist medications (including prazosin, terazosin, doxazosin, and tamsulosin) for the treatment of benign prostatic hyperplasia, as they are strongly associated with intraoperative floppy iris syndrome (IFIS) and with fluctuations in pupil size during cataract surgery. All $α_{1a}$-blockers can bind to postsynaptic nerve endings of the iris dilator muscle for a prolonged period, causing excessive iris mobility. This effect may occur after only one dose of the medication and may persist indefinitely, even after discontinuation of the drug. Anecdotal reports document other medications, including certain antipsychotics and antihypertensives, that may possess some $α_{1a}$-antagonist properties and also may be associated with IFIS. See Chapter 8 for further discussion of IFIS.

The ophthalmologist should document medication allergies and question patients and their families about sensitivity to sedatives, narcotics, anesthetics, povidone-iodine, and latex. Factors limiting the patient's ability to cooperate in the operating room or to lie comfortably on the operating room table (eg, deafness, language barriers, dementia, claustrophobia, restless legs syndrome, head tremor, or musculoskeletal disorders) will influence the choice of topical, local, or general anesthesia.

The extent of the formal medical preoperative evaluation should be based on the patient's overall health and may be guided by requirements of the facility where the procedure is to take place. Screening with self-reported information gained from health questionnaires may help identify patients who are at higher risk for medical difficulties related to surgery, although this method should not be the only form of evaluation. Certainly, for all patients with possible risk factors related to their ability to undergo surgery, a history should be obtained and a physical examination along with relevant laboratory work performed. However, routine medical testing before cataract surgery has not been shown to increase the safety of the procedure.

Chang DF, Braga-Mele R, Mamalis N, et al. ASCRS White Paper: clinical review of intraoperative floppy iris syndrome. *J Cataract Refract Surg*. 2008;34(12):2153–2162.

Chang DF, Campbell JR. Intraoperative floppy iris syndrome associated with tamsulosin. *J Cataract Refract Surg*. 2005;31(4):664–673.

Marcus EN, Gayer S, Anderson DR. Medical evaluation of patients before ocular surgery. *Am J Ophthalmology*. 2003;136(2):338–339.

Schein OD, Katz J, Bass EB, et al. The value of routine preoperative medical testing before cataract surgery. Study of Medical Testing for Cataract Surgery. *N Engl J Med*. 2000;342(3):168–175.

Wykoff CC, Flynn HW Jr, Han DP. Allergy to povidone-iodine and cephalosporins: the clinical dilemma in ophthalmic use. *Am J Ophthalmol*. 2011;151(1):4–6.

Pertinent Ocular History

The ocular history will help the ophthalmologist identify conditions that could affect the surgical approach and the visual prognosis. Trauma, inflammation, amblyopia, glaucoma, optic nerve abnormalities, or retinal disease might affect the visual outcome after cataract removal.

Active uveitis should be controlled before cataract surgery so that the risk of complications from postoperative inflammation, such as macular edema and iris adhesion to the lens implant, can be minimized. Ideally, the eye should be quiet without the use of topical corticosteroids for at least 3 months before surgery. Systemic immunomodulation may be necessary to achieve remission. The presence of zonular abnormalities, fibrin membranes, and posterior synechiae will require the surgeon to adjust his or her surgical technique, as discussed in Chapter 9.

A family history of retinal detachment or a history of retinal pathology in either of the patient's eyes is a risk factor for postoperative retinal detachment. Previous vitrectomy for the treatment of retinal disease or vitreous hemorrhage may cause intraoperative chamber fluctuations that increase the risk of posterior capsule disruption and loss of nuclear fragments posteriorly.

In glaucoma patients, optimal control of the intraocular pressure (IOP) should be achieved prior to cataract surgery. If this cannot be accomplished, the surgeon may wish to consider a combined operation (cataract surgery along with an intervention to lower IOP). See Chapter 9 in this volume and BCSC Section 10, *Glaucoma*.

Past records document the patient's visual acuity before the development of cataract. If the patient has had cataract surgery in the fellow eye, it is important to obtain information about the operative and postoperative course. If problems such as elevated IOP, vitreous loss, cystoid macular edema, endophthalmitis, or hemorrhage occurred during or after the first operation, the surgical approach and postoperative follow-up could be modified for the second eye in order to reduce the risk of similar complications.

If the patient previously had refractive surgery, it is helpful to know the following: the type of procedure that was performed, the original refraction, the original keratometry readings, whether any intraoperative complications occurred, and whether the postoperative refraction before cataract development was stable. This information is useful for both calculating the lens implant power and determining the surgical approach.

> Foster CS. Cataract surgery and uveitis. *Current Insight*. San Francisco: American Academy of Ophthalmology; 2006: Q3. Available at http://one.aao.org/CE/News/CurrentInsight.aspx.

Social History

As discussed earlier, the decision to undertake cataract surgery is based not only on the patient's visual acuity but also on the ramifications of reduced vision on the individual's quality of life. The surgeon should be aware of the patient's occupation, hobbies, lifestyle, and any possible chemical dependencies, including nicotine and illicit (recreational) drugs, as all of these may affect postoperative recovery. Any surrogate decision makers must be identified and included in preoperative planning.

Measurements of Visual Function

Visual Acuity Testing

It is useful to measure Snellen acuity under lighted and darkened examination conditions. Although visual acuity testing in the ophthalmologist's office is commonly performed in a darkened room, diminished Snellen acuity from a symptomatic cataract may sometimes be demonstrated only in a lighted room. Distance and near visual acuity must be tested and a careful refraction performed, so that best-corrected visual acuity can be determined. Visual acuity may improve after pupillary dilation, especially in patients with PSCs.

Refraction

Careful refraction must be performed on both eyes. This assessment is useful for calculating the intraocular lens (IOL) power necessary to obtain the desired postoperative refraction, as well as for determining whether a myopic shift has occurred. If the fellow eye has a clear lens and a high refractive error that requires correction, achieving emmetropia in the surgical eye might cause problems with postoperative anisometropia. The ophthalmologist should inform the patient specifically about this possibility. Aiming for a similar myopic refractive result in the fellow eye is one option, but this will ensure long-term dependence on refractive correction. A planned monovision outcome may optimize spectacle independence, but the patient either must have experience with monovision or must be tested to find out whether adapting to unequal refractive errors will be tolerated. Alternatively, the patient can be given the option to wear a contact lens in the phakic eye.

Rigid contact lens overrefraction is a useful technique to assess the degree to which irregular astigmatism or other corneal irregularity is contributing to a patient's visual disability.

Glare Testing

Glare testing attempts to measure the degree of visual impairment caused by the presence of a light source located in the patient's visual field. Testing can be done with a nonprojected eye chart in ambient light conditions or with a projected eye chart and an off-axis bright light directed at the patient. Various instruments are available to standardize and facilitate this measurement. Patients with significant cataracts commonly show a decrease of 3 or more lines under these conditions, compared with results obtained when visual acuity is tested in a darkened room. Performing this assessment before the patient's pupils are dilated is recommended, as studies have shown that visual acuity decreases significantly when testing is performed after dilation. Results of any testing done after pupillary dilation must be adjusted to account for the related decrease in acuity.

Wiggins MN, Irak-Dersu I, Turner SD, Thostenson JD. Glare testing in patients with cataract after dilation. *Ophthalmology.* 2009;116(7):1332–1335.

Contrast Sensitivity

Patients with cataracts may experience diminished contrast sensitivity even when Snellen acuity is preserved. Various specialized charts have been developed to test contrast sensitivity in the ophthalmologist's office. Some charts are mounted on a wall; others are handheld or incorporate the use of a monitor. Certain contrast sensitivity charts feature sine wave gratings to evaluate different spatial frequencies. However, no instrument is currently considered the standard for contrast sensitivity testing. Of note, contrast sensitivity may be decreased by a wide variety of ophthalmic conditions affecting the cornea, optic nerve, and retina. It is therefore essential that the ophthalmologist identify any comorbidities before attributing an irregularity in test results solely to cataract.

> Pesudovs K, Hazel CA, Doran RM, Elliott DB. The usefulness of Vistech and FACT contrast sensitivity charts for cataract and refractive surgery outcomes research. *Br J Ophthalmol.* 2004;88(1):11–16.

External Examination

The preoperative evaluation of a patient with cataract should include the body habitus and any abnormalities of the external eye and ocular adnexa. Such conditions as extensive supraclavicular fat, kyphosis, ankylosing spondylitis, generalized obesity, or head tremor may affect the surgical approach. The presence of enophthalmos or prominent brow may affect not only the surgical approach but also the chosen route of anesthesia.

Entropion, ectropion, or eyelid-closure abnormalities, as well as abnormalities in the tear film, may have an impact on the ocular surface and thus adversely affect postoperative recovery if not addressed preoperatively. Severe blepharitis and acne rosacea may pose an increased risk of endophthalmitis and should likewise be treated before cataract surgery. Active nasolacrimal disease should also be treated, particularly if there is a history of inflammation, infection, or obstruction.

Motility

The ophthalmologist should evaluate ocular alignment and test the range of movement of the extraocular muscles. Cover testing should be performed to document any muscle deviation. Abnormal motility may suggest preexisting strabismus with amblyopia as a cause of vision loss. Patients must be made aware that they may experience diplopia after cataract surgery if they have a significant tropia resulting in disruption of fusion. Also, removal of a dense cataract may improve vision but make the patient aware of ocular misalignment.

Pupils

In addition to checking direct and consensual constriction of the pupil to light, the ophthalmologist should perform the swinging flashlight test to detect a *relative afferent pupillary defect (RAPD;* also known as a *Marcus Gunn pupil),* the presence of which indicates extensive retinal disease or optic nerve dysfunction. (See also BCSC Section 5, *Neuro-Ophthalmology.*) Although the vision of a patient with RAPD in the cataractous eye may improve after cataract surgery, the visual outcome may be limited by optic nerve dysfunction. The patient must be made aware of the possibility of less than complete restoration of vision.

It is important to measure the size of the pupil under different lighting conditions, because this information may affect selection of the IOL. For example, small-optic lenses may be inappropriate for a patient who has a large pupil in moderate or dim illumination. The edge of the optic can fall inside the pupil border, allowing light to pass around the optic edge, with resultant glare or dysphotopsias. Also, the function of a multifocal IOL will be affected by a small pupil or one that does not adequately constrict. It is helpful to assess pupil size before and after dilation, because small pupils that do not dilate adequately (eg, in patients with diabetes, posterior synechiae, exfoliation syndrome, or a history of systemic α_{1a}-adrenergic antagonist or long-term topical miotic use) may increase the risk of surgical complications and require that the surgeon use expansion techniques. These techniques are discussed in Chapters 7 and 9.

Slit-Lamp Examination

Conjunctiva

Vascularization or scarring of the conjunctiva due to previous inflammation, injury, or ocular surgery may indicate compromised healing and limit surgical exposure. Symblepharon or shortening of the fornices may be associated with underlying systemic or ocular surface diseases. Infectious processes should receive appropriate treatment before cataract surgery in order to ensure optimal postoperative healing.

Cornea

The clinician should assess corneal thickness and look for the presence of corneal dystrophy, as abnormalities could increase the risk of poor healing and decompensation postoperatively. Specular reflection with the slit lamp may provide an estimate of the endothelial cell count and provide information regarding cell morphology. Irregularity of the Descemet membrane associated with corneal guttae, as well as any central opacity, may affect the surgeon's view of the lens during surgery and limit visual acuity after surgery. In patients with pannus due to long-term contact lens wear or other conditions, the surgeon should plan to avoid making corneal incisions in areas of vascularization, if possible. Also, weakened or thinned areas in the cornea should be identified so that they can be avoided during surgery.

Areas of scarring possibly consistent with a history of herpetic eye disease should prompt further questioning of the patient, as prophylactic antiviral medication and avoidance of steroid therapy in the perioperative period may be advisable to prevent reactivation.

If the patient has undergone previous corneal refractive surgery, the surgeon should document the placement of radial or astigmatic incisions, as well as any apparent problems with healing. If the patient has undergone previous radial keratotomy (RK), the surgeon must take care to develop a surgical plan that avoids corneal splitting at the site of the RK incisions. See also BCSC Section 13, *Refractive Surgery*.

Anterior Chamber and Iris

Knowing the depth of the anterior chamber and the axial thickness of the lens aids in surgical planning. A shallow anterior chamber may indicate anatomically narrow angles, nanophthalmos, short axial length, an intumescent lens, or forward displacement of the lens–iris diaphragm due to posterior pathology (eg, a ciliary body tumor).

The clinician should perform gonioscopy preoperatively to rule out suspected angle abnormalities, including peripheral anterior synechiae, neovascularization, or a prominent major arterial circle. Use of a 3-mirror lens helps in the evaluation of the lens zonule for traumatic or congenital dehiscence. Gonioscopy is essential if anterior chamber IOL implantation is anticipated.

The presence of iridodonesis or exfoliation at the margin of the undilated pupil indicates weakened or absent zonular attachments and may affect the surgical plan.

Crystalline Lens

The clinician should carefully note the appearance of the lens both before and after dilation of the pupil. The impact of "oil droplet" nuclear cataracts and small PSCs is best correlated with visual symptoms before pupil dilation. After dilation, nuclear density can be evaluated, exfoliation syndrome can be detected, and opacities and distortion of the retinoscopic reflex can be visualized more easily.

To assess the lenticular contribution to the visual deficit, the clinician should evaluate the clarity of the media in the visual axis. During the slit-lamp examination, a thin slit beam of white light is focused on the posterior capsule. The light is then changed to cobalt blue. If the posterior capsule is no longer illuminated (as a result of blue-light scatter), the contribution to visual acuity is significant, with visual acuity usually being 20/50 or worse. Dense, brunescent nuclear sclerotic cataracts may permit remarkably good vision, especially at near, whereas vacuolar cataracts detected through the red reflex can cause surprisingly severe vision loss. When dense cortical opacification is present, the intraoperative use of capsular dye to enhance visualization of the capsulorrhexis should be considered. A congenital posterior polar opacity is associated with a significant risk of capsule rupture and should be identified before surgery.

The position of the lens and the integrity of the zonular fibers should also be evaluated. Lens decentration, phacodonesis, or excessive distance between the lens and the pupillary margin indicates zonular disruption due to conditions such as lens subluxation as a result of previous trauma, metabolic disorders, or hypermature cataract. An indentation or flattening of the lens periphery may indicate focal loss of zonular support. For patients with these types of zonular disruption, the surgeon should be prepared to alter surgical technique, including using capsular tension rings or other capsular or iris support devices intraoperatively.

Ozturk F, Osher RH. Capsular staining: recent developments. *Curr Opinion Ophthalmol.* 2006;17(1):42–44.

Pandey SK, Werner L, Escobar-Gomez M, Roig-Melo EA, Apple DJ. Dye-enhanced cataract surgery. Part 1: anterior capsule staining for capsulorrhexis in advanced/white cataract. *J Cataract Refract Surg.* 2000;26(7):1052–1059.

Limitations of Slit-Lamp Examination

Some visually significant cataracts may appear minimal on slit-lamp biomicroscopy. However, examination of the lens with the retinoscope may clarify the lenticular contribution to the patient's vision changes. By examining the retinoscopic reflex, the clinician may detect posterior subcapsular opacities, refractile nuclear changes, or even diffuse cataracts. Similarly, examination using the direct ophthalmoscope through a +10 D lens at a distance of 2 ft will enhance the portions of the cataractous lens that are producing optical aberrations. This technique is particularly useful for identifying "oil droplet" cataracts.

Fundus Evaluation

Ophthalmoscopy

The ophthalmologist must perform a full fundus examination to evaluate the macula, optic nerve, vitreous, retinal vessels, and retinal periphery. Particular attention should be paid to early macular degeneration or other maculopathy that may limit vision rehabilitation after an otherwise uneventful cataract extraction. The indirect ophthalmoscope is not useful for judging the visual significance of cataract. Although the direct ophthalmoscope, retinal contact lens, and noncontact fundus lens are more useful in judging media clarity, the ophthalmologist must keep in mind that they, too, provide light that is more intense than that available to the patient under ambient lighting conditions.

Patients with diabetes should be examined carefully for the presence of macular edema, retinal ischemia, and background and proliferative retinopathy. Even in uncomplicated cataract surgery and in patients with minimal or no retinopathy, diabetic eye disease can progress postoperatively. Retinal ischemia may potentiate posterior or anterior neovascularization postoperatively, especially if the surgeon uses an intracapsular technique or ruptures the posterior capsule during extracapsular cataract extraction. Careful examination of the retinal periphery may reveal the presence of vitreoretinal traction or preexisting retinal holes and lattice degeneration that may warrant preoperative treatment.

> Hong T, Mitchell P, de Loryn T, Rochtchina E, Cugati S, Wang JJ. Development and progression of diabetic retinopathy 12 months after phacoemulsification cataract surgery. *Ophthalmology.* 2009;116(8):1510–1514.

Optic Nerve

The ophthalmologist should examine the optic nerve for cupping and pallor, as well as other abnormalities. Visual acuity, measurement of IOP, and the results of confrontation testing and the pupillary examination will help determine whether other adjunctive testing is warranted.

Fundus Evaluation With Opaque Media

B-scan ultrasonography of the posterior segment of the eye is useful whenever a dense cataract makes visualization of the retina impossible. Ultrasonography can elucidate whether a retinal detachment, vitreous opacity, posterior pole tumor, or staphyloma is present.

(See also BCSC Section 3, *Clinical Optics*.) Tests such as light projection, 2-point discrimination, gross color vision, photostress recovery, blue-light entoptoscopy, or Maddox rod may also be useful in detecting retinal pathology. Electroretinography and visually evoked response testing are warranted when other modalities are inconclusive and the surgeon must decide whether cataract removal would provide any benefit.

See BCSC Section 12, *Retina and Vitreous*, for discussion of these tests.

Special Tests

Potential Acuity Estimation

Potential acuity estimation can be helpful in assessing the lenticular contribution to vision loss. The potential acuity pinhole test is a simple but accurate method of evaluation for patients who do not have other ocular pathology and whose visual acuity is better than 20/200. For this test, the patient is asked to read a brightly illuminated near card through a pinhole aperture. The Retinal Acuity Meter, or RAM (AMA Optics, Miami Beach, FL), functions in a similar manner.

In laser interferometry, twin sources of monochromatic helium–neon laser light create a diffraction fringe pattern on the retinal surface. Transmission of this pattern is mostly independent of lens opacities. It is possible to estimate retinal visual acuity by varying the spacing of the pattern; however, the area of the pattern subtending the retina is considerably larger than the fovea. For this reason, small foveal lesions that limit vision may not be detected.

The Potential Acuity Meter (PAM) (Mentor/Marco, Jacksonville, FL) is one of several instruments that project a numerical or Snellen vision chart through a small entrance pupil. The image can be projected onto the retina, around lenticular opacities, allowing for an estimate of best visual acuity if the media abnormality were absent.

It is important to note that these tests can be misleading in the presence of several disorders, including age-related macular degeneration, amblyopia, macular edema, glaucoma, small macular scars, and serous retinal detachment. An accurate clinical examination of the eye is often the best predictor of visual outcome.

In rare cases in which the results of other testing are inconclusive, electroretinography or visually evoked response testing can be performed to evaluate retinal and/or optic nerve function.

> Hofeldt AJ, Weiss MJ. Illuminated near card assessment of potential acuity in eyes with cataract. *Ophthalmology*. 1998;105(8):1531–1536.
> Melki SA, Safar A, Martin J, Ivanova A, Adi M. Potential acuity pinhole: a simple method to measure potential visual acuity in patients with cataracts, comparison to potential acuity meter. *Ophthalmology*. 1999;106(7):1262–1267.

Visual Field Testing

Confrontation field testing should be performed in all cataract patients, although formal visual field testing is not indicated for every patient with lens opacity. Visual field testing may help the ophthalmologist identify vision loss resulting from disease processes other than cataract. Patients with a history of glaucoma, optic nerve disease, or retinal abnormality may benefit from static or kinetic visual field evaluation to document the degree of visual field loss. Preoperative visual field loss does not preclude improvement in visual function following cataract surgery. Progressive cataracts may induce diffuse visual field depression that disappears after cataract removal.

Objective Tests of Macular Function

Optical coherence tomography (OCT) is not routinely done as part of the preoperative testing regimen for cataract surgery. However, it may be useful in the assessment or detection of macular pathology, including neovascularization, edema, holes, and traction. OCT should be considered when the vision is poorer than the degree of cataract would suggest, as subtle macular traction or edema can be accurately identified with this test.

Fluorescein angiography can be used to assess microvascular retinopathy, macular edema, and neovascularization.

Preoperative Measurements

Accurate preoperative measurements of the eye are essential to achieving the desired postoperative refractive result.

Biometry

Ocular axial length (AL) is a key component of IOL power calculations, discussed later in this chapter. Several techniques are available to measure AL. No matter which is used, it is helpful to obtain data for both eyes, even if surgery is planned for only one eye. The difference in AL between the two eyes should be no greater than 0.3 mm, unless there is a refractive difference or there are other relevant ocular findings. The clinician should know the cause of any significant disparity in AL.

A-scan ultrasonography measures AL by using either an immersion technique (Fig 6-1) or a contact applanation method. With the immersion technique, a shell is placed on the eye between the eyelids to provide a watertight seal over the cornea. An ultrasound transducer is mounted in the shell. With the contact applanation method, the examiner must be careful not to compress the cornea, because corneal compression results in an artificially shortened AL measurement. Though generally not clinically significant in the patient with an "average" refraction, such errors become more important in the patient with high hyperopia (AL of 20 mm or less), in whose short eyes each millimeter of error results in up to 3.75 D of inaccuracy in IOL power. The immersion technique avoids this problem.

It should be noted that ultrasonographic measurement of AL is actually determined by calculation. The ultrasonic biometer measures the transit time of the ultrasound pulse. Using an estimated average velocity through the various ocular media (cornea, aqueous, lens, and vitreous), the biometric software calculates the AL. This value should be altered when velocities differ from the norm. For example, in performing AL measurements in a patient with silicone oil in the posterior chamber, the clinician must take into account the different transit times for silicone oil and vitreous, which are 980 m/sec and 1532 m/sec,

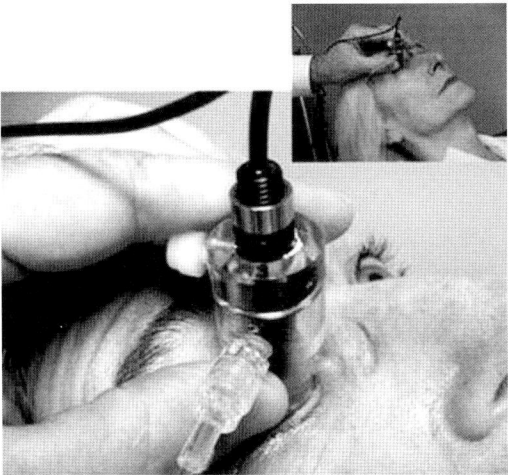

Figure 6-1 Immersion shell (Prager design). *(Courtesy of ESI, Inc.)*

respectively. In addition, the index of refraction of silicone oil is significantly less than that of vitreous, and thus the refractive index of the oil (as well as the design of the IOL) must be figured into IOL calculations for these eyes.

Optical biometers are noncontact instruments that use optical coherence reflectometry instead of ultrasound to measure multiple parameters, such as AL, corneal curvature, anterior chamber depth, and horizontal white-to-white distance (corneal diameter). Because the level of patient cooperation varies, the technician or physician performing biometry should be adept at working with patients to obtain the most accurate measurements. Biometers are optical devices; therefore, measurements may be confounded by corneal scarring, mature or posterior subcapsular cataracts, or vitreous hemorrhage. Examples of optical biometers are the IOLMaster (Carl Zeiss Meditec, Dublin, CA) and the Lenstar LS 900 (Haag-Streit, Koeniz, Switzerland).

> Bjeloš RM, Bušić M, Cima I, Kuzmanović EB, Bosnar D, Miletić D. Intraobserver and interobserver repeatability of ocular components measurement in cataract eyes using a new optical low coherence reflectometer. *Graefes Arch Clin Exp Ophthalmol.* 2011; 249(1):83–87. Epub 2010 Oct 28.
>
> Hill WE. The IOLMaster. *Techniques in Ophthalmology.* 2003;1:62–67.
>
> Packer M, Fine IH, Hoffman RS, Coffman PG, Brown LK. Immersion A-scan compared with partial coherence interferometry: outcomes analysis. *J Cataract Refract Surg.* 2002;28(2):239–242.
>
> Roessler GF, Huth JK, Dietlein TS, et al. Accuracy and reproducibility of axial length measurement in eyes with silicone oil endotamponade. *Br J Ophthalmol.* 2009; 93(11):1492–1494.

Corneal Topography

Topography provides a map of the corneal contour. Using a method similar to that of the Placido disk or Scheimpflug imaging, it provides additional information about the corneal surface and power. Corneal topography is particularly helpful if the patient has irregular astigmatism or early keratoconus, has previously undergone keratorefractive surgery, may desire a toric IOL, or may require limbal relaxing incisions.

Additional Evaluation of the Cornea

In patients with a history of endothelial dystrophy, previous ocular surgery, or trauma, additional corneal measurements may be useful. These data may aid the surgeon in counseling the patient regarding the possibility of postoperative corneal decompensation. In some cases, consideration of a combined surgery incorporating removal of the cataract and transplantation of corneal tissue may be in order.

Corneal pachymetry, a method used to measure corneal thickness, is useful for indirectly assessing the function of the endothelium. In general, significantly increased central corneal thickness in patients with endothelial dysfunction is associated with a greater risk of postoperative corneal decompensation.

Specular microscopy is used to determine the number of corneal endothelial cells per square millimeter and evaluate their regularity. Because cataract surgery results in some loss of endothelial cells, the risk of postoperative corneal decompensation is increased if the preoperative endothelial cell count is low. Abnormal endothelial cell morphology, including enlargement (polymegathism) and irregularity (pleomorphism), may limit the cornea's ability to withstand stress. (See also BCSC Section 8, *External Disease and Cornea.*)

IOL Power Determination

Formulas used for calculating the appropriate IOL power are based on the refracting power of the cornea, the anticipated postoperative distance between the anterior surface of the cornea and the anterior surface of the IOL (anterior chamber depth), and the AL of the eye. The refracting power of the cornea is determined by keratometry (manual or automatic) or by optical coherence biometry. Anterior chamber depth is estimated from measurements made on eyes with implants similar to the style of IOL to be used, or it is measured using biometry. The AL is the distance between the anterior surface of the cornea and the fovea as measured by A-scan ultrasonography or optical coherence reflectometry (see the earlier discussion on determining AL by A-scan ultrasonography and optical coherence biometry). For every IOL, an "*A* constant," a theoretical value relating the lens power to AL and keratometry, is specified by the manufacturer. This constant is not expressed in units, and it is specific to the design of the IOL and its intended location and orientation within the eye.

Preventing Errors in IOL Calculation, Selection, and Insertion

The A-scan transducer should be calibrated before each day's use. Several scans should be done on each patient, and the measurements should cluster around a value with no more than 0.2-mm variance. Both eyes should be checked, especially if the first eye measures longer or shorter than anticipated. The intereye difference should be no greater than 0.3 mm unless there is a refractive or other anatomical explanation. The surgeon should make sure that the correct patient name and K readings, as well as AL and white-to-white measurements, are written on an IOL form. Also, the appropriate lens power and manufacturer's model number should be specified on this form. In addition, lenses and powers for placement in the bag, sulcus, or anterior chamber angle should be selected and carefully distinguished.

This information should be accessible to the surgeon in the operating room, and the lenses should be pulled preoperatively. The surgeon should check the IOL calculations to verify that the lenses are correct and should perform a final check before opening the lens just prior to insertion.

IOL Calculation

Regression formulas are empiric formulas that are generated by averaging large numbers of postoperative clinical results. These formulas are used to predict the appropriate IOL power for emmetropia. The following formula, developed by Sanders, Retzlaff, and Kraff in the 1980s (SRK formula), will serve as illustration of IOL calculation.

$$P = A - (2.5L) - 0.9K$$

where

P = lens implant power for emmetropia (diopters)
L = axial length (mm)
K = average keratometric reading (diopters)
A = constant specific to the lens implant to be used

Newer versions of regression formulas have been developed that are helpful in IOL power calculation for eyes outside the range of 22–25 mm in axial length (eg, SRK/T, Holladay 2, Hoffer Q, Haigis). These later generations of IOL formulas are also more complex. For example, they incorporate the concept that the postoperative anterior chamber depth is not identical to preoperative measurements but varies with factors such as corneal curvature and IOL position. In addition, the formulas allow the ophthalmologist to adjust IOL calculations based on personal experience with a particular lens.

> Fang JP, Hill WE, Wang L, Chang V, Koch DD. Advanced intraocular lens power calculations. In: Kohnen T, Koch DD, eds. *Cataract and Refractive Surgery*. Berlin: Springer-Verlag; 2006:31–48.
>
> Hoffer KJ. Modern IOL power calculations: avoiding errors and planning for special circumstances. *Focal Points: Clinical Modules for Ophthalmologists*. San Francisco: American Academy of Ophthalmology; 1999, module 12.
>
> Narváez J, Zimmerman G, Stulting RD, Chang DH. Accuracy of intraocular lens power prediction using the Hoffer Q, Holladay 1, Holladay 2, and SRK/T formulas. *J Cataract Refract Surg*. 2006;32(12):2050–2053.
>
> Prager TC, Hardten DR, Fogal BJ. Enhancing intraocular lens outcome precision: an evaluation of axial length determinations, keratometry, and IOL formulas. *Ophthalmol Clin North Am*. 2006;19(4):435–448.

Improving Outcomes

The cataract surgeon should track his or her refractive outcomes, asking questions such as the following: Are there overcorrections or undercorrections, and do they occur more often with longer eyes, shorter eyes, or both? Does the incision routinely induce cylinder? Are toric lenses correcting as calculated? If limbal relaxing incisions have been used intraoperatively for the correction of astigmatism, have they been effective? Commercially available programs may be useful for tracking outcomes.

After the surgeon has analyzed these factors, he or she may make adjustments to improve refractive outcomes, such as including a "surgeon factor" (a modification of the parameters used that reflects the surgeon's experience) in lens power calculation, changing the calculation software, or using immersion or optical biometry. Improving outcomes is important for increasing not only patient satisfaction but also surgeon confidence.

IOL Calculation Following Refractive Surgery

Calculating the IOL power for eyes that have undergone refractive surgery presents problems for both patients and surgeons. These patients were initially motivated to have refractive surgery because they did not want to be dependent on glasses. They do not want to wear glasses after cataract surgery. However, determining the central keratometric power, a key element in lens power calculation, is complicated because of the corneal change that occurred as a result of the original refractive procedure. For example, the refractive outcomes of cataract surgery patients who had previous radial keratotomy (RK) were often fraught with undercorrections.

Manual keratometers and corneal topography units (videokeratography) do not measure corneal curvature directly but rather calculate the curvature of the anterior cornea. Following corneal refractive surgery, the cornea becomes aspheric and does not maintain a spherocylindrical contour. This asphericity invalidates the anterior corneal curvature measurements obtained by either type of instrument.

In addition, although RK did not alter the relative positions of the anterior and posterior corneal surfaces, such is not the case following photorefractive keratectomy (PRK) or laser in situ keratomileusis (LASIK). For these reasons, different techniques must be employed to accurately estimate the anterior corneal surface curvature following these types of refractive surgery. Newer corneal topography systems that measure both anterior and posterior corneal curvatures can improve the accuracy of IOL power calculation.

Patients who have undergone previous corneal refractive surgery should be informed of potential problems with accurate IOL selection. The surgeon should mention that "refractive surprise" due to overcorrections and undercorrections and potentially requiring IOL exchange is a possibility; that further corneal refractive surgery may be needed, if feasible; and that spectacle or contact lens correction may be necessary postoperatively. Documenting this discussion is extremely important.

A variety of methods have been developed to better estimate the central corneal power after refractive surgery. As each method has advantages and disadvantages, the ophthalmic surgeon should use more than one method to calculate the corneal power. Selecting the highest IOL value of a tightly clustered group may avoid undercorrection. See also BCSC Section 13, *Refractive Surgery*.

Contact lens method

The contact lens method uses a plano hard contact lens with a known base curve to determine the corneal power. Corneal power is calculated as the sum of the contact lens base curve, power, and overrefraction minus the spherical equivalent of the manifest refraction without a contact lens. This method is applicable only to those patients with a best-corrected visual acuity of at least 20/80; and, although it is logical, it has not yet been validated through clinical studies.

Topographical method

This method (after Maloney) uses a topography machine to select the apical axial curvature:

Central keratometric power = (Central topographic power × 376/337.5) − 4.9

Smith RJ, Chan WK, Maloney RK. The prediction of surgically induced refractive change from corneal topography. *Am J Ophthalmol.* 1998;125(1):44–53.

Historical methods

If the patient's pre–refractive surgery data are available, the surgeon can use the clinical history method to calculate the IOL power.

One such method (after Hoffer) involves calculating the corneal power from the refractive and keratometry measurements made before and after the patient's refractive surgery. Thus, it is critical that the pre–refractive surgery data are accurate. The formula is

$K1$ + (sph equiv 1) − (sph equiv 2) = $K2$

where

$K1$ = average corneal power before refractive surgery
sph equiv 1 = spherical equivalent refractive error before refractive surgery
sph equiv 2 = spherical equivalent refractive error after refractive surgery but prior to cataract development
$K2$ = estimated corneal power after refractive surgery

Another historical method (after Feiz and Mannis) calculates the IOL power from the pre–refractive surgery data and then increases this power by a factor related to the amount of refractive change in the spectacle plane produced by the refractive surgery:

IOL pre–refractive surgery − (change in refraction/0.7) = IOL desired for patient

A potential problem with using certain regression formulas in post–refractive surgery cases is that reduced central corneal power may be linked in the formula to an anterior chamber depth that is assumed to be less than it actually is, resulting in the calculation of a lower IOL power than is really required. The Holladay 2 formula includes pre-refractive corneal data that may correct for this error. Otherwise, the keratometric value may be modified so that undercorrections are reduced.

Aramberri J. Intraocular lens power calculation after corneal refractive surgery: Double-K method. *J Cataract Refract Surg.* 2003;29(11):2063–2068.

Feiz V, Mannis MJ, Garcia-Ferrer F, et al. Intraocular lens power calculation after laser in situ keratomileusis for myopia and hyperopia: a standardized approach. *Cornea.* 2001; 20(8):792–797.

Hamed AM, Wang L, Misra M, Koch DD. A comparative analysis of five methods of determining corneal refractive power in eyes that have undergone myopic laser in situ keratomileusis. *Ophthalmology.* 2002;109(4):651–658.

Seitz B, Langenbucher A, Nguyen NX, Kus MM, Küchle M. Underestimation of intraocular lens power for cataract surgery after myopic photorefractive keratectomy. *Ophthalmology.* 1999;106(4):693–702.

Wang L, Booth MA, Koch DD. Comparison of intraocular lens power calculation methods in eyes that have undergone LASIK. *Ophthalmology.* 2004;111(10):1825–1831.

Patient Preparation and Informed Consent

When planning cataract surgery, the surgeon must evaluate the patient's ability to comply with the postoperative care regimen. The surgeon should inform the patient (and caregivers, if appropriate) of the importance of using prescribed medication, maintaining proper ocular hygiene, and keeping required appointments. It is helpful to provide written instructions, along with appropriate illustrations or video presentations, and include a family member or friend in preoperative discussions in order to reinforce the patient's memory. The patient should understand that there are activity restrictions during the immediate postoperative period, although the advent of small-incision surgery has significantly minimized these limitations. The surgeon should also assess the patient's ability to function with only the fellow eye in the event that vision rehabilitation of the surgical eye is prolonged.

The surgeon must obtain informed consent preoperatively. Before deciding to proceed with cataract surgery, the patient should have a clear understanding of the indications for surgery, the risks and benefits, and the alternatives to surgical intervention. The surgeon should identify any known reason for potentially decreased visual outcome or prolonged healing. In addition, the surgeon and patient should discuss the anticipated postoperative refractive status, the limitations of pseudophakic correction, and the proposed date for providing the final optical correction.

Any costs associated with the surgery (eg, those related to medications or the use of premium IOL implants) should also be clearly outlined preoperatively. In addition, if co-management with an optometrist or another ophthalmologist is planned, the patient must be explicitly notified and must give consent in writing.

American Academy of Ophthalmology and American Society of Cataract and Refractive Surgery. Joint Position Paper. Ophthalmic Postoperative Care. San Francisco: American Academy of Ophthalmology; 2000. Available at http://one.aao.org/CE/PracticeGuidelines/ClinicalStatements.aspx.

American Academy of Ophthalmology Cataract and Anterior Segment Panel. Preferred Practice Pattern Guidelines. *Cataract in the Adult Eye.* San Francisco: American Academy of Ophthalmology; 2011. Available at: www.aao.org/ppp.

Moseley TH, Wiggins MN, O'Sullivan P. Effects of presentation method on the understanding of informed consent. *Br J Ophthalmol.* 2006;90(8):990–993.

CHAPTER **7**

Surgery for Cataract

In this chapter, we will briefly review the past, examine the present, and look to the future of cataract surgery.

The Remote Past

Ancient and Medieval Techniques

The first documented treatment of cataract is couching (from the French verb *coucher*, to put to bed), which has a colorful history starting from about the fifth century BC and which physicians in parts of the developing world continue to use today (Fig 7-1). Couching was practiced in India, and its use spread throughout the Roman Empire, medieval Europe, and sub-Saharan Africa. The procedure was an outgrowth of the limited understanding of ocular anatomy. The "crystalloides" (or lens) was thought to rest in the middle of the eye, in front of which was a clear space. An abnormal "humor" developed and flowed in front of the lens (the word *cataract* also means waterfall). The couching procedure sought to displace the abnormal material from its position in front of the crystalloides.

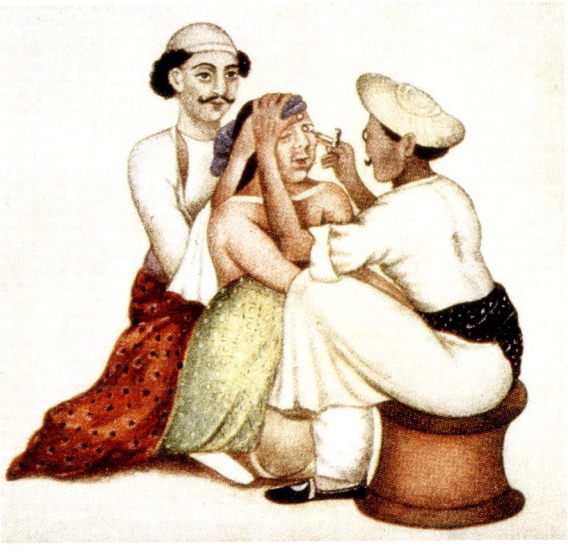

Figure 7-1 Couching. *(Reproduced from Duke-Elder S.* Diseases of the Lens and Vitreous; Glaucoma and Hypotony. *St Louis: Mosby; 1969. System of Ophthalmology; vol II.)*

Couching was performed most commonly on patients with mature cataracts. The patient was seated and positioned so that sunlight would stream over the surgeon's shoulder, illuminating the patient's head. Techniques involved the use of 1 or 2 instruments. Basically, an incision was made somewhere posterior to the corneoscleral junction. A knife or needle (Fig 7-2) was used for the entry, and a needle or rod was used to push the cataractous lens inferiorly. An assistant to the physician restrained the patient. The speed of dislocation was related to both the skill of the surgeon and the status of the zonule. "Patching" with soft wool soaked either in egg white, breast milk, or clarified butter was applied postoperatively.

How miraculous it must have seemed, particularly to the patient, who began the day as a blind person needing to be led to the procedure area, and who, by procedure's end, was able to see enough to walk in familiar surroundings. Not only was the patient rehabilitated, but the burden on the patient's family was reduced significantly. This immediate outcome was responsible for the procedure's popularity. The lack of sterilization and the inflammation that would occur from the retained lens with its disrupted capsule resulted in complications that developed after the surgeon had gone on to another town.

A variant technique, described by the Iraqi ocularist Ammar (AD 996–1020), involved suction aspiration of the cataract through a hollow needle. Syrians in the 12th and 13th centuries also tried this method but abandoned it because of lack of efficacy.

> Corser N. Couching for cataract: its rise and fall. In: *Proceedings from the Ninth Annual History of Medicine Days*. Calgary: University of Calgary; 2000:35–41.
>
> Sood NN, Ratnaraj A. Couching for cataract: hazards and management. *Am J Ophthalmol*. 1968;66(4):687–693.

Early Extracapsular Cataract Extraction

By 1600, anatomists had correctly identified the true position of the lens, and opacification of the lens had become the new definition of the word *cataract*. This simple statement belies the controversies that these new understandings generated between anatomists

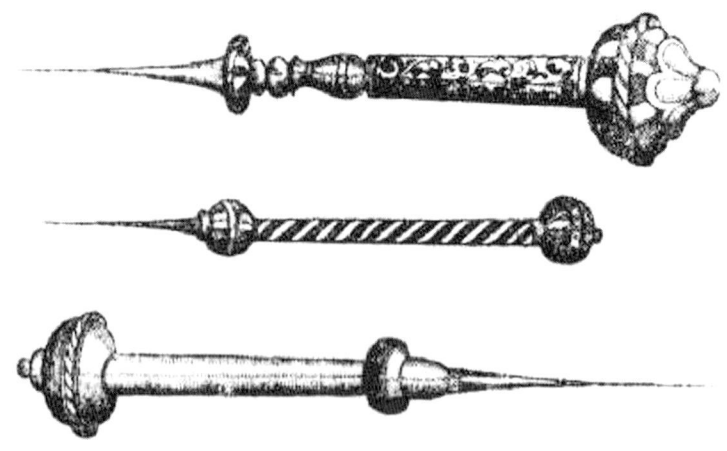

Figure 7-2 Couching needles. *(Courtesy of the Royal College of Ophthalmologists.)*

and surgeons; however, that more modern view required an equally modern therapeutic response.

Daviel (1696–1762) is justifiably credited with propelling cataract surgery toward the modern era. He restricted his practice to ophthalmology, and his decision to remove rather than displace the cataract was followed by the development of instruments to allow this revolutionary procedure. In Daviel's method of cataract extraction, an incision was made through the inferior cornea and enlarged with scissors. The cornea was elevated, the lens capsule incised, the nucleus expressed, and the cortex removed by curettage (Fig 7-3). Each operation took a few minutes and was performed without either anesthesia or aseptic technique. Presciently, Daviel's writings mention removal of the anterior lens capsule after creation of a circular opening.

Daviel's extracapsular cataract extraction (ECCE) was an innovation and an improvement over couching. But the technique, burdened by its moment in time, raised the following issues: wound healing; uveal, vitreous, or retinal prolapse; lens remnant–induced inflammation; and infection. Secondary procedures were common, particularly opening pupillary membranes that resulted from capsular opacification (discission). In fact, all the complications of cataract surgery that occur in small numbers in our era (as discussed in Chapter 8, Complications of Cataract Surgery) occurred with greater frequency in Daviel's era; he reported a 50% success rate with his method.

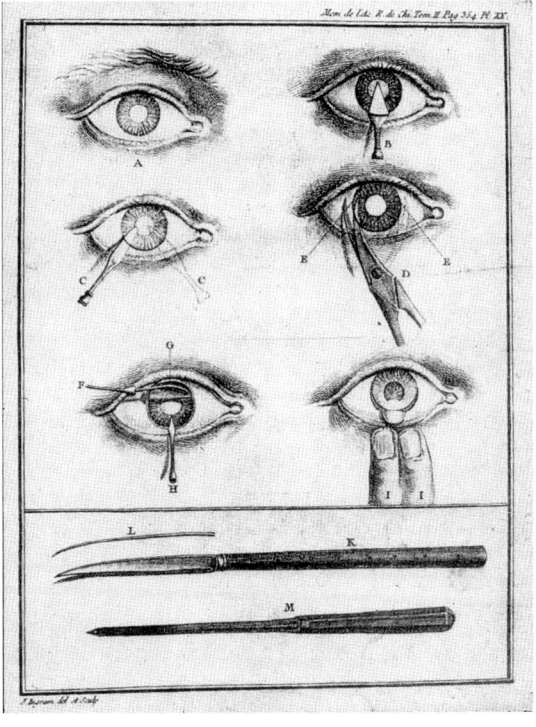

Figure 7-3 Daviel J. Sur une nouvelle methode de guérir la cataracte par l'extraction du cristalin. *(From Louis M, et al.* Memoires de l'Académie Royale de Chirurgie. *Paris: Théophile Barrois Lejeune; 1787.)*

Extracapsular surgery became the new standard of care, and technological developments improved surgical outcomes. Von Graefe (1828–1870) improved upon extracapsular technique by developing a knife that created a better-apposed incision. This innovation decreased the rate of infection and uveal prolapse. But problems related to retention of lens material and opacification of the posterior capsule persisted.

Rucker CW. Cataract: a historical perspective. *Invest Ophthalmol.* 1965;4:377–383.

Early Intracapsular Cataract Extraction

Samuel Sharp first performed a successful intracapsular cataract extraction (ICCE) in 1753 by removing a cataractous lens, capsule intact, through a limbal incision, using pressure from his thumb. ICCE had arrived.

One of the chief problems to be solved in the development of ICCE was how to lyse or break the zonular fibers. Lieutenant Colonel Henry Smith, an Englishman stationed in India, used external manipulation with a muscle hook to break the inferior attachments mechanically and expel (express) the cataractous lens from the eye through a limbal incision. The lens would "tumble": the inferior pole of the lens would exit the eye before the superior pole. His technique, called the *Smith-Indian operation,* was used in 50,000 cases over a 25-year period at the end of the 19th and beginning of the 20th century.

Another method of lens removal was direct extraction. Toothless forceps, developed by ophthalmologists such as Verhoeff and Kalt, were used to grasp the lens capsule (Fig 7-4). The cataract was then gently pulled from the eye with a side-to-side motion that broke the zonular insertion. Suction cup–like devices called *erysiphakes* were devised by Stoewer and by Ignacio Barraquer (1884–1965) to remove the lens with traction or tumbling (Fig 7-5).

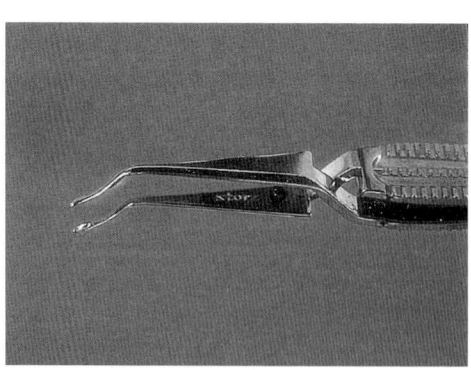

Figure 7-4 Kalt forceps.

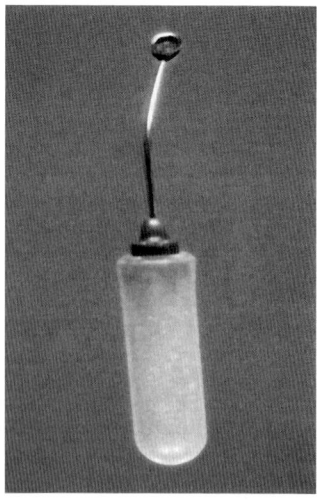

Figure 7-5 Barraquer erysiphake.

The Recent Past

Modern Advances in Intracapsular Surgery

In relatively short order, fine suture material, the binocular operating microscope, and modern sterilization techniques increased surgical success and reduced the number and severity of complications. Chemical dissolution of the zonular fibers with the enzyme α-chymotrypsin was first reported by Joaquin Barraquer in 1957. The traditional capsule forceps and erysiphake had given way to the cryoprobe for lens extraction. The *cryoprobe* is a hollow metal-tipped probe that is cooled by compressed nitrous oxide and then applied to the lens surface. As the temperature of the metal drops below freezing, an iceball forms; the lens then adheres to the probe (Fig 7-6). Gentle to-and-fro maneuvers during delivery of the lens help strip anterior vitreous membrane attachments from the lens, break remaining zonular adhesions, and reduce vitreous loss.

ICCE evolved into a very successful operation. Modern ICCE still plays a role in less-advantaged parts of the world because it requires less sophisticated instrumentation (operating loupes instead of operating microscopes; nonautomated extraction devices such as cryoprobes, capsular forceps, or erysiphakes), allowing ICCE to be performed in a wide range of conditions. In addition, vision rehabilitation with the use of temporary aphakic spectacles is usually possible soon after surgery. Even in the best of surgical facilities, ICCE may be advantageous for patients with subluxed or dense brunescent lenses or for those with exfoliation.

Absolute contraindications include cataracts in children and young adults and cases of traumatic capsule rupture. Relative contraindications include high myopia, Marfan syndrome, morgagnian (hypermature) cataracts, and vitreous presenting in the anterior chamber. For a general description of modern ICCE, see the appendix.

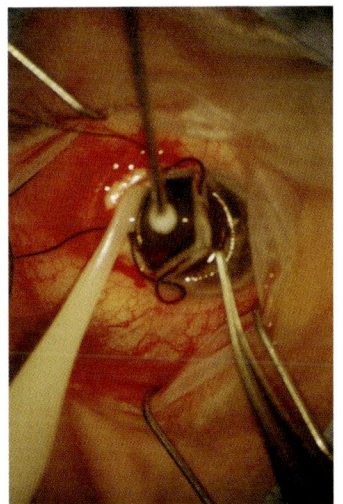

Figure 7-6 Cryoextraction of cataract (ICCE). Lens lifted out of the eye. *(Courtesy of Lisa F. Rosenberg, MD.)*

Problems after ICCE are related to the following:

- *Size of the incision.* Consequences include delayed healing, greater induced astigmatism, and delayed dispensing of final refractive correction. Problems include wound leaks, suture irritation, suture abscess, filtering blebs, and iris or vitreous incarceration as a result of elevated internal pressure on the incision.
- *Bending of the cornea or inadvertent corneal touch with the cryoprobe or cataractous lens during extraction.* Endothelial cell loss and corneal edema can occur as a result.
- *Loss of a barrier between the anterior and posterior segments.* Forward movement of the vitreous plays a role in the development of postoperative cystoid macular edema (CME) and rhegmatogenous retinal detachment, both of which are more common after ICCE than after ECCE or phacoemulsification.
- *Limitations of intraocular lens (IOL) choice and position.* An anterior chamber lens can be used. There is no capsular bag or capsule remnant to which to secure a posterior chamber lens. A posterior chamber lens would have to be secured either to the iris or transsclerally.

Because of these drawbacks, ECCE again became the preferred technique in the late 1960s.

> Blodi FC. Cataract surgery. In: Albert DM, Edwards DD, eds. *The History of Ophthalmology.* Cambridge, MA: Blackwell Scientific; 1996:165–177.
>
> Gorin G. *History of Ophthalmology.* New York: Raven Press; 1982.

The Renaissance of Extracapsular Extraction

The shift from ICCE procedures to new ECCE techniques was driven by developments that decreased the rate of complications that might lead to blindness. One such development was leaving the posterior lens capsule intact, which enabled anterior and posterior compartments of the eye to maintain their separation, thus eliminating forward movement of the vitreous. This development reduced the risk of potentially blinding complications such as aphakic retinal detachment, CME, and decompensation of the cornea.

To avoid the complications previously seen with ECCE, modern extracapsular surgery required complete removal of cortical lens material that remained after the nucleus was removed. Technology once again responded, with the introduction of irrigation and aspiration of cortical material, first with manual systems and then with systems that provided variable suction and gravity flow of fluid to keep the anterior chamber formed. Increased knowledge of aqueous humor composition and corneal endothelial metabolism led to the development of balanced salt solution and to this solution's importance as a tool for the extracapsular surgeon. Ophthalmic viscosurgical devices (OVDs), a most important advance for the surgeon using phacoemulsification, aided the extracapsular surgeon as well.

The Modern ECCE Procedure

The rediscovery of ECCE by nucleus expression was a major leap forward in 20th-century cataract surgery. Selection of this technique depends on the instrumentation available, the surgeon's level of experience, the size of the pupil, the density of the lens, and the status of the zonule.

ECCE involves removal of the lens nucleus and cortex through an opening in the anterior capsule, with the capsular bag left in place. This technique has a number of advantages over ICCE. Because it is performed through a somewhat smaller incision, it results in less trauma to the corneal endothelium, less induced astigmatism, and a more stable and secure incision. In addition, the posterior capsule remains intact, which reduces the risk of intraoperative vitreous loss and the incidence of CME, retinal detachment, corneal edema, and bacterial access to the vitreous cavity. ECCE also provides a barrier that restricts the exchange of some molecules between aqueous and vitreous, allows better anatomical position for the IOL, and eliminates the short-term and long-term complications associated with vitreous adherence to the iris, IOL, cornea, and incision. Primary (concomitant) or secondary (subsequent) IOL implantation, filtration surgery, corneal transplantation, and wound repair are all technically easier and safer when an intact posterior capsule is present.

Equipment

A wide range of instruments is available for each step of modern ECCE, from opening the capsule to dissecting and extracting the lens nucleus, removing the lens cortex, and polishing the lens capsule. The *cystitome* is an instrument used for anterior capsulotomy, the opening of the anterior capsule of the lens. Cystitomes can be fashioned from 23- to 27-gauge needles: the needle is bent at its hub and at the place where the beveled tip begins. Prefabricated cystitomes are also commercially available.

Blunt cannulas are used to irrigate and aspirate fluid, as well as to aspirate cortical lens material during surgery; they are available in various sizes and configurations. Cannulas have an opening at the side or end of the tip to direct fluid flow. The intended function of the instrument helps determine the gauge of the opening. Smaller ports develop high suction and adhesion and are better for grasping and withdrawing material, whereas larger ports allow irrigation and aspiration of thicker substances such as OVDs and lens cortex. A coaxial, double-lumen cannula is commonly used for extracapsular surgery: one lumen irrigates balanced salt solution into the chamber while the second lumen aspirates lens material from the chamber (Fig 7-7). Irrigation is gravity-fed from a solution bottle; fluid flow is regulated with adjustment of the bottle height and the flow restrictor slide. The infusion may be constant, or the surgeon can employ a foot switch connected to a pinch valve. Aspiration may simply involve a syringe connected to the cannula, or it may be

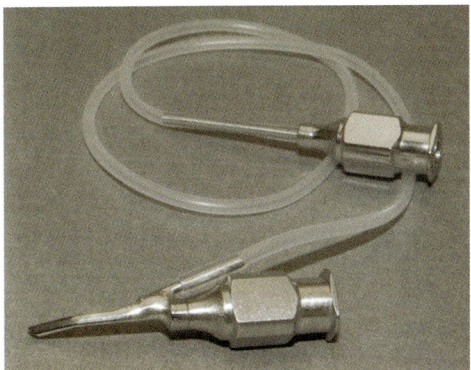

Figure 7-7 Simcoe irrigating/aspirating cannula. *(Photo by Carol Everhart Roper. Courtesy of Accutome, Inc.)*

part of a pump system controlled by a foot pedal. Such automated systems are discussed further in the section on phacoemulsification later in this chapter.

For a general description of the ECCE surgical procedure, see the appendix at the end of the book.

Manual small-incision cataract surgery

Manual small-incision cataract surgery (MSICS) is a recent nonphacoemulsification technique that is a variant of manual ECCE. In ECCE, a 12–14-mm scleral groove is made 2 mm posterior and parallel to the limbus. The anterior chamber is entered through the groove with a paracentesis stab incision, which the surgeon then enlarges with corneoscleral scissors in each direction. In contrast, a 7–8-mm straight or frown scleral groove is made 2 mm posterior to the limbus in MSICS. A scleral tunnel is then created from the scleral groove. The anterior chamber is then entered with a 3.2-mm keratome. Whereas ECCE generally entails a can-opener capsulotomy, a continuous curvilinear capsulorrhexis is often used in MSICS, sometimes with relaxing incisions at the 3- and 9-o'clock positions (if the frown incision has been made at the superior limbus). The final main procedural difference occurs in lens removal. Whereas the lens nucleus is expressed intact in ECCE, it may be removed in whole or in fragments in MSICS. Suturing of the wound is always required in ECCE, but suturing is optional in certain cases with MSICS. Because phacoemulsification equipment is not necessary, MSICS is gaining popularity in developing countries, but the procedure requires both coaxial illumination and an operating microscope. It is also being taught in academic centers as an alternative to a traditional ECCE procedure for dense nuclei.

> Ang GS, Wheelan S, Green FD. Manual small incision cataract surgery in a United Kingdom university teaching hospital setting. *Int Ophthalmol.* 2010;30(1):23–29. Epub 2009 Jan 8.
>
> Gogate PM, Deshpande M, Wormald RP, Deshpande R, Kulkarni SR. Extracapsular cataract surgery compared with manual small incision cataract surgery in community eye care setting in western India: a randomised controlled trial. *Br J Ophthalmol.* 2003;87(6): 667–672.

Ophthalmic Viscosurgical Devices

Ophthalmic viscosurgical devices (OVDs) are also referred to as *viscoelastic agents.* Their use in anterior segment surgery beginning in 1979 has had a profound influence on the evolution of extracapsular and phacoemulsification (phaco) surgery and has decreased the incidence of corneal edema as a complication of phaco surgery.

OVDs contain one or more of the following substances in varying concentrations: sodium hyaluronate, chondroitin sulfate, or hydroxypropyl methylcellulose.

Sodium hyaluronate is a biopolymer that occurs in many connective tissues throughout the body. It has a high molecular mass (2.5–4 million) and low protein content, and it carries a single negative charge for the disaccharide unit. Hyaluronate has a half-life of approximately 1 day in aqueous and 3 days in vitreous.

Chondroitin sulfate is a viscoelastic biopolymer similar to hyaluronate but possessing a sulfated group with a double-negative charge. Chondroitin sulfate is commonly obtained from shark cartilage.

Hydroxypropyl methylcellulose (HPMC) does not occur naturally in animal tissues, but cellulose is widely distributed in plant fibers such as cotton and wood. The commercial product is a cellulose polymer modified by the addition of hydroxypropyl and methyl groups to increase the hydrophilic property of the material. *Methylcellulose* is a nonphysiologic compound that does not appear to be metabolized intraocularly. It is eventually eliminated in the aqueous but can easily be irrigated from the eye.

Physical Properties

The physical properties of OVDs are the result of chain length and molecular interactions both within chains and between chains and ocular tissue.

Viscosity describes a resistance to flow or shear force. The higher the molecular mass, the more the compound resists flow. A compound with high viscosity holds its shape better than does a compound with low viscosity. The viscosity of an OVD at rest is a function of concentration, molecular mass, and the size of the flexible molecules in the material.

Viscoelasticity means that the substance reacts as an elastic compound or gel when energy is transmitted at a high frequency. At low-frequency energy, the substance reacts primarily as a viscous compound. OVD can be slowly introduced into the eye with a 23-gauge cannula and yet can maintain the intraocular space even if the incision is open while manipulations occur in the anterior chamber. The degree of elasticity increases with increasing molecular mass and chain length.

Pseudoplasticity is the ability of an OVD to transform from a gel to a liquidlike substance when under pressure. In clinical terms, at 0 shear force, an OVD is a lubricant and coats tissues well, but when it is forced through a small-gauge cannula, an OVD functions like a liquid.

Surface tension relates to the coating ability of an OVD. Lower surface tension provides better coating and a low contact angle. However, OVDs with lower surface tensions are harder to remove from the eye.

Cohesive and *dispersive* describe the general behaviors of any OVD (Table 7-1). Cohesive OVDs adhere to themselves and are generally high-molecular-mass agents with high surface tensions and high pseudoplasticity. Dispersive agents, conversely, are substances with little tendency for self-adherence, generally low molecular masses, and good coating abilities (low surface tension). Practically speaking, cohesive agents tend to be easily aspirated and are rapidly removed from the eye, whereas dispersive agents are removed less rapidly. Cohesive agents include, for example, Healon, Healon GV (Abbott Medical Optics [AMO], Santa Ana, CA); Amvisc, Amvisc Plus, and OcuCoat (Bausch & Lomb, Rochester, NY); and Provisc (Alcon, Ft Worth, TX). Dispersive agents include OcuCoat (Bausch & Lomb, Rochester, NY); and Viscoat and CelluGel (Alcon, Ft Worth, TX).

Table 7-1 Properties of Ophthalmic Viscosurgical Devices

	Self-Adherence	Molecular Mass	Surface Tension	Ease of Aspiration
Cohesive	High	High	High	Easy
Dispersive	Low	Low	Low	Difficult

Some additional OVDs may need separate classification, such as the visco-adaptive agent Healon 5 (AMO, Santa Ana, CA) and the viscous-dispersive agent DisCoVisc (Alcon, Ft Worth, TX). These OVDs offer surgeons more choices in OVD properties and may be useful in complex cases. The removal of these OVDs requires more time and attention to avoid postoperative intraocular pressure (IOP) elevations.

Characteristics of OVDs

The *space-maintenance ability* of OVDs keeps the anterior chamber formed despite the presence of one or more incisions. With expansion of the chamber, manipulations can be made away from the corneal endothelium and posterior lens capsule. A cohesive OVD can be used to enlarge a marginally dilated pupil (viscomydriasis). It can also be used to keep the plane of the anterior capsule flat to assist a controlled continuous curvilinear capsulorrhexis (discussed later in this chapter). Lens implantation is less traumatic to the zonular fibers and the posterior capsule when the capsular bag is inflated with an OVD. In the presence of an open posterior lens capsule, a dispersive OVD can be injected over the tear to keep the vitreous from moving anteriorly. Injection of an OVD through the pars plana can elevate lens fragments that have fallen into the anterior vitreous through a posterior capsule tear; the surgeon can then emulsify these fragments or remove them manually.

Because of its dispersive nature, the OVD can be used for coating the endothelium in cases that require more time, phaco power, or both. Care must be taken to remove the intraocular OVD completely to reduce the risk of an ocular hypertensive period related to angle outflow obstruction.

The *optical clarity* of an OVD has allowed surgeons to use a layer of OVD on the surface of the cornea. When slightly moistened with balanced salt solution, the agent coats the epithelium. This maneuver prevents drying and eliminates the need to irrigate the corneal surface. It also provides a slightly magnified view of anterior segment structures.

 Buratto L, Giardini P, Bellucci R. *Viscoelastics in Ophthalmic Surgery.* Thorofare, NJ: Slack; 2005:5.
 Lane SS, Lindstrom RL. Viscoelastic agents: formulation, clinical applications, and complications. In: Steinert RF, ed. *Cataract Surgery: Technique, Complications, and Management.* Philadelphia: Saunders; 1995:37–45.
 Oshika T, Eguchi S, Oki K, et al. Clinical comparison of Healon 5 and Healon in phacoemulsification and intraocular lens implantation: randomized multicenter study. *J Cataract Refract Surg.* 2004;30(2):357–362.
 Pape LG, Balazs EA. The use of sodium hyaluronate (Healon) in human anterior segment surgery. *Ophthalmology.* 1980;87(7):699–705.
 Riedel PJ. Ophthalmic viscoelastic devices (OVDs). *Focal Points: Clinical Modules for Ophthalmologists.* San Francisco: American Academy of Ophthalmology; 2012, module 8.

Anesthesia for Cataract Surgery

Historically, cataract surgery was performed without anesthesia. Koller used topical cocaine anesthesia applied at the limbus in the late 1800s. Retrobulbar anesthesia was first described in 1884 by Knapp, who injected 4% cocaine for ocular anesthesia prior to

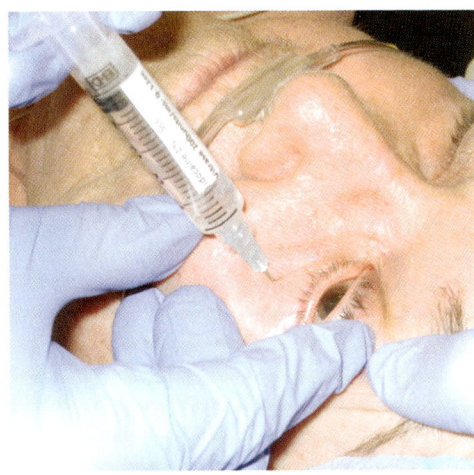

Figure 7-8 Retrobulbar injection. *(Courtesy of Michael N. Wiggins, MD.)*

enucleation surgery. The modern technique of retrobulbar anesthesia, described in 1945 by Atkinson, allowed the evolutionary advances of peribulbar and sub-Tenon anesthesia.

Retrobulbar anesthesia (Fig 7-8), used with or without regional anesthesia of cranial nerve VII (facial nerve), provides excellent ocular akinesia and anesthesia. Complications of retrobulbar anesthesia are uncommon but include the following: retrobulbar hemorrhage; globe penetration; optic nerve trauma; extraocular muscle toxicity; inadvertent intravenous injection associated with cardiac arrhythmias; and inadvertent intradural injection with associated seizures, respiratory arrest, and brainstem anesthesia (these complications are discussed more fully in BCSC Section 1, *Update on General Medicine*). A surgeon should know how to perform a *lateral cantholysis* to release a tense retrobulbar hemorrhage (see BCSC Section 7, *Orbit, Eyelids, and Lacrimal System*).

In *peribulbar anesthesia,* a shorter (2.5 mm or 1″) 25- or 27-gauge needle is used to introduce anesthetic solution external to the muscle cone, underneath the Tenon capsule, via single or multiple injection sites (Fig 7-9). Theoretically, peribulbar anesthesia eliminates the risk of complications such as optic nerve injury and central nervous system spread of anesthesia from intradural injection (Fig 7-10; also see Fig 7-9B). However, the risk of globe penetration is not eliminated, and the peribulbar method is slightly less effective than the retrobulbar method for providing akinesia and anesthesia. In addition, the onset of effect is slower.

Topical anesthesia has evolved as a natural extension of phacoemulsification with foldable IOLs. Advantages of topical anesthesia include no risk of ocular perforation, extraocular muscle injury, or central nervous system depression. Vision returns almost immediately, and patients are able to leave the operating room without being patched because no eyelid block is used. Disadvantages of topical anesthesia include increased extraocular motility, blepharospasm, and patient discomfort.

Topical anesthesia is administered as topical proparacaine or tetracaine drops, cellulose pledgets, or lidocaine jelly. Topical anesthetic agents are used with or without intravenous sedation. Topical anesthesia may be supplemented with the *intracameral* use of preservative-free lidocaine. Only nonpreserved lidocaine, generally 1% to 2%, should be

100 • Lens and Cataract

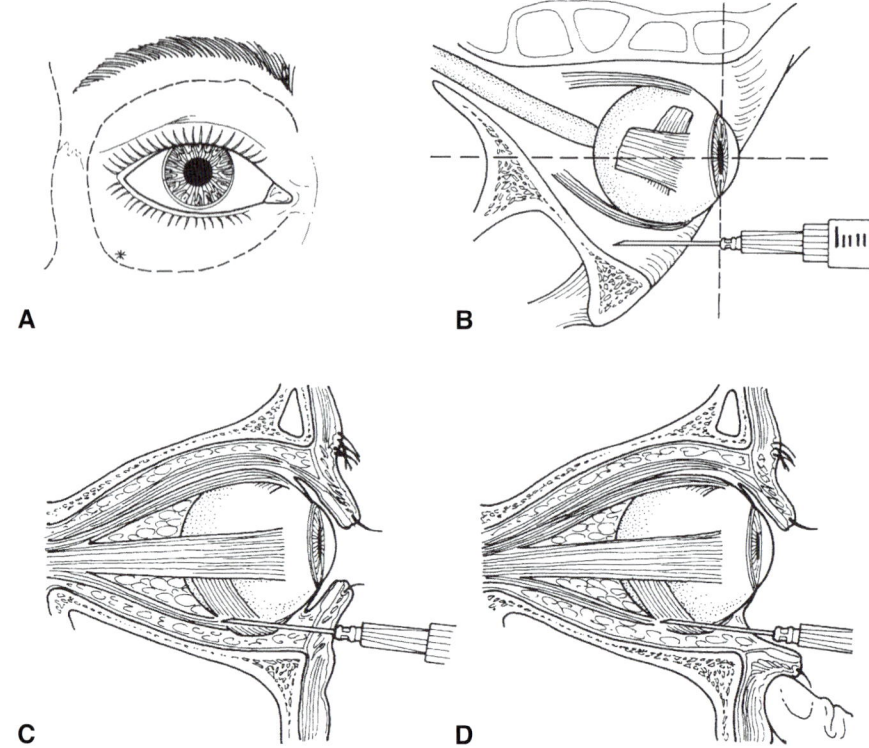

Figure 7-9 Peribulbar anesthesia. **A,** A 27-gauge 20- to 25-mm sharp disposable needle enters the orbit at the lower temporal orbital rim *(asterisk),* slightly up from the orbital floor and very close to the bone. **B,** The needle passes backward in a sagittal plane and parallel to the orbit floor **(C and D),** passing the globe equator to a depth controlled by observing the needle/hub junction reaching the plane of the iris **(B).** The technique is equally applicable to the transcutaneous **(C)** or transconjunctival **(D)** route. *(Reproduced with permission from Jaffe NS, Jaffe MS, Jaffe GF. Cataract Surgery and Its Complications. 6th ed. St Louis: Mosby; 1997.)*

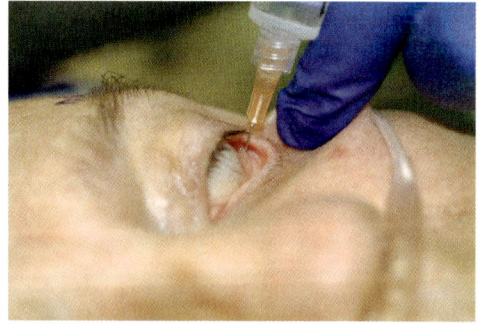

Figure 7-10 Peribulbar injection via conjunctiva. *(Courtesy of Ken Mitchell, MD, and Dan Skufca, MD.)*

used for anterior chamber instillation, as some preservative agents can be toxic to intraocular structures. Transient amaurosis due to a direct retinal effect has been reported following the use of intracameral anesthetics, more commonly in patients with open posterior capsules or previous vitrectomy. Topical anesthesia should be reserved for the cooperative cataract patient who, with a dilated pupil, can tolerate the microscope light.

The type of anesthesia appropriate for the individual patient should be considered carefully. A general discussion of the advantages and risks of the different types of anesthesia should accompany the informed-consent process. A discussion of what the patient will experience in the operating room will increase the likelihood that the patient will be more relaxed on the day of surgery.

Subconjunctival lidocaine can be used to augment topical anesthesia in patients who experience sensation after administration of topical tetracaine or intracameral lidocaine. A 30-gauge needle is used to inject the lidocaine subconjunctivally posterior to the phaco incision.

Sub-Tenon (Fig 7-11) infusion of lidocaine can be used to provide anesthesia and moderate akinesia during surgery. Lidocaine is administered through a cannula or catheter placed into a small posterior incision, under the conjunctiva and Tenon capsule.

A *facial nerve block* (Fig 7-12), common in the era of large-incision ICCE and ECCE, is not generally needed with small-incision surgery. However, patients with essential or reactive blepharospasm may require a facial block.

General anesthesia, with clearance from the patient's primary care physician or an anesthesiologist, is appropriate to consider for pediatric patients and for patients who have any condition that would prevent their cooperation during surgery, including dementia, head tremor, deafness, neck or back problems, restless legs syndrome, or claustrophobia.

> Boulton JE, Lopatatzidis A, Luck J, Baer RM. A randomized controlled trial of intracameral lidocaine during phacoemulsification under topical anesthesia. *Ophthalmology.* 2000; 107(1):68–71.

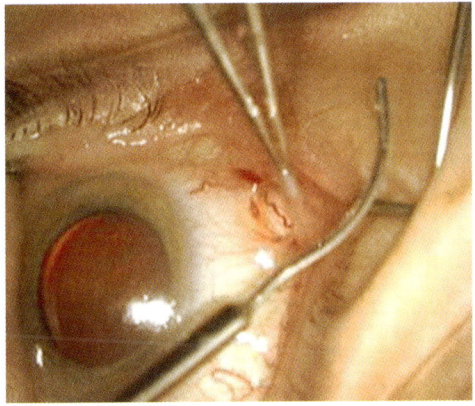

Figure 7-11 Sub-Tenon injection. *(Courtesy of University of Iowa, Dept of Ophthalmology.)*

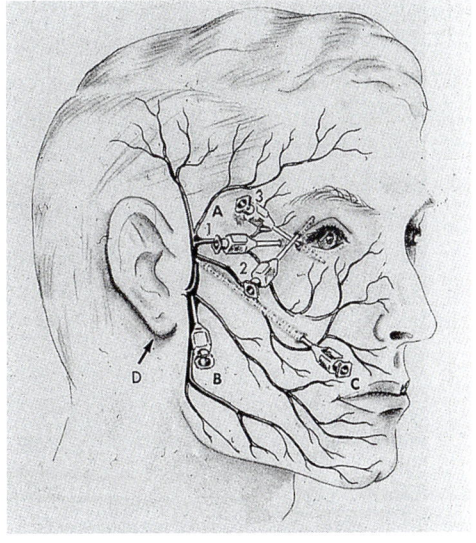

Figure 7-12 Akinesia of orbicularis oculi. *A,* Van Lint akinesia. *B,* O'Brien akinesia. *C,* Atkinson akinesia. *D,* Nadbath-Ellis akinesia. *(Reproduced with permission from Jaffe NS, Jaffe MS, Jaffe GF. Cataract Surgery and Its Complications. 5th ed. St Louis: Mosby; 1990.)*

Hunter DG, Lam GC, Guyton DL. Inferior oblique muscle injury from local anesthesia for cataract surgery. *Ophthalmology.* 1995;102(3):501–509.

Pang MP, Fujimoto DK, Wilkens LR. Pain, photophobia, and retinal and optic nerve function after phacoemulsification with intracameral lidocaine. *Ophthalmology.* 2001;108(11): 2018–2025.

Phacoemulsification

Originally, all extracapsular techniques involved nuclear expression. In 1967, Kelman developed phacoemulsification surgery, which differed from conventional ECCE with nuclear expression by the size of the incision and the method of nucleus removal. Initially, Kelman met with considerable resistance from his colleagues.

Phacoemulsification uses an ultrasonically driven tip to fragment the nucleus of the cataract and to emulsify these fragments. The technique also uses a surgeon-controlled automated aspiration system to remove the cortical material through a small needle introduced through a very small incision. Phacoemulsification results in a lower incidence of wound-related complications, faster healing, and more rapid vision rehabilitation than procedures that require larger incisions. This technique also creates a relatively closed system during both phacoemulsification and aspiration, thereby controlling anterior chamber depth and providing safeguards against positive vitreous pressure and choroidal hemorrhage.

One problem for the early phaco surgeon was related to the proximity of the phaco needle to the corneal endothelium. Coaxial irrigation sleeves and the development of OVDs allowed space to be maintained between the phaco needle's tip and the endothelium. Another stumbling block was that after the nucleus was emulsified and the cortical material was aspirated, the incision had to be opened to accommodate rigid polymethylmethacrylate anterior chamber and posterior chamber lenses, which required an opening slightly larger than the optic. In the 1980s, Mazzocco developed and implanted the first foldable IOL made of silicone; other designs followed, with IOLs in both silicone and acrylic. The development of foldable IOLs that could be inserted through sub-4.0-mm incisions enabled the phaco surgeon to keep the incision small. Many more surgeons transitioned to phaco and small-incision surgery, and phacoemulsification of cataract with insertion of a foldable IOL has become the predominant technique for cataract surgery in the developed world.

Ultrasonics Terminology

The following are terms commonly used in phaco surgery.

Cavitation The formation of gas bubbles arising from the aqueous in response to pressure changes at the tip of the phaco needle; these bubbles expand and contract. Implosion of the bubbles causes localized intense heat and pressure liberation at the tip, resulting in emulsification of lens material. Continuous cavitation, produced by continuous ultrasound, is less efficient than the transient cavitation of pulsed ultrasound delivery.

Chatter Chatter occurs when the ultrasonic stroke overcomes the vacuum, or "holding power." This causes the nuclear fragments to be repelled by the ultrasonic tip until the vacuum reaches high-enough levels to neutralize the ultrasonic tip's repulsive energy and once again attracts the material. This back-and-forth movement of lens material from the tip inhibits followability (defined in Vacuum Terminology). A reduction in phaco power can diminish chatter by decreasing the stroke length of the tip excursion, thereby reducing forces that push the fragment away from the tip.

Duty cycle During pulsed phacoemulsification, the period when phaco power is being delivered. If the time of "power on" equals the time of "power off," the duty cycle is 50%.

Energy Energy and power are not the same but are related directly with time (energy = power × time). This concept is important as phaco surgeons may reduce the amount of energy released inside the eye by decreasing either the phaco power or the time that the phaco power is on. The concept is also useful in understanding the reduction in energy delivered with changes in duty cycles.

Frequency In phacoemulsification, the speed at which the phaco needle moves back and forth. The frequency of ultrasonic handpieces is between 27,000 hertz (Hz) and 60,000 Hz.

Inflow The infusion of balanced salt solution into the eye through the tubing and handpiece by depressing the foot pedal to position 1 (see Phaco Instrumentation).

Load In ultrasonics, the mass of nuclear material in contact with the phaco tip. Responding to the load requires that the system and the ultrasonic tip maintain constant stroke length or power. Because the load is constantly changing, the system must be able to adapt to changing conditions. If the system cannot adapt, then the cutting efficiency will be compromised.

Piezoelectric crystal A type of transducer used in ultrasonic handpieces that transforms electrical energy into mechanical energy. Linear motion is generated when a tuned, highly refined crystal is deformed by the electrical energy supplied by the console.

Power The ability of the phaco needle to vibrate and cavitate the adjacent lens material. Power is noted as a linear percentage of the maximum stroke length of which the needle is capable. Phaco power is produced when the foot pedal is depressed to position 3.

Stroke The linear distance that the tip traverses to produce an impact on lens material. This impact is measured by the velocity of tip movement at an ultrasonic frequency between 27,000 Hz and 60,000 Hz, and by the stroke length, which varies among the various devices from 2 to 4 mils (0.05–0.10 mm or 0.002"–0.004").

Tuning The method used to match the optimum driving frequency of the ultrasonic board within the console with the operating frequency of the phaco handpiece in a specific medium (eg, balanced salt solution).

Ultrasonic Frequencies above the range of human audibility, or greater than 20,000 Hz. In phacoemulsification, the term *ultrasonic* is used because the phaco needle moves back and forth in excess of 20,000 Hz.

Vacuum Terminology

A review of the following terms may help the reader to understand concepts related to the removal of nuclear and cortical material.

Aspiration The withdrawal of fluid and lens material from the eye; produced by depressing the foot pedal to position 2 and continuing in position 3.

Aspiration flow rate The flow of fluid through the tubing, measured in milliliters per minute (mL/min). Other factors influencing flow include compliance, venting, and size of the tubing.

Followability The ability of a fluidic system to attract and hold nuclear or cortical material on the distal end of an ultrasonic or irrigation/aspiration handpiece until vacuum forces achieve evacuation.

Occlusion An obstruction of the aspiration port or aspiration tubing. When lens material occludes the tip of the phaco needle, vacuum builds until the material is evacuated.

Rise time The rate at which vacuum builds once the aspiration port has been occluded. Rise time is directly related to the aspiration flow rate, which is related to the pump speed. The faster the aspiration flow rate (or pump speed), the faster the rise time.

Surge A phenomenon that occurs when a vacuum has built up because of an occlusion and the occlusion is suddenly broken, causing the fluid in the higher-pressure (positive) anterior chamber to rush into the lower-pressure (negative) phaco tip. If the negative surge exceeds the inflow capability of the irrigation line, anterior chamber depth fluctuations may occur; and the iris or posterior capsule may be drawn into the tip. Changes made in phaco equipment in order to limit surge include the following: higher fluid inflow, lower vacuum, low-compliance tubing of smaller diameter, a smaller tip, coiled aspiration tubing, and occlusion mode software. In addition, improvements in software allow automatic modification of aspiration and flow.

Vacuum Aspiration level, or *vacuum*, is a parameter measured in millimeters of mercury (mm Hg) or inches of water and defined as the magnitude of negative pressure created in the tubing. Vacuum determines how well particulate material that has occluded the phaco tip will be held to it.

Venting Also known as "exposing to the air," the process whereby negative pressure or vacuum is equalized to atmospheric levels to minimize surge.

Phaco Instrumentation

All current phaco machines have in common foot-pedal controls with at least 3 positions. Position 1 allows entry of fluid into the handpiece through the irrigation port. Position 2 engages the aspiration mode at a constant or variable rate, depending on the settings that each surgeon selects. Position 3 adds the phaco power at a variable or fixed level.

The instruments used in phacoemulsification involve both ultrasonics and vacuum and fluid dynamics. The phaco handpiece is an instrument that has been likened to a jackhammer, vacuum, or garden hose that allows breaking the nucleus of the crystalline lens into fragments and aspirating them from the eye. Irrigation both cools the handpiece and keeps the anterior chamber formed.

The mechanical energy is produced by a to-and-fro oscillation of the tip at a frequency that is preset for each machine. The amplitude of the movement, or stroke length, is variable; it is measured in mils (1 mil = 0.001″ or 0.025 mm). It is the stroke length of the phaco tip that is changed when the power is changed. As the tip moves forward, compression of gas atoms in solution occurs; as the tip moves backward, expansion of gas atoms occurs, and bubbles of gas form. The bubbles are subject to the same compression and expansion. When the bubbles implode, they release heat and shock waves (cavitation) that contribute at the tip to activity that disassembles the nucleus. Cavitation can be enhanced by changes in the needle shape. For example, the distal bend in the angled Kelman tip adds a nonaxial vibration to the primary oscillation. The nonaxial vibration augments the axial vibration and produces at the cutting tip an elliptical motion that increases the mechanical breakdown of nuclear material (Fig 7-13).

Phaco tips vary according to the angle of the tip and the size of the lumen. Phaco tips are available in 0°, 15°, 30°, 45°, 60°, and combined 30°/60° (turbo) beveled tips (Fig 7-14). In general, the surgeon chooses the bevel angle of the phaco tip based on personal preference. The angle also influences the direction of spread of the cavitation force. Tips with steeper bevels are better for cutting nuclear material (eg, using continuous phacoemulsification during sculpting). A tip with a greater bevel has an oval-shaped port with a larger

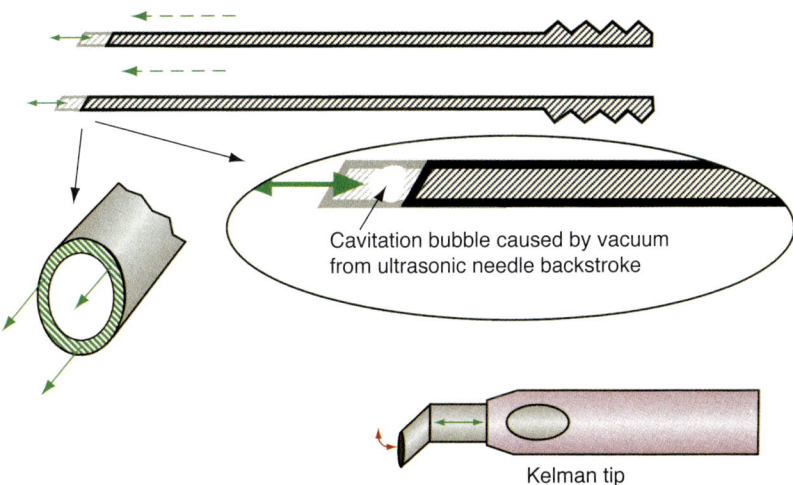

Figure 7-13 Cavitation is affected by the angle of the phaco tip as well as by different needle shapes. *(Reprinted with permission from Seibel BS. Phacodynamics: Mastering the Tools and Techniques of Phacoemulsification Surgery. 3rd ed. Thorofare, NJ: Slack; 1999.)*

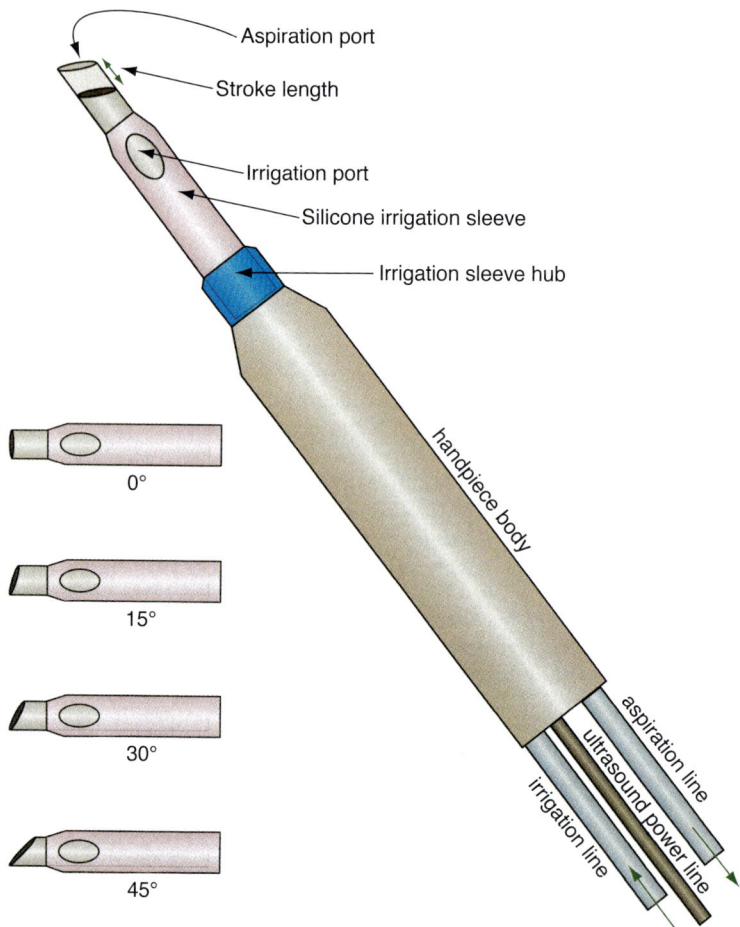

Figure 7-14 Parts of a phaco handpiece; smaller drawings depict the different tip bevels available. *(Reprinted with permission from Seibel BS.* Phacodynamics: Mastering the Tools and Techniques of Phacoemulsification Surgery. *3rd ed. Thorofare, NJ: Slack; 1999.)*

surface area. Because pressure is defined as force per unit area, the tips with the greater surface area can generate greater adherence of nuclear material (Fig 7-15).

Phaco Power Delivery

Continuous phacoemulsification describes the constant delivery of phaco power when the machine is in foot-pedal position 3. *Panel control* ultrasound allows the power to be set from 0% to 100%; the set level of power is delivered when the foot pedal is depressed throughout the position 3 excursion. With linear ultrasound, the surgeon controls the amount of phaco power delivered by varying the excursion of the foot pedal while it is in position 3. Continuous phaco power delivery may be used for sculpting deep grooves in the lens nucleus (eg, for "divide and conquer" or phaco "stop and chop" techniques).

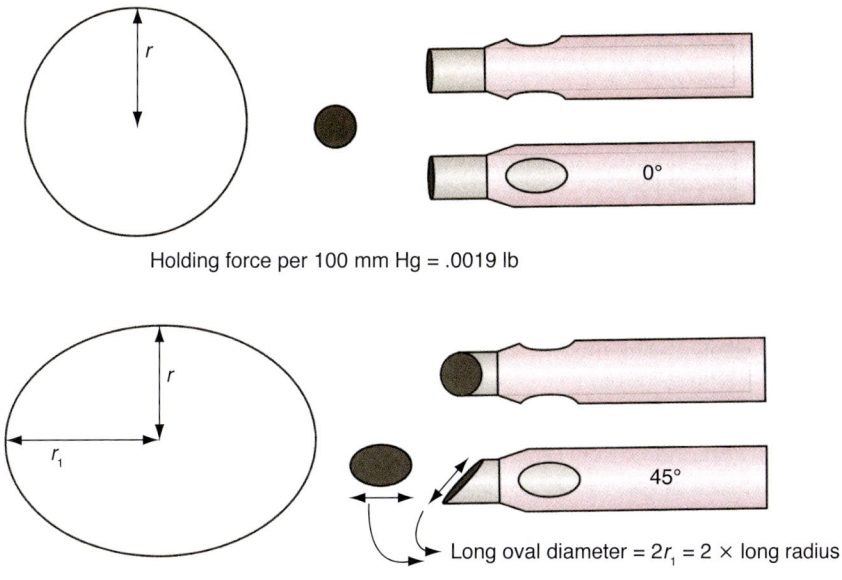

Figure 7-15 Drawing depicts the relationship between the phaco tip bevel and holding force. *(Reprinted with permission from Seibel BS.* Phacodynamics: Mastering the Tools and Techniques of Phacoemulsification Surgery. *3rd ed. Thorofare, NJ: Slack; 1999.)*

The delivery of phaco power is a double-edged sword. Certainly, cavitation, shock waves, shear forces, and heat buildup at the tip may all facilitate nucleus disassembly. However, the classic longitudinal stroke of the phaco tip tends to push nuclear fragments away even as the aspiration attracts them (chatter). In addition, continuous cavitation is less energy-efficient than is intermittent cavitation. Lastly, heat buildup from phaco power delivery may cause wound burns.

In an attempt to deliver phaco power more efficiently, modes such as pulse and burst were developed.

- Pulsed phacoemulsification involves setting the number of pulses per second while in position 3. The term *pulse* describes an interval of phaco power turned on alternating with the same interval during which phaco power is off. The amount of power delivered depends on the foot-pedal excursion in position 3. The delivery of phaco power for only a portion of the cycle reduces repulsion of material by the vibrating tip and improves followability.
- *Burst*-mode phacoemulsification involves delivery of preset power (0%–100%) in single bursts that are separated by decreasing intervals as the foot pedal is depressed through position 3. At the end of the position 3 excursion, the power is no longer delivered in bursts but is continuous. Burst mode allows the phaco needle tip to bury into the lens, an essential step for chopping techniques.

Additional advances in the control of phaco power delivery are discussed in the section Advances in Energy Delivery.

Irrigation

The fluid dynamics of phacoemulsification require constant irrigation through the irrigation sleeve around the ultrasound tip, with some egress of fluid through the incisions. Balanced salt solution was designed to resemble aqueous humor. Its biocompatibility, along with its sterility, was a major impetus for the development of automated irrigation and aspiration.

Constant irrigation maintains anterior chamber depth and cools the phaco probe, preventing heat buildup and consequent damage to adjacent tissue. Some advocate the use of chilled irrigation fluid, claiming that the cold fluid cools the probe more effectively, constricts blood vessels, maintains corneal clarity better, and may even stabilize the blood–aqueous barrier. Some surgeons put epinephrine in the balanced salt solution irrigating bottle to maintain pupillary dilation. Others put antibiotics in the bottle as prophylaxis against endophthalmitis (see the section Antimicrobial Prophylaxis).

> Devgan U. Basic principles of phacoemulsification and fluid dynamics. *Focal Points: Clinical Modules for Ophthalmologists.* San Francisco: American Academy of Ophthalmology; 2010, module 8.
>
> Liou SW, Yang CY. The effect of intracameral adrenaline infusion on pupil size, pulse rate, and blood pressure during phacoemulsification. *J Ocul Pharmacol Ther.* 1998;14(4): 357–361.
>
> Seibel BS. *Phacodynamics: Mastering the Tools and Techniques of Phacoemulsification Surgery.* 4th ed. Thorofare, NJ: Slack; 2005.

Aspiration

The aspiration system of phaco machines varies according to pump design. The 3 types of pumps are peristaltic, diaphragm, and Venturi.

The *peristaltic pump* consists of a set of rollers that move along flexible tubing, forcing fluid through the tubing and creating a relative vacuum at the aspiration port of the phaco tip (Fig 7-16). Vacuum response time with this type of pump is relatively rapid; linear control is achieved as the speed of the rollers is increased. Vacuum is flow-based and does not build up until the tip is occluded.

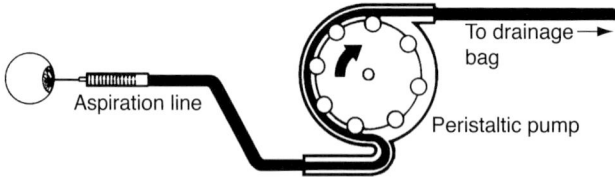

Figure 7-16 The peristaltic pump. *(Redrawn with permission from* Practical Phacoemulsification: Proceedings of the Third Annual Workshop. *Montreal, Quebec: Medicopea International; 1991:43–48.)*

The *diaphragm pump* consists of a flexible diaphragm overlying a fluid chamber with 1-way valves at the inlet and outlet. The diaphragm moves out, creating a relative vacuum in the chamber that shuts the exit valve, causing the fluid to flow into the chamber. The diaphragm then moves in, which increases the pressure in the chamber and closes the intake valve while opening the exit valve (Fig 7-17). This type of pump system produces a slower rise in vacuum. With continued occlusion of the aspiration port, however, the vacuum will continue to increase in an exponential manner.

The *Venturi pump* (Fig 7-18) creates a vacuum based on the Venturi principle: a flow of gas or fluid across a port creates a vacuum proportional to the rate of flow of the gas. This system produces a rapid, linear rise in vacuum and allows for instantaneous venting to the atmosphere that immediately stops the flow through the port. The vacuum is not flow-based and builds according to the machine setting.

In general, all of these pumps are effective. The vacuum rise time (the amount of time required to reach a given level of vacuum) varies among the different pump designs (Fig 7-19). In planning a specific technique, the surgeon should consider the relationship between the aspiration flow rate and the rise time of the instrument. The vacuum rise time is inversely proportional to the aspiration flow rate. As the aspiration flow rate is decreased by half, from 40 to 20 mL/minute, the vacuum rise time is doubled, from 1 to 2 seconds (Fig 7-20).

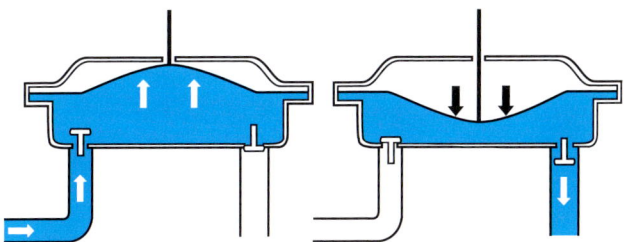

Figure 7-17 The diaphragm pump. *(Redrawn with permission from* Practical Phacoemulsification: Proceedings of the Third Annual Workshop. *Montreal, Quebec: Medicopea International; 1991:43–48.)*

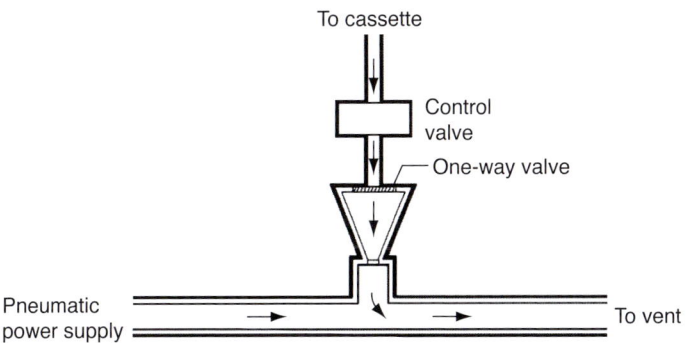

Figure 7-18 The Venturi pump. *(Redrawn with permission from* Practical Phacoemulsification: Proceedings of the Third Annual Workshop. *Montreal, Quebec: Medicopea International; 1991:43–48.)*

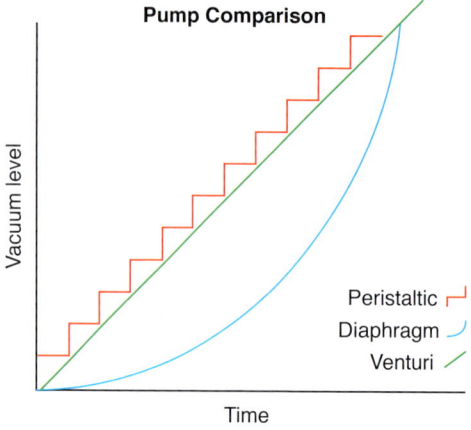

Figure 7-19 Comparison of vacuum rise times in the peristaltic, diaphragm, and Venturi pumps. *(Redrawn with permission from* Practical Phacoemulsification: Proceedings of the Third Annual Workshop. *Montreal, Quebec: Medicopea International; 1991:43–48.)*

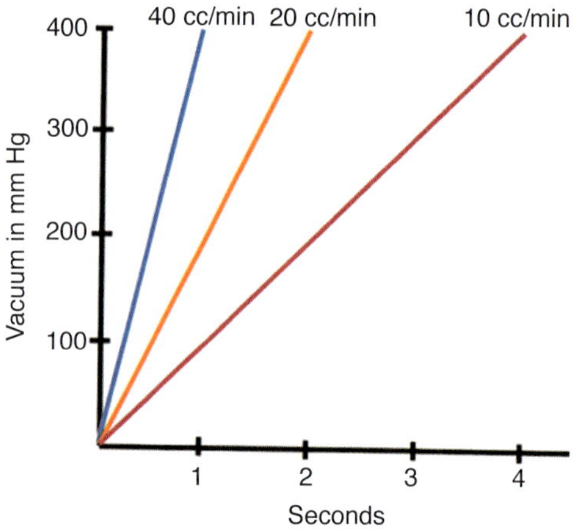

Figure 7-20 Graph depicts the relationship between aspiration flow rate and vacuum rise time. *(Modified with permission from Seibel BS.* Phacodynamics: Mastering the Tools and Techniques of Phacoemulsification Surgery. *3rd ed. Thorofare, NJ: Slack; 1999.)*

A Basic Outline of the Phaco Procedure

As with conventional ECCE, pupillary dilation with mydriatic/cycloplegic drops is essential. The experienced phaco surgeon can use pupil-stretching techniques or special iris retractors to open miotic pupils that are unresponsive to pharmacologic dilation (see Chapter 9).

Exposure of the Globe

During surgery, the eyelids are usually held apart with a lid speculum. When selecting the speculum, the surgeon should make sure that it will accommodate the phaco handpiece and other instruments. For a surgeon seated for phacoemulsification from a superior approach, a bridle suture may be placed to help position the globe. The bridle suture is especially helpful to the beginning phaco surgeon for stabilizing the globe and exposing the bulbar conjunctiva to create a conjunctival flap.

Paracentesis

A sharp blade is used to create a small paracentesis, placed approximately 2 or 3 clock-hours away from the site where an incision will be made for the phaco handpiece. A straight entry plane is made parallel to the iris and to the left for a right-handed surgeon or to the right for a left-handed surgeon. An OVD is then instilled to protect intraocular structures and allow more control during creation of the phaco incision. The paracentesis provides access for multiple purposes, such as the introduction of a second instrument.

Scleral Tunnel Incisions

A scleral tunnel incision with an internal corneal lip may reduce the incidence of both early and late surgically induced astigmatism. A limited conjunctival peritomy is created over the intended wound site. The surgeon then clears the overlying Tenon capsule from the sclera and applies light bipolar cautery to achieve hemostasis. Excessive cautery is to be avoided because it may cause scleral shrinkage and postoperative astigmatism.

The initial scleral step incision should be made depending on the style of IOL that the surgeon intends to implant. Foldable IOLs can be inserted through smaller incisions, whereas polymethylmethacrylate (PMMA) IOLs require openings slightly larger than the diameter of the optic. The scleral incision is usually linear (tangential to the limbus), but it may be curvilinear (following the limbus or following the curve opposite the limbus) or chevron shaped. The surgeon then uses a blade to enter the scleral groove at a chosen depth and dissects anteriorly, parallel to the corneoscleral surface and into clear cornea, developing a tunnel incision (Fig 7-21). The tunnel incision is carried forward, just anterior to the vascular arcade. If the scleral groove is entered too deeply, the scleral flap will be very thick, and the blade may penetrate the anterior chamber earlier than anticipated,

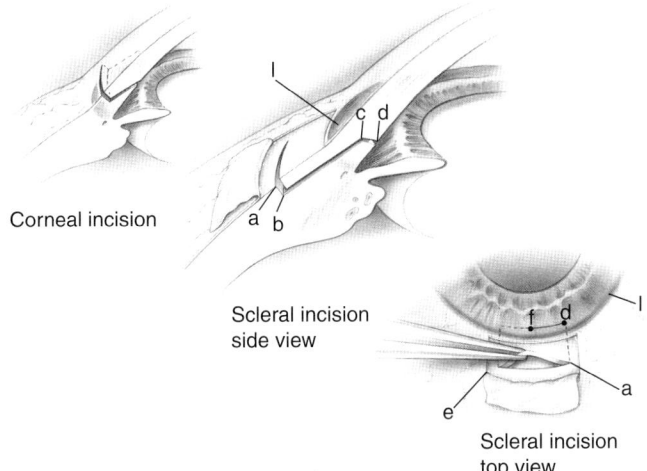

Figure 7-21 Two types of phaco incisions. Detail for scleral incision, side view: *a to b:* Initial groove is ⅓ to ½ of scleral depth; if groove is too deep, bleeding may increase and entry into anterior chamber is likely to be too posterior, causing iris prolapse. *a to l:* Incision is traditionally 2–3 mm posterior to limbus. *b to c:* Tunnel is traditionally dissected past vascular arcade; if too long, ultrasound tip mobility is restricted and corneal striae decrease visibility. *c to d:* Short third plane is made by changing angle of blade prior to entering anterior chamber. In scleral incision, top view: *e to a:* Length of incision is determined by size of IOL. *f to d:* Initial opening into anterior chamber is usually 3.00–3.25 mm; after phacoemulsification, it is fully opened for IOL insertion. If opening is too small, irrigation flow is decreased, chamber tends to shallow, and heat buildup may cause burn. If opening is too large, excessive fluid egress causes chamber shallowing and iris may prolapse. *(Reproduced with permission from Johnson SH. Phacoemulsification. Focal Points: Clinical Modules for Ophthalmologists. San Francisco: American Academy of Ophthalmology; 1994, module 6. Illustration by Christine Gralapp.)*

closer to the vascular iris root. If the scleral groove is entered superficially, the scleral flap will be very thin and prone to tears or buttonholes. Either metal or diamond knives may be used for fashioning the scleral tunnel, but beginning surgeons may benefit from the added resistance and the tactile feedback provided by a metal blade.

To enter the anterior chamber from beneath the scleral flap, the surgeon uses a keratome sized to match the phaco tip width. The keratome is inserted into the corneal stroma until the tip reaches the clear cornea beyond the vascular arcade. The heel of the keratome is elevated, and the tip of the keratome is pointed posteriorly, aiming toward the center of the lens and creating a dimple in the peripheral cornea. The keratome is then slowly advanced in this posterior direction, creating an internal corneal lip as it enters the anterior chamber. The stepped incision creates a valve that allows the incision to be self-sealing once the anterior chamber is re-formed. If the scleral tunnel incision is too long, the surgeon may have problems manipulating the phaco tip within the anterior chamber. In addition, corneal striae and distortion may reduce visibility as the surgeon manipulates the phaco tip. If the tunnel is too short, the valve may not seal the incision. The phaco tip may also abrade the iris, causing atrophy of the surface and possible pupil distortion.

The closure of a step, or tunnel, incision at the end of the case depends not on radial compression of the anterior and posterior lips of the incision but rather on reapproximation of the surfaces of the tunnel flap. Various suture closures of scleral incisions are illustrated in Figure 7-22.

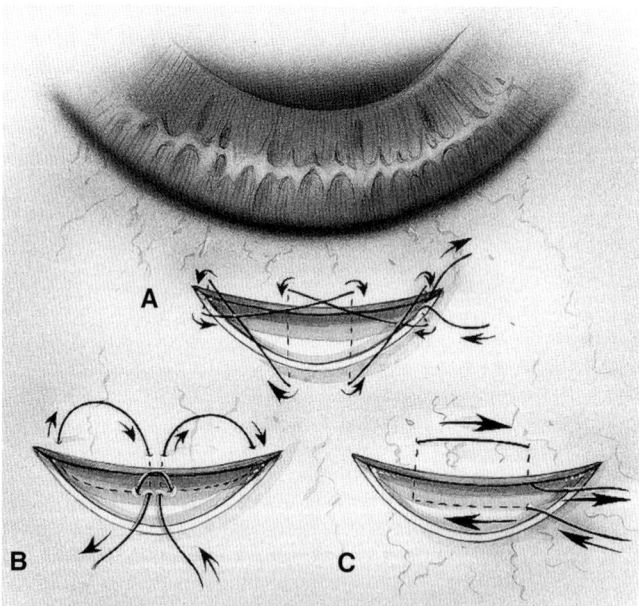

Figure 7-22 Incision closure techniques. **A,** Classic radial running x-closure must be keratometrically monitored (preferably quantitatively rather than qualitatively) during tying to avoid undesired postoperative astigmatism. Alternatively, horizontal suturing techniques using multiple bites **(B)** or a single bite **(C)** have been devised to try to decrease the induced astigmatism. *(Reproduced with permission from Johnson SH. Phacoemulsification. Focal Points: Clinical Modules for Ophthalmologists. San Francisco: American Academy of Ophthalmology; 1994, module 6. Illustration by Christine Gralapp.)*

With the continuing evolution of techniques for self-sealing incisions and the use of foldable IOLs, many surgeons have elected not to suture the incision at all in small-incision cases. Long-term evaluation of the results and stability of this type of incision closure have shown that small scleral tunnel and clear corneal incisions, both with and without suture closure, heal quickly, are relatively stable, and induce minimal astigmatism. Even though no-stitch cataract surgery has many advantages, the surgeon should always be ready to place a suture if the incision closure appears to be inadequate.

Clear Corneal Incision

Phaco surgeons most often use a clear corneal incision (Fig 7-23). These small incisions are typically 3.2 mm wide or less and just large enough to accommodate the phaco handpiece. They usually have little or no effect on preexisting astigmatism. Globe stabilization is important in clear corneal incisions, especially if the procedure is performed with topical anesthesia. Fixation rings, 0.12-mm toothed forceps, or instruments supplying counterpressure can be used to stabilize the globe as the incisions are made. The incisions can be made superiorly, temporally, or at the steepest axis of the cornea, depending on the surgeon's preference.

One approach for the clear corneal incision is a multiplanar incision using a vertical corneal groove. In the technique introduced by Langerman, a diamond or metal knife is used to create a 0.3-mm-deep groove perpendicular to the corneal surface. Another blade is inserted into the groove, and its tip is then directed tangentially to the corneal surface, thereby creating a 1.5-mm tunnel through clear cornea into the anterior chamber. This

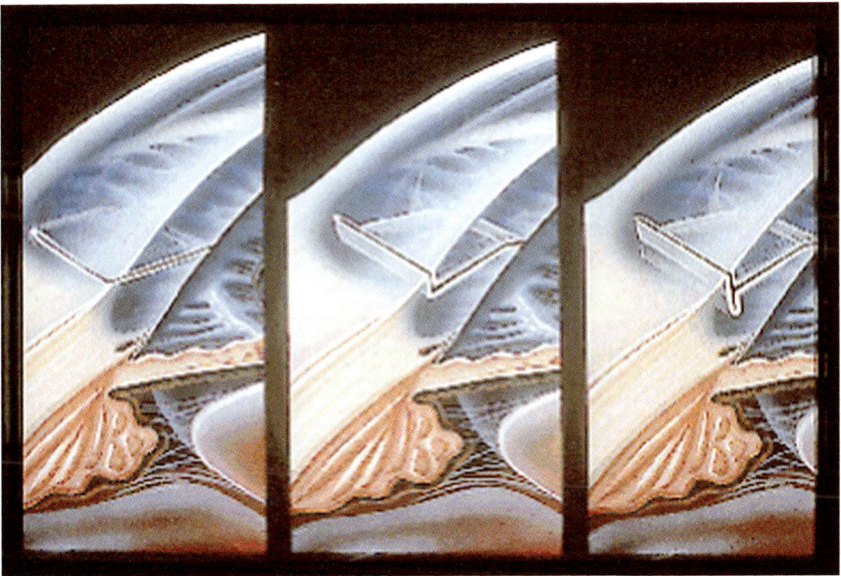

Figure 7-23 Architecture of clear corneal incisions. Single plane *(left)*, shallow groove *(center)*, and deep groove *(right)*. *(Reprinted with permission from Fine IH. Clear Corneal Lens Surgery. Thorofare, NJ: Slack; 1999.)*

multiplanar incision architecture is usually watertight. A variation on the multiplanar incision involves making a deeper vertical groove and creating a hinge.

Another approach is the beveled, multiplanar self-sealing incision, as advocated by Shimuzu and Fine. A beveled 3-mm diamond blade is flattened against the eye, and the tip is used to enter the cornea just anterior to the vascular arcade. The blade is advanced tangentially to the corneal surface until the shoulders of the blade are fully buried in the stroma. The point of the blade is then redirected posteriorly so that the point and the rest of the blade enter the anterior chamber parallel to the iris. This technique ideally creates a 3 × 2-mm corneal incision that is watertight. Disposable steel blades of varying dimensions can also be used to create these incisions. Newer beveled, trapezoidal diamond blades (Fig 7-24) have been developed for self-sealing clear corneal incisions. Such blades can be advanced in one motion and in one plane, from clear cornea into the anterior chamber. The blade is oriented parallel to the iris (0°), and the tip is placed at the start of the clear cornea, just anterior to the vascular arcade. The blade is tilted up and the heel down so that the blade is angled 10° from the iris plane and then advanced into the anterior chamber in one smooth, continuous motion. Regardless of which type of clear corneal incision is used, the goal is to keep the incision just large enough to accommodate the folded IOL with its inserter, generally 2.7–3.2 mm.

A third type is the "near clear" approach, in which the incision begins within the vascular arcade. Proponents of this approach cite better closure and reduced incidence of induced astigmatism. However, slight bleeding may occur during surgery; conjunctival ballooning may occur; and a subconjunctival hemorrhage may be present postoperatively.

A temporal approach for the clear (or near-clear) technique has the following advantages:

- avoids dissection of Tenon capsule and of conjunctiva, which decreases the risk of bleeding (eg, in patients on anticoagulants)
- creates a self-sealing incision that does not usually require sutures and allows for rapid vision rehabilitation
- offers better accessibility because brow obstruction is eliminated with a temporal approach
- offers an excellent red reflex
- spares the superior conjunctiva for subsequent surgery (eg, glaucoma filtering procedures or glaucoma drainage device implantation)
- avoids the need for a traction suture

However, the surgeon should also be aware of the disadvantages of temporal approach surgery, which include the following:

- need for the surgeon to adapt to a different surgical position
- difficulty in converting to a manual expression ECCE technique
- possible corneal thermal burns
- higher incidence of endophthalmitis in some studies (thought to be related to inadequate incision closure)

Ernest PH, Neuhann T. Posterior limbal incision. *J Cataract Refract Surg.* 1996;22(1):78–84.

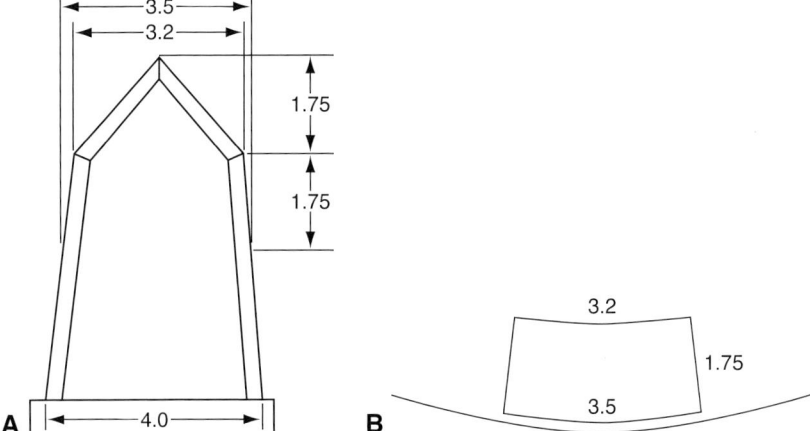

Figure 7-24 A, Dimensions and shape of a beveled trapezoidal diamond blade used in clear corneal incisions. **B,** Contour of the incision made with this knife. All dimensions are in millimeters. *(Modified with permission from Fine IH, Fichman RA, Grabow HB.* Clear-Corneal Cataract Surgery and Topical Anesthesia. *Thorofare, NJ: Slack; 1993.)*

Fine IH. Corneal tunnel incision with a temporal approach. In: Fine IH, Fichman RA, Grabow HB, eds. *Clear-Corneal Cataract Surgery and Topical Anesthesia.* Thorofare, NJ: Slack; 1993:50–51.

Langerman DW. Architectural design of a self-sealing corneal tunnel, single-hinge incision. *J Cataract Refract Surg.* 1994;20(1):84–88.

Masket S. Cataract incision and closure. *Focal Points: Clinical Modules for Ophthalmologists.* San Francisco: American Academy of Ophthalmology; 1995, module 3.

Masket S. Horizontal anchor suture closure method for small incision cataract surgery. *J Cataract Refract Surg.* 1991;17(suppl):689–695.

Nagaki Y, Hayasaka S, Kadoi C, et al. Bacterial endophthalmitis after small-incision cataract surgery: effect of incision placement and intraocular lens type. *J Cataract Refract Surg.* 2003;29(1):20–26.

Shepherd JR. Induced astigmatism in small incision cataract surgery. *J Cataract Refract Surg.* 1989;15(1):85–88.

Yeu E, Rubenstein JB. Management of astigmatism in lens-based surgery. *Focal Points: Clinical Modules for Ophthalmologists.* San Francisco: American Academy of Ophthalmology; 2008, module 2.

Continuous Curvilinear Capsulorrhexis

After the incision has been made, the next step is to open the capsule. Although a can-opener capsulotomy can be used with phacoemulsification, continuous curvilinear capsulorrhexis (CCC) is the capsular opening that allows a wider range of safer phaco techniques (Fig 7-25). CCC resists radial tears that could extend around and open the posterior capsule, setting the stage for complications. In addition, CCC stabilizes the nucleus, allowing maneuvers to disassemble the nucleus within the capsular bag. Disassembling the nucleus in the capsular bag decreases endothelial trauma. CCC also helps stabilize and center the

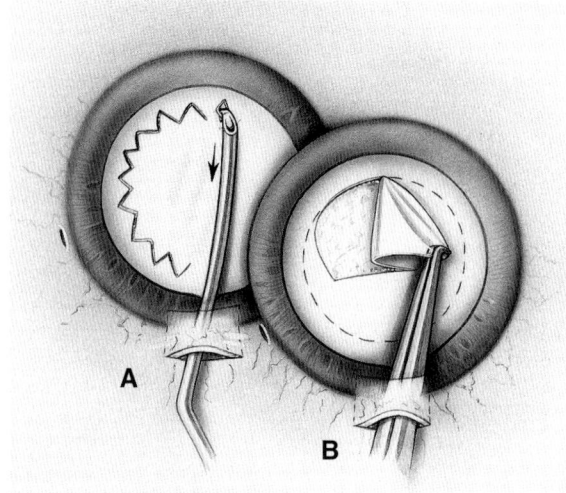

Figure 7-25 Anterior capsulotomy techniques. **A,** In the can-opener incision, punctures are made peripherally and pulled centrally so that the torn edges connect. Each puncture site has the potential for a radial tear if stressed. **B,** In the capsulorrhexis, tearing is begun within the area to be excised and finished from the outside in. When stress lines in the free flap appear between forceps and the tear site, best control is maintained by regrasping the flap near the tear site. Positive vitreous pressure makes the tear travel peripherally; filling the anterior chamber with an OVD will counteract the posterior vitreous pressure and make it easier to complete the capsulorrhexis tear. *(Reproduced with permission from Johnson SH. Phacoemulsification.* Focal Points: Clinical Modules for Ophthalmologists. *San Francisco: American Academy of Ophthalmology; 1994, module 6. Illustration by Christine Gralapp.)*

lens implant. Further, CCC transfers the haptic forces circumferentially and prevents lens implant decentration if Nd:YAG posterior capsulotomy is performed. A CCC sized just smaller than the IOL optic may allow a tighter contact between the posterior surface of the posterior chamber IOL and the posterior capsule, possibly reducing posterior capsule opacification. Lastly, certain lens implants designed to provide multifocality require a CCC of a certain size.

The surgeon begins a CCC with a central radial cut in the anterior capsule, using a cystitome needle or capsulorrhexis forceps with special tips for grasping and tearing the anterior capsule. At the end of the radial cut, the needle is either pushed or pulled in the direction of the desired tear, allowing the anterior capsule to fold over on itself. The surgeon then engages the free edge of the anterior capsule with either forceps or the capsulotomy needle, and the flap is carried around in a circular manner as the surgeon directs the tension toward the center of the lens.

The tear should not be allowed to turn either inward, as this results in a central opening that is too small, or outward, as this leads to an opening that is too large or to extension of the tear to the posterior capsule. An opening that is too small complicates most nucleus disassembly techniques and may contract postoperatively (capsular phimosis). The overlapping anterior capsule is prone to opacification, especially in diabetic patients. A capsulorrhexis that is too large complicates endocapsular phaco techniques and may allow the IOL optic or haptic to dislocate anteriorly. For these reasons, many surgeons advocate a size that allows the capsular rim to cover the optic edge to reduce posterior capsule opacification.

For maximum control of the size, frequent regrasping of the flap near the tear is helpful. The forceps or cystitome can be used to change the direction of the tear and prevent a CCC that is too small or too large. OVD should be added to keep the lens surface flat to avoid extension peripherally. Any factor that causes shallowing of the chamber will also make the lens move forward, directing the tear "downhill" toward the periphery. The surgeon should check for pressure on the globe caused by the capsulotomy instrument, the surgeon's fingers, or the eyelid speculum. Inserting a second instrument (such as an iris spatula) through the paracentesis to press posteriorly on the lens may also help control the direction of the tear.

If the capsulorrhexis seems too small after phacoemulsification is completed, the surgeon must decide whether to enlarge it before or after IOL implantation. If a foldable lens is to be used, the capsular bag can be expanded with a cohesive OVD; the lens may then be inserted. The cystitome or microscissors can be used to cut the anterior capsule edge of the CCC and extend the new tear around so that it enlarges the original CCC.

In cases with loose zonular fibers, creation of a CCC may be hampered by the lens nucleus and bag rotating along with the tear, dehiscing more zonular fibers and setting the stage for complications. Use of capsular hooks may stabilize the bag to allow completion of the tear.

If a CCC cannot be completed, conversion to a can-opener anterior capsulotomy is an acceptable strategy. However, this type of anterior capsulotomy makes hydrodissection, hydrodelineation, and endocapsular phacoemulsification more challenging because of a higher likelihood of an anterior capsule extension. If the surgeon encounters a fibrotic capsule, small-incision scissors may be used to cut the capsule to complete the capsulotomy.

Mackool RJ. Capsule stabilization for phacoemulsification [letter]. *J Cataract Refract Surg.* 2000;26(5):629.

Hydrodissection

Hydrodissection is performed to separate the peripheral cortex from the underlying posterior lens capsule. In addition to loosening the lens nucleus/cortex complex, this procedure facilitates nuclear rotation during phacoemulsification and hydrates the peripheral cortex, making it easier to aspirate after nucleus removal.

The surgeon places a bent, blunt-tipped 25- to 30-gauge cannula or flattened hydrodissection cannula attached to a 3–5-mL syringe under the anterior capsule flap. While carefully lifting the capsular flap, the surgeon injects balanced salt solution in a radial direction. Gentle posterior pressure centrally on the nucleus will express posterior fluid and prevent fluid pressure from rupturing the posterior capsule. Gentle irrigation should continue until the surgeon sees a wave of fluid moving under the nucleus and across the red reflex. In mature cataracts or in cases without a red reflex, careful hydrodissection should continue until nuclear rotation can be performed. Irrigation in the subincisional area may require a right-angled or J-shaped hydrodissection cannula.

If the nucleus is displaced into the anterior chamber, it can be reposited into the posterior chamber with OVD and application of slight posterior pressure. Alternatively, a supracapsular phaco technique may be selected in this situation. Hydrodissection is riskier after a can-opener capsulotomy has been performed, with zonular fibers that are weakened, or in a patient who has posterior polar cataracts.

Hydrodelineation

Some surgeons also inject balanced salt solution into the substance of the nucleus to hydrodelineate, or separate, the various layers of the nucleus after hydrodissection. This technique separates the harder central endonucleus from the softer outer epinucleus, which can remain behind to act as a cushion to protect the underlying posterior capsule from inadvertent trauma during nucleus removal. In less brunescent cataracts, a fluid wave can be seen to separate the endonucleus from the epinucleus and produce the "golden ring" sign. Hydrodelineation is not effective in white or densely brunescent nuclei.

Nuclear Rotation

If hydrodissection has succeeded in breaking attachments between posterior cortex and posterior capsule, the surgeon should be able to rotate the endonucleus and epinucleus within the capsular bag. Phaco techniques are easier to perform when the lens rotates freely within the bag. Therefore, surgeons should confirm nuclear rotation before proceeding with phacoemulsification.

Difficulty in rotating the nucleus may occur with soft nuclei or may suggest either inadequate hydrodissection (which can be repeated) or loose zonular fibers. If the zonular fibers are loose, attempted rotation will weaken the attachment of the capsular bag instead of the nucleus. Use of bimanual techniques through 2 paracenteses may allow rotation.

Instrument Settings for Phacoemulsification

Most methods of nucleus removal consist of several distinct steps, including sculpting, cracking or chopping, grasping, and emulsifying. With contemporary phaco machines, all the phaco parameters—power levels and intervals of delivery, aspiration flow rate, and vacuum—can be adjusted for each step of the procedure, giving the surgeon maximum control of the process. The vacuum is set to a level appropriate for the hardness of the nucleus. For example, harder cataracts require higher vacuum. If vacuum is set too low, lens chatter can occur, with large and small nuclear fragments bouncing around the anterior chamber. Higher vacuum improves the purchase of the phaco tip on the nuclear material and allows techniques with lower ultrasound power and shorter ultrasound time. Of course, higher vacuum might attract and tear the iris and anterior or posterior capsule. It is suggested that the beginning phaco surgeon start with power, pulse, burst, and vacuum levels recommended in courses or by surgical mentors.

Sculpting, the process of debulking the central nucleus, involves a shaving maneuver in which the tip of the phaco needle is never fully occluded. Without occlusion, only incidental vacuum is generated. Only a portion of the phaco needle is in contact with the nucleus with each forward pass; thus, lens material can be removed in a controlled fashion. Aspiration is responsible for bringing the nuclear particles into the aspiration port and out of the eye. Sculpting is usually performed with modest vacuum, low aspiration flow, and high phaco power.

After the nucleus has been sculpted and cracked or chopped, the nuclear fragments are grasped and emulsified. Vacuum is essential at this point in the procedure to grasp the nuclear fragments and pull them to a safe zone, between the posterior capsule and endothelium, before emulsification. Full occlusion of the phaco tip allows the vacuum to build up to its maximum preset level. Full vacuum draws nuclear material into the tip and allows it to be molded as it enters. The ultrasound power then emulsifies the material into smaller pieces. Vacuum drives the emulsified nuclear material farther into the tip, and it also helps feed additional nuclear material into the tip. If the repulsive action of the ultrasound tip oscillating against the nuclear material is counterbalanced by the vacuum and the flow pulling the material inward, chatter is reduced.

A low flow rate is considered desirable because it provides greater stability to the anterior chamber. After each nuclear fragment is completely emulsified and aspirated and occlusion is broken, low flow is immediately resumed. With low flow, emulsification and aspiration occur at a slower, more controlled rate; with high flow, events occur more quickly, and the iris and other intraocular tissue can be aspirated inadvertently. Once the nucleus is removed, the epinuclear material may be removed with lower flow and aspiration settings with either the phaco handpiece or with the irrigation/aspiration (I/A) instrument.

Location of Emulsification

The nucleus may be emulsified at various locations within the eye, including the anterior chamber, iris plane, and posterior chamber. The location chosen for emulsification will determine which techniques the surgeon employs for nucleus management.

Anterior chamber

The earliest technique of phacoemulsification involved emulsifying the lens in the anterior chamber. This technique has the benefits of excellent visibility and reduced risk of rupturing the posterior capsule. However, the risk of corneal endothelial trauma and resultant corneal edema increases because of the proximity of the phaco needle to the endothelium.

Iris plane

A later development was to perform phacoemulsification at the iris plane. In this location, the superior pole of the nucleus is prolapsed anteriorly (Fig 7-26A); and emulsification occurs halfway between the corneal endothelium and the posterior capsule, thereby reducing the risk of damage to either structure. Once prolapsed, the nucleus can be manipulated (Fig 7-26B) with less stress on the posterior capsule and zonular fibers. In patients with small pupils, this technique permits placement of the nucleus within the pupil, thus maintaining visualization and allowing for safe emulsification.

The iris plane location is often desirable for the beginning phaco surgeon and in patients who have small pupils or compromised capsular or zonular integrity. The disadvantages of this technique include the difficulty in prolapsing the nucleus and the risk of potential damage to the corneal endothelium if the surgeon emulsifies the superior pole of the nucleus too close to the cornea.

Posterior chamber

The posterior chamber is now the most common region for dismantling the nucleus (Fig 7-27). Removing the nucleus from this location requires capsulorrhexis, hydrodissection, and nuclear rotation. The advantages of posterior chamber phacoemulsification are the reduced risk of corneal endothelial trauma and the ability to minimize the size of the capsulorrhexis opening, which is useful with suboptimal dilation. The disadvantages include the need to emulsify close to the posterior capsule, the greater stress placed on the posterior capsule and zonular fibers when the nucleus is being manipulated, the technical difficulty in small-pupil cases, and the need to employ more-sophisticated methods of nuclear splitting.

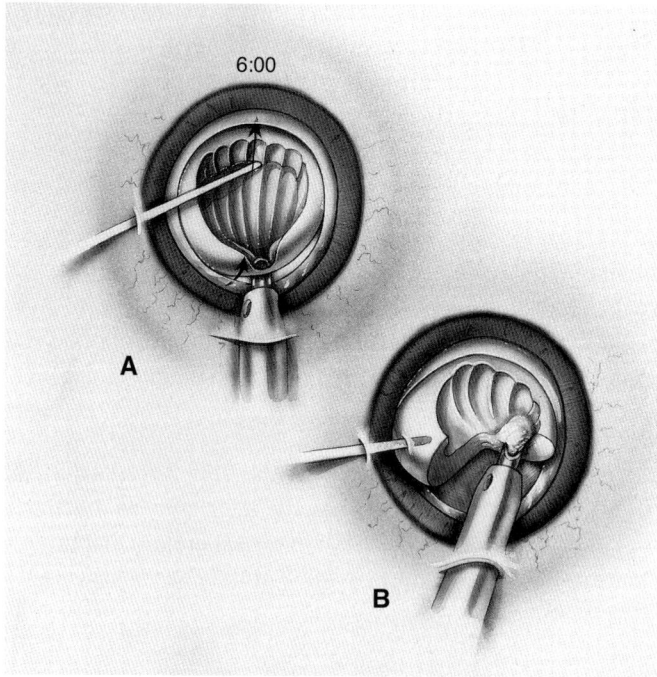

Figure 7-26 Emulsification of the nucleus as a whole at the iris plane, following central sculpting. **A,** Lens is subluxed by pushing the spatula against the ledge to move the lens toward the 6-o'clock position, leaving the anterior-posterior plane of the spatula unchanged. The anterior chamber is shallowed by stopping irrigation, allowing the superior lens equator to present anteriorly as the lens rotates around the stable spatula. The ultrasound tip is partially withdrawn to catch the posterior surface of the superior lens equator and help lift the lens. **B,** Nucleus is stabilized by sticking it with the spatula, and the ultrasound tip debulks the lens by quadrants. Both instruments are used to rotate the lens counterclockwise as the process continues. *(Reproduced with permission from Johnson SH. Phacoemulsification. Focal Points: Clinical Modules for Ophthalmologists. San Francisco: American Academy of Ophthalmology; 1994, module 6. Illustration by Christine Gralapp.)*

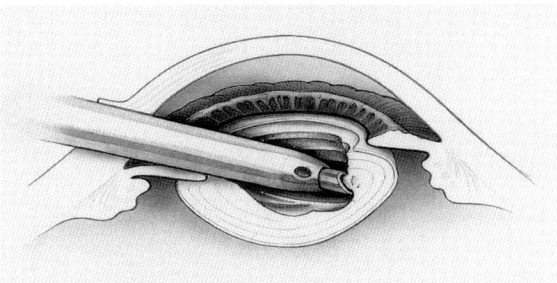

Figure 7-27 Central sculpting of the nucleus when managed as a whole. If the surgeon uses the iris plane approach, the nucleus is sculpted to $\frac{1}{2}-\frac{2}{3}$ its depth, leaving an inferior ledge; with a posterior chamber approach, the nucleus is sculpted deep centrally and thinned inferiorly to weaken the remaining lens material. *(Reproduced with permission from Johnson SH. Phacoemulsification.* Focal Points: Clinical Modules for Ophthalmologists. *San Francisco: American Academy of Ophthalmology; 1994, module 6. Illustration by Christine Gralapp.)*

Supracapsular technique

This technique involves prolapsing the nucleus through the capsulorrhexis during hydrodissection and then either repositing the nucleus in the posterior chamber on top of the capsular bag or leaving a pole anterior to the iris. Both positions require medium to large capsulorrhexes. This approach theoretically reduces the stress on the zonular fibers during nucleus manipulation.

The risks of this technique include a greater chance of aspirating and damaging the iris in the phaco tip and the inability to maintain control of the nuclear pieces as they are separated.

Techniques of Nucleus Disassembly

A popular approach of nucleus disassembly usually requires 2 instruments to subdivide the nucleus prior to its emulsification. This process allows for removal of the hard endonucleus first, within the capsular bag, using the epinucleus and cortex as a cushion to protect the underlying posterior capsule. The endonucleus is divided into several small pieces. This division process allows for a more controlled removal using less phaco power and time. This technique requires a CCC to provide an intact and very resilient capsular opening.

Phaco fracture technique

The most widely used 2-handed technique, developed by Gimbel (nucleofractis) and Shephard ("divide and conquer"), effectively removes all but very soft cataracts. After having performed adequate hydrodissection and hydrodelineation, the surgeon uses continuous ultrasound to sculpt a deep central linear groove or trough in the nucleus. Any groove must be deep enough to allow subsequent cracking. Clues that the groove depth is adequate include smoothing of the striations in the groove, brightening of the red reflex in the groove, and sculpting to a depth of 2 to 3 phaco tip diameters.

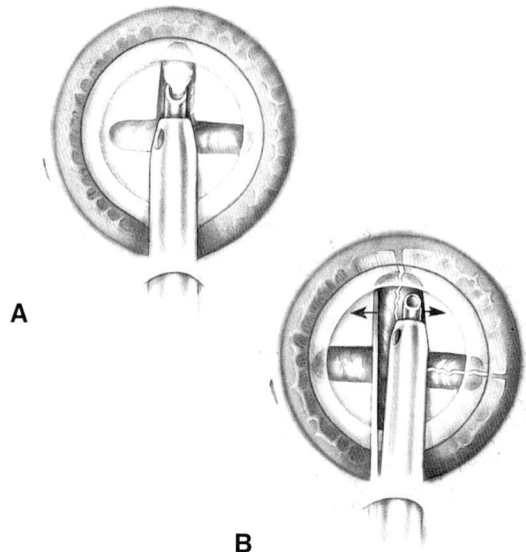

Figure 7-28 **A,** Sculpting grooves. **B,** Cracking with phaco needle and second instrument. *(Reproduced with permission from Johnson SH. Phacoemulsification. Focal Points: Clinical Modules for Ophthalmologists. San Francisco: American Academy of Ophthalmology; 1994, module 6. Illustration by Christine Gralapp.)*

At this point, the surgeon can use nuclear cracking to separate the nucleus into 2 pieces, or the surgeon can rotate the nucleus halves after separation to create 2 additional troughs to divide each half into 2 quadrants. The phaco tip and second instrument are inserted into each groove and spread apart, with a cross action or parallel action, thereby achieving the complete separation of the pieces (Fig 7-28).

The surgeon can then use the second instrument to present either the peripheral rim or the apex of the quadrant to the phaco needle (Fig 7-29). This piece is engaged by the phaco tip; and after adequate vacuum is attained, the nuclear quadrant is pulled toward the center of the capsular bag and emulsified. Each quadrant is sequentially removed in the same manner.

Chopping techniques

The *horizontal phaco chop* technique originally described by Nagahara does not entail creation of a central groove but instead advocates use of the natural fault lines in the lens nucleus for creation of a fracture plane. After burying the phaco tip in the center of the nucleus by using high vacuum, the surgeon inserts a phaco chop instrument under the anterior capsule flap, deeply engages the endonucleus in the periphery, and draws it toward the phaco tip, thereby cracking the nucleus into 2 pieces. The phaco tip is then buried in one of the nuclear halves, and the surgeon uses the phaco chop instrument in the same fashion to create multiple small wedges of nucleus for emulsification.

Koch and Katzen modified this procedure by making a central groove and starting with division of the nucleus into 2 pieces through sculpting and cracking, with subsequent chopping of heminuclei ("stop and chop" phaco; Fig 7-30). The groove affords the surgeon more room to manipulate the nuclear pieces in the capsular bag. High levels of

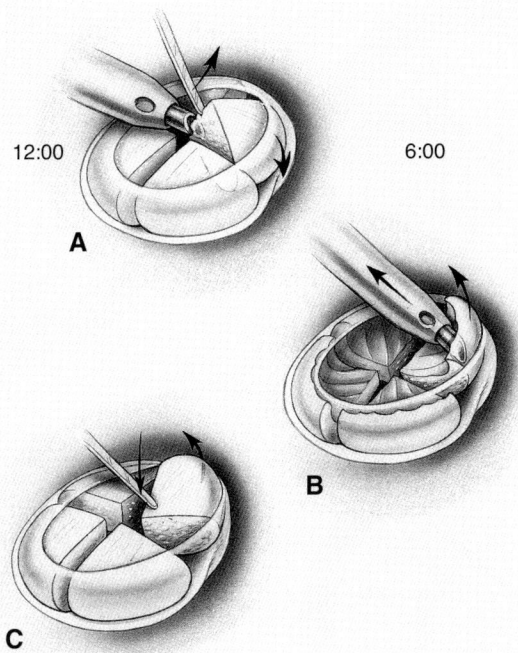

Figure 7-29 Quadrant removal techniques. **A,** Spatula lifts the apex of the quadrant; the ultrasound tip is embedded into the posterior edge; and aspiration centralizes the quadrant for emulsification. **B,** Quadrants are debulked centrally after splitting; the ultrasound tip is embedded into the cortical rim and aspiration is maintained to tumble the rim and remainder of the quadrant centrally. **C,** Spatula pushes the apex of the quadrant posteriorly so the rim moves to front and center. *(Reproduced with permission from Johnson SH.* Phacoemulsification. *Focal Points: Clinical Modules for Ophthalmologists. San Francisco: American Academy of Ophthalmology; 1994, module 6. Illustration by Christine Gralapp.)*

vacuum are necessary to maintain a firm grasp on the nucleus as it is being fragmented; in addition, the high vacuum allows more controlled removal of the pieces and reduces the use of ultrasound energy. Any remaining epinucleus and cortex are removed in standard fashion.

Classic horizontal chop entailed the challenge of placing the chopper under the capsular rim and around the equatorial nucleus without direct visualization, and "stop and chop" phaco required creation of a groove. *Vertical chopping* techniques that eliminate both of these challenges have been developed. After the center of the nucleus is impaled with the phaco tip using high vacuum and burst mode, a chopper with a sharp tip is buried within the nucleus, just adjacent to the phaco tip. The phaco tip lifts while the chopper depresses, and the surgeon separates the instruments to effect the chop, which occurs along natural fault lines in the nucleus.

In practice, either the vertical or the horizontal chopping technique can be used with almost any other strategy for disassembly of the nucleus. Chopping is not appropriate for soft nuclei, such as pure posterior subcapsular cataracts. Other techniques, such as hydrodelamination and aspiration with minimal phaco power, may be more appropriate in these cases.

124 • Lens and Cataract

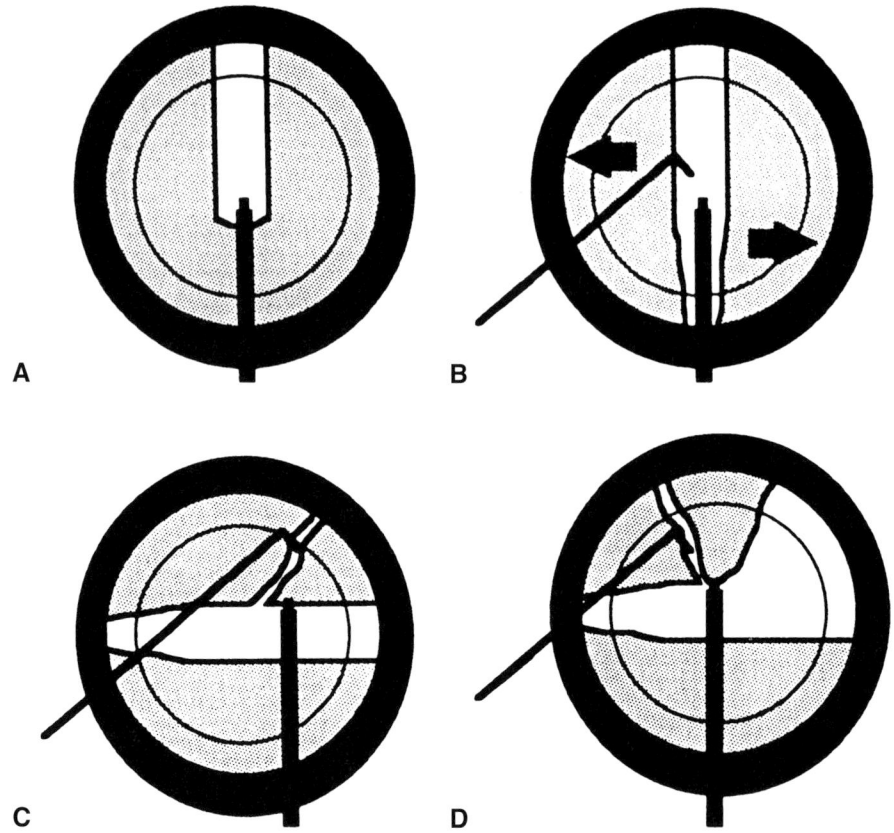

Figure 7-30 "Stop and chop" techniques. **A,** Soft cataracts are prepared by sculpting a trench in the middle of the cataract, providing space for later manipulation. **B,** After sculpting is complete, the nucleus is fractured into halves with the phaco tip and the chopper. **C,** The phaco tip is driven into the nuclear half about a third of the way across from right to left. The chopper is buried in the periphery of the nucleus and pulled toward the phaco tip. When the instruments are close to each other, they are separated, and a small segment of the nucleus is chopped off. It is already impaled on the phaco tip and can be emulsified without further manipulation. **D,** The phaco tip is driven into the remaining nucleus and the same steps are repeated: bury the chopper, pull it toward the phaco tip, chop, separate, remove. This sequence is repeated until the entire nucleus is emulsified. *(Reproduced with permission from Koch PS, Katzen LE. Stop and chop phacoemulsification.* J Cataract Refract Surg. *1994;20:566–570. © American Society of Cataract and Refractive Surgery.)*

Chang DF. *Phaco Chop: Mastering Techniques, Optimizing Technology, and Avoiding Complications.* Thorofare, NJ: Slack; 2004.

Koch PS. *Mastering Phacoemulsification: A Simplified Manual of Strategies for the Spring, Crack, and Stop and Chop Technique.* 4th ed. Thorofare, NJ: Slack; 1994.

One-handed technique of nucleus disassembly

This technique involves an adequate capsulorrhexis and one surgical incision. Because no OVD is present before keratome entry, a diamond blade may be useful for its exquisite sharpness and ease in entering the anterior chamber. The surgeon performs hydrodissection, hydrodelineation, and nuclear rotation within the capsular bag. The phaco needle is used to shave layer by layer through the nucleus from edge to edge, and the nucleus is rotated to access thicker regions (Fig 7-31). When the nucleus has been removed, the phaco needle can be used to remove the epinuclear envelope, with low phaco power and medium vacuum settings. Any residual cortex is removed with I/A.

> Gimbel HV. Divide and conquer nucleofractis phacoemulsification: development and variations. *J Cataract Refract Surg.* 1991;17(3):281–291.
> Koch PS. *Converting to Phacoemulsification: Making the Transition to In-the-Bag Phaco.* 3rd ed. Thorofare, NJ: Slack; 1992.
> Koch PS, Davison JA, eds. *Textbook of Advanced Phacoemulsification Techniques.* Thorofare, NJ: Slack; 1991.
> Shepherd JR. In situ fracture. *J Cataract Refract Surg.* 1990;16(4):436–440.
> Steinert RF, ed. *Cataract Surgery: Technique, Complications, and Management.* 2nd ed. St Louis: Mosby; 2004.

Strategies for Irrigation and Aspiration

In phacoemulsification and in ECCE with manual expression, the same instruments and techniques are used for I/A of cortical material.

A plate of soft epinucleus (or transitional cortex) may rest on the posterior capsule. The surgeon can use the phaco needle to accomplish I/A without ultrasound; reduced vacuum and flow settings can be used to aspirate this material from the capsular fornix or posterior capsule. The I/A system straight tip can be used with the port down and low vacuum to strip this material carefully from the posterior capsule.

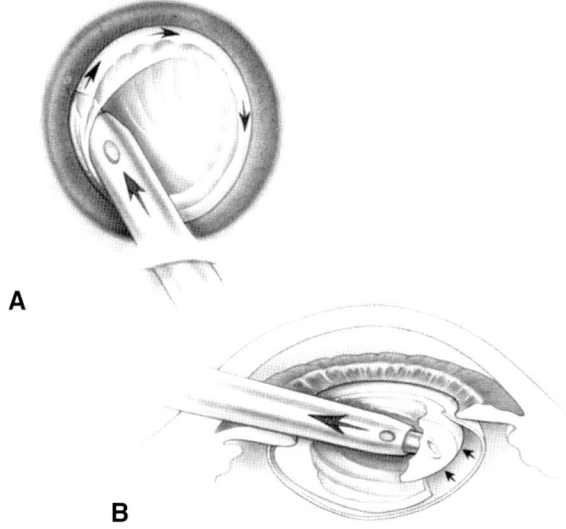

Figure 7-31 One-handed nuclear rotation **(A)** and nuclear rim removal **(B)**. *(Reproduced with permission from Johnson SH. Phacoemulsification. Focal Points: Clinical Modules for Ophthalmologists. San Francisco: American Academy of Ophthalmology; 1994, module 6. Illustration by Christine Gralapp.)*

The surgeon can remove peripheral cortical material by first rotating the port toward the equator of the lens capsule. The cortical material should be engaged under low suction and dragged to the center of the inflated capsular bag. The surgeon rotates the port so that it is fully visible, and the cortex can be stripped under greater suction. In an alternative technique, the cortex is engaged with mild suction at the tip of the cannula. The cortex is then stripped from the fornix and released by manual irrigation into the anterior chamber. This procedure is repeated until all the cortex is free.

Sometimes the surgeon finds it difficult to reach the subincisional cortex. In these cases, a 45°, right-angled (90°), or U-shaped (180°) aspiration cannula may be useful to engage and strip this cortical material. The I/A functions may also be separated, and the aspiration port may be introduced through the paracentesis while irrigation through the phaco incision or a second sideport maintains the chamber. Another technique involves filling the anterior chamber with OVD and aspirating subincisional cortex with a J-shaped aspiration cannula attached to a handheld syringe.

Cortex resistant to aspiration can be separated from the capsular bag with OVD (ie, viscodissected) to allow easier access with the I/A handpiece. Another strategy is to put off removal of subincisional cortex until after implantation of the IOL. The IOL can be rotated within the bag so the haptics will further loosen the cortex. The surgeon must weigh the benefits of attempting to remove small amounts of residual cortex against the risk of damaging the posterior capsule. Very small amounts of retained fine cortical strands may easily be resorbed postoperatively.

After removing the cataract and inserting the IOL, the surgeon should remove the OVD from the anterior segment. Some surgeons remove the OVD from behind the optic; others push the optic down to release the OVD from the bag and allow its aspiration from the anterior chamber.

To produce a slightly firm eye, balanced salt solution is used, via the paracentesis, to re-form the anterior chamber. The incision is examined for leakage. If the incision leaks, both sides of the corneal tunnel incision can be hydrated with balanced salt solution injected through a syringe with a blunt 25- to 26-gauge irrigating tip. Hydration of the corneal incision causes temporary stromal swelling and increases the wound apposition between the roof and the floor of the tunnel, thereby reducing the risk of leakage. Some surgeons hydrate the stroma in all cases. If the incision leaks after stromal hydration, it requires a suture. Larger incisions that are used to allow insertion of a lens generally require suture closure.

Advances in Energy Delivery

Technological advances have reduced the total amount of phaco energy delivered to achieve emulsification. Examples of these technologies include the OZil torsional technology on the Alcon Infiniti (Ft Worth, TX), the WhiteStar Cold Phaco technology on the AMO Sovereign (Santa Ana, CA), the Custom Control Software in the Bausch & Lomb Millennium Microsurgical System (Rochester, NY), and the Sonic WAVE Ultrasound Alternative Phacoemulsification System from the STAAR Surgical Company (Monrovia, CA).

Alternative Technologies for Nucleus Removal

Laser Photolysis

Currently, the only laser system that the Food and Drug Administration (FDA) has approved for cataract extraction is the Dodick Photolysis, Q-switched Nd:YAG system (A.R.C. Laser Corp, Salt Lake City, UT). It generates laser shock waves at 200 to 400 nanoseconds that strike a titanium target at the end of the aspirating handpiece. The system includes Venturi fluidics and a touch-screen control panel; it also includes an ultrasound handpiece port for emulsifying cataracts that are too dense for laser phacoemulsification.

Fluid-Based Phacolysis

The AquaLase Liquefaction Device is an instrument that has been in use since 2000 and commercially available from Alcon (Ft Worth, TX) in the Infiniti Vision System since 2003. With this system, 4-µL boluses of warmed balanced salt solution are delivered through a polymer tip to delaminate lens material without longitudinal or rotary mechanical movement of the instrument. The polymer tip is soft and is less likely to rupture the posterior capsule than are metal phaco tips. Unlike with ultrasonic phacoemulsification, there has been no reported incisional burn with this system. This technology has been used to remove nuclei of all grades of density.

Femtosecond Laser Cataract Extraction

The FDA approved femtosecond lasers for cataract extraction in 2010. Well known to refractive surgeons, this technology has the potential to provide precise corneal incisions as well as being used for capsulotomies and lens disassembly.

> He L, Sheehy K, Culbertson W. Femtosecond laser-assisted cataract surgery. *Curr Opin Ophthalmol.* 2011;22(1):43–52. Epub 2010 Dec 9.

Antimicrobial Prophylaxis

Because endophthalmitis remains one of the worst complications of cataract surgery (see Chapter 8), one goal of the preoperative preparation and intraoperative management of the patient is to reduce the introduction of pathogenic organisms into the anterior chamber.

Before Surgery

Before the day of surgery, the surgeon should identify and reduce infectious risk factors as much as possible through preoperative treatment of coexisting eyelid disorders such as conjunctivitis, blepharitis, hordeolum, or chalazion. An ocular prosthesis in the fellow eye may harbor bacteria, warranting evaluation of the socket and cleaning of the prosthesis before surgery. Systemic infections should be identified and treated before elective surgery.

Cataract surgery is not considered to be an invasive procedure that induces transient bacteremia, and antibiotic prophylaxis is not required. If questions arise about whether antibiotic prophylaxis is advisable in the perioperative period, the surgeon should consult with the physicians involved in the patient's systemic care.

Although no studies convincingly demonstrate the efficacy of topical antibiotics in reducing the risk of endophthalmitis in routine cataract surgery, some evidence supports an association between the use of preoperative topical antibiotics and a reduction in ocular surface bacterial counts, as well as a lower incidence of positive aqueous cultures after surgery. Many cataract surgeons give their patients topical antibiotics as prophylaxis before surgery; the dosage varies from administration for 2 to 3 days preoperatively to frequent dosing just prior to surgery.

> Carrim ZI, Mackie G, Gallacher G, Wykes WN. The efficacy of 5% povidone-iodine for 3 minutes prior to cataract surgery. *Eur J Ophthalmol.* 2009;19(4):560–564.
>
> He L, Ta CN, Miño de Kaspar H. One-day application of topical moxifloxacin 0.5% to select for fluoroquinolone-resistant coagulase-negative *Staphylococcus. J Cataract Refract Surg.* 2009;35(10):1715–1718.

In Surgery

In the operating room, sterilization of the fornix has become an important goal. A 5% solution (not scrub or soap) of povidone-iodine placed in the conjunctival fornix prior to surgery has been associated with a reduction in bacterial colony counts cultured from the ocular surface at the time of surgery and a decreased risk of culture-proven endophthalmitis. In addition, preparation of the skin around the eye with a 5% to 10% povidone-iodine solution reduced bacterial counts on the eyelid margins. Because eyelid margins may harbor pathogens, care should be taken to drape the eyelashes out of the operative field (Fig 7-32).

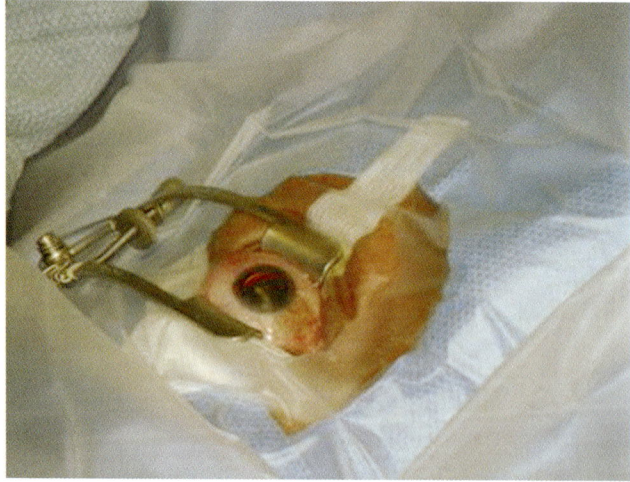

Figure 7-32 Sterile draping with eyelid margin coverage. *(Courtesy of Ken Mitchell, MD.)*

It is important not only to limit the number of times that the surgeon introduces instruments into the eye but also to check for signs of lint, cilia, and other debris on the tips of all instruments inserted. It is wise to reduce intraoperative manipulation as well. Meticulous wound closure is imperative. Despite all of these efforts, the conjunctiva may harbor residual bacteria. Studies have documented that 7% to 35% of cataract surgeries result in bacterial inoculation of the anterior chamber. That endophthalmitis is infrequent is a testament to the ability of the anterior chamber to clear itself of a potentially pathologic inoculum.

The surgeon should also recognize that the risk of endophthalmitis increases with a torn posterior lens capsule, vitreous loss, and prolonged surgery. Some surgeons place antibiotics in the irrigating solution or inject them into the anterior chamber at the end of surgery. Some have reported a significant reduction in endophthalmitis with the use of intracameral cefuroxime. The injection of antibiotics under the conjunctiva or Tenon capsule is also an option.

Conflict surrounds the possibility of an increased risk of endophthalmitis after non-sutured clear corneal temporal-approach cataract surgery. It has been shown that hypotony may cause the nonsutured incision to allow inflow of tear contents into the eye. For this reason, hydrating the stroma and leaving a slightly firm eye at the end of the case may reduce the risk of wound separation. Any question about wound leakage should prompt the use of suture closure.

After Surgery

Use of antibiotic eyedrops is often continued or instituted after routine cataract surgery. Although reduced bacterial counts have been documented with the administration of topical antibiotics, no clear-cut evidence has yet confirmed that their use reduces the incidence of endophthalmitis. The studies cited here indicate the complexity of the issues involved in avoiding postoperative infection.

> Cooper BA, Holekamp NM, Bohigian G, Thompson PA. Case-control study of endophthalmitis after cataract surgery comparing scleral tunnel and clear corneal wounds. *Am J Ophthalmol.* 2003;136(2):300–305.
>
> Endophthalmitis Study Group, European Society of Cataract & Refractive Surgeons (ESCRS). Prophylaxis of postoperative endophthalmitis following cataract surgery: results of the ESCRS multicenter study and identification of risk factors. *J Cataract Refract Surg.* 2007; 33(6):978–988.
>
> Liesegang TJ. Intracameral antibiotics: questions for the United States based on prospective studies. *J Cataract Refract Surg.* 2008;34(3):505–509.
>
> Miller JJ, Scott IU, Flynn HW Jr, Smiddy WE, Newton J, Miller D. Acute-onset endophthalmitis after cataract surgery (2000–2004): incidence, clinical settings, and visual acuity outcomes after treatment. *Am J Ophthalmol.* 2005;139(6):983–987.
>
> Sharifi E, Porco TC, Naseri A. Cost-effectiveness analysis of intracameral cefuroxime use for prophylaxis of endophthalmitis after cataract surgery. *Ophthalmology.* 2009;116(10): 1887–1896.
>
> Wykoff CC, Flynn HW Jr, Han DP. Allergy to povidone-iodine and cephalosporins: the clinical dilemma in ophthalmic use. *Am J Ophthalmol.* 2011;151(1):4–6.

Modification of Preexisting Astigmatism

Cataract surgery has been called the most commonly performed refractive procedure in ophthalmology. Certainly, elimination of spherical refractive error through meticulous lens implant calculations is possible. Multiple methods of astigmatism reduction are available to the cataract surgeon.

Because a cataract can induce refractive astigmatism, it is important for the surgeon to compare the preoperative refractive cylinder with K readings. If the refractive cylinder matches the power and axis by keratometry, cataract-induced astigmatism is negligible, and the refractive cylinder can be considered for reduction through surgery. Any discrepancy may be analyzed through computerized corneal imaging. If questions remain, it is wiser to defer astigmatism reduction until stable refractions are obtained in the postoperative period.

Surgical planning for refractive cataract surgery includes consideration of incision size and location, postoperative astigmatism reduction with photorefractive corneal surgery, intraoperative and postoperative limbal relaxing incisions, and use of toric IOLs. (Also see BCSC Section 13, *Refractive Surgery*.)

Over time in aging eyes, there tends to be a natural against-the-rule drift of corneal astigmatism as a result of flattening of the superior meridian. Corneal burns from the phaco tip may also induce postoperative astigmatism. Modification of preexisting corneal astigmatism through incision architecture and location on the steeper meridian, combined with peripheral corneal relaxing incisions, may reduce the astigmatism.

Incision Size and Location

One prerequisite to modifying preexisting astigmatism is to create a small incision that does not induce any corneal astigmatism. If a larger incision is required, placing it across the steeper meridian may reduce preoperative astigmatism.

Astigmatic Keratotomy

Astigmatic keratotomy (AK) is a technique surviving from the era of refractive keratotomy. Within the cornea, paired incisions were placed at varying distances from the apex of the steepest corneal meridian in order to decrease the curvature of that meridian and to increase the curvature of the meridian 90° away (a technique known as *coupling*). Glare from the incisional scar is a potential problem for the cataract surgical patient, for whom postoperative quality of vision is paramount. Any infection near the center of the cornea has serious consequences. For these reasons, AK has largely been supplanted by limbal relaxing incisions. (See also BCSC Section 13, *Refractive Surgery*.)

Limbal Relaxing Incisions

Limbal relaxing incisions (LRIs) have been advocated as an effective method for reducing 0.5–3.0 diopters (D) of astigmatism. Because of their placement at the limbus, LRIs have the potential advantage of preserving the optical qualities of the cornea, inducing less postoperative glare, minimizing discomfort, reducing overcorrections, and allowing quicker recovery of vision.

Surgeons planning to use a surgical technique that is unfamiliar to them should consider taking courses and performing practice surgeries. To improve outcomes, the surgeon should select a nomogram and track postoperative refractive results.

Before any injected anesthetic is given to the patient, the 6- and 12-o'clock meridians are marked with the patient sitting upright. Marks are made at the limbus with either a sterile skin marker or other technique, such as a 25-gauge needle in the corneal epithelium. The steep meridian is then identified with use of these landmarks or other natural landmarks if they exist. An incision is made at the limbus circumferentially across the steep meridian. One or more incisions are made depending on the nomogram of the surgeon's choosing. Some surgeons place the cataract incision within the LRI; others prefer to use a separate location. LRIs may also be done postoperatively in an office setting. Use of the femtosecond laser to make incisions prior to cataract surgery shows promise for increasing the precision and reproducibility of these modifications of the corneal curvature.

> Budak K, Freidman NJ, Koch DD. Limbal relaxing incisions with cataract surgery. *J Cataract Refract Surg*. 1998;24(4):503–508.
> Gills JP. *A Complete Guide to Astigmatism Management*. Thorofare, NJ: Slack; 2003.
> Nichamin LD. Opposite clear corneal incisions. *J Cataract Refract Surg*. 2001;27(1):7–8.
> Palanker DV, Blumenkranz MS, Andersen D, et al. Femtosecond laser-assisted cataract surgery with integrated optical coherence tomography. *Sci Transl Med*. 2010;2(58):58ra85.

Toric IOLs

Toric IOLs are designed to correct astigmatism without corneal incisions, which helps avoid extra incisional complications. In addition, better standardization of correction occurs with these IOLs than with incisional correction. The disadvantages of the toric IOL relate to possible lens rotation away from the desired axis. Rotation may be more likely when the IOL is implanted in a larger capsular bag. Each degree of rotation reduces the effect of astigmatism correction by approximately 3% and may induce higher-order aberrations. If needed, a second procedure to rotate the lens to the correct axis should be done early in the postoperative period, before complete capsular fixation of the lens occurs. Examples of these lenses include the STAAR Toric IOL (STAAR Surgical Company, Monrovia, CA) and the AcrySof IQ Toric IOL by Alcon (Ft Worth, TX). These lenses are reported to correct up to 6.00 D (AcrySof IQ Toric IOL) and 2.3 D (STAAR Toric IOL) at the corneal plane. Higher levels of correction from the AcrySof IQ Toric IOL are now available.

> Ahmed II, Rocha G, Slomovic AR, et al; Canadian Toric Study Group. Visual function and patient experience after bilateral implantation of toric intraocular lenses. *J Cataract Refract Surg*. 2010;36(4):609–616.
> Holland E, Lane S, Horn JD, Ernest P, Arleo R, Miller KM. The AcrySof Toric intraocular lens in subjects with cataracts and corneal astigmatism: a randomized, subject-masked, parallel-group, 1-year study. *Ophthalmology*. 2010;117(11):2104–2111.
> Sun XY, Vicary D, Montgomery P, Griffiths M. Toric intraocular lenses for correcting astigmatism in 130 eyes. *Ophthalmology*. 2000;107(9):1776–1782.

Pars Plana Lensectomy

The posterior approach to lens extraction is performed through the pars plana, generally in combination with vitrectomy. See also BCSC Section 12, *Retina and Vitreous*.

Indications

The presence of a significant cataract with the urgent need for pars plana vitrectomy and/or retinal surgery is the general indication for this approach. Following trauma with lens rupture and vitreous disruption, this single approach is the best way to clean all of the vitreous and lens material from the eye. A pars plana approach may also facilitate removal of retained foreign bodies and management of perforating injuries. Clear lens removal may be essential in procedures for anterior proliferation of the hyaloid and in cases requiring anterior dissection of the vitreous for detachments with proliferative vitreoretinopathy. A posterior approach may be desirable in cases of symptomatic lens subluxation.

Contraindications

The most common contraindication for this approach is a nucleus too hard to be removed by this technique. A dense brunescent lens may be unsuitable for fragmentation through the pars plana; it may be preferable for the cataract surgeon to use an anterior approach and remove the lens first. Either combined surgery or sequential surgery may be performed.

Intraocular Lens Implantation

Historical Perspectives

Before 1949, cataract surgery resulted in aphakia, and patients were destined (unless highly myopic) to wear high-hyperopic spectacles that were of considerable weight and that caused image magnification and distortion to the sides. When they became available and their use was possible, scleral contact lenses and eventually corneal contact lenses were used.

The development of modern IOL implantation began in 1949. Harold Ridley, an English ophthalmologist, observed that PMMA fragments from airplane cockpit windshields were well tolerated in the anterior segment of the eyes of injured World War II pilots. He placed a disc-shaped PMMA lens into the posterior chamber of a 45-year-old woman after he performed an ECCE (Fig 7-33).

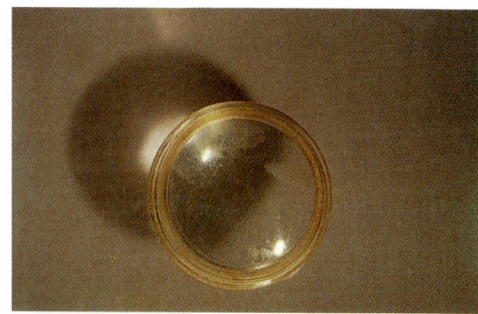

Figure 7-33 Original Ridley lens, first implanted by Harold Ridley in November 1949. *(Courtesy of Robert C. Drews, MD.)*

Ridley's lens corrected aphakic vision, but a high incidence of postoperative complications such as glaucoma, uveitis, and dislocation caused him to abandon his lens design. Though frustrated in his attempts, Ridley showed foresight in 3 important areas. First, he constructed his original lens of PMMA in a biconvex design. Second, he used extracapsular surgery for implantation of the lens. Third, he placed the lens in the posterior chamber. Ridley set the stage for a period of advances in cataract surgery that continues to this day, and he was knighted for his contributions.

Ophthalmologists in the 1950s were troubled by the serious complications associated with early IOL styles and by the fact that nearly all of the investigative work was done in humans, occasionally with very little scientific basis. Uncertainty concerning the long-term success and stability of these lenses limited their use. Yet the desire to manage aphakia without the problems and inconvenience of aphakic spectacles or contact lenses continued to inspire investigation into IOL implantation.

Extracapsular cataract surgery in the 1950s was crude by modern standards and was generally associated with retained lens cortex, which caused fibrosis and adhesions between iris and capsule. ICCE eliminated residual cortical material and became the preferred procedure. Because ICCE was more commonly performed in the early days of lens implantation, IOLs of that period featured optics with loops, struts, or holes for sutures required for fixation to the iris for support (Fig 7-34).

The anterior chamber angle was an alternate site for support of an IOL. The first anterior chamber IOLs (ACIOLs) of Barraquer, Strampelli, and others (Fig 7-35) were crude and ultimately required explantation because of severe inflammatory reactions. Later models by Choyce and others were better made, though still rigid; and some patients complained of tenderness postoperatively.

Fitting the length of the lens to the width of the chamber was difficult. The IOL length was selected by estimating anterior chamber width based on the horizontal corneal diameter. Because such estimation is crude even with modern instruments, complications arose. Oversized lenses and closed-loop IOLs caused pupillary distortion and contributed to uveitis-glaucoma-hyphema (UGH) syndrome. ACIOLs that were too short would spin, decenter, and come into contact with the corneal endothelium.

Complications associated with rigid ACIOLs spurred the development of the flexible-loop ACIOL. Additional advances included open support arms with 4-point fixation (Fig 7-36); these modifications have allowed ACIOLs to remain a treatment choice for cases with compromised capsular bags or for secondary IOL insertion.

As a result of the conversion to modern ECCE, IOL designs changed to allow placement in the posterior chamber and support from the lens capsule. ACIOLs were largely relegated to a backup role when capsule support was absent or when other problems precluded implantation of a posterior chamber IOL (PCIOL).

> Apple DJ, Mamalis N, Olson RJ, et al. *Intraocular Lenses: Evolution, Designs, Complications, and Pathology.* Baltimore: Williams & Wilkins; 1989.

Posterior Chamber IOLs

The desire to place the IOL in the lens capsule was the impetus to expand research into posterior chamber lens implantation. Shearing took a flexible version of a 3-piece IOL

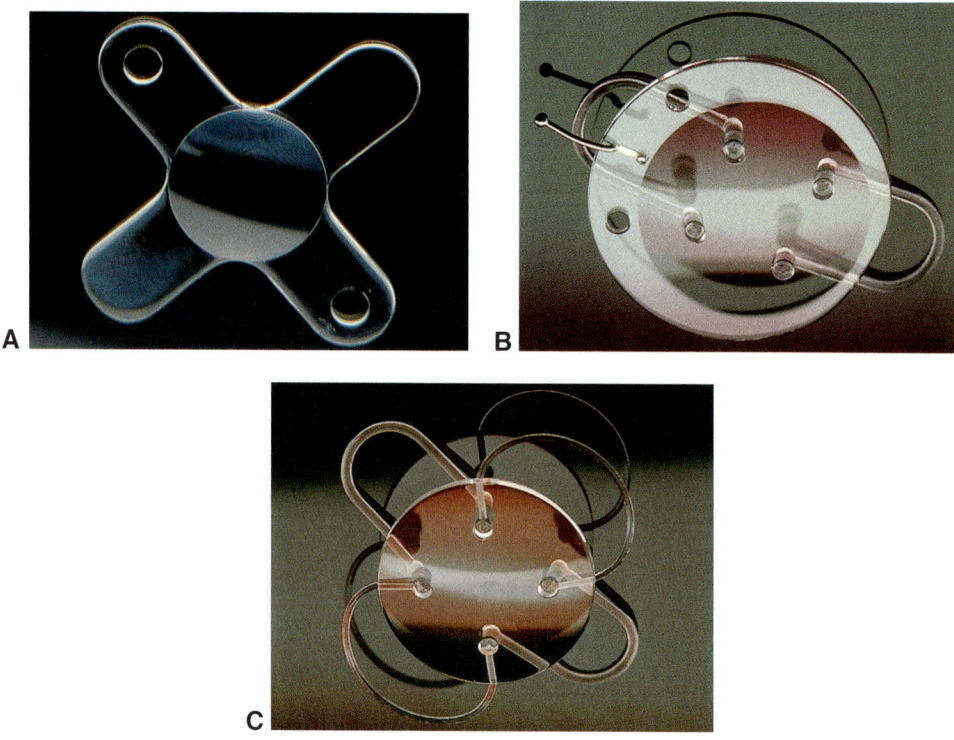

Figure 7-34 IOL styles for intracapsular surgery. **A,** Epstein lens made by Copeland; iris supported with 2 opposing haptics placed anterior and posterior to the iris. **B,** Medallion lens with platinum clip designed by Worst; lens was implanted with polypropylene haptics posterior to the iris at the 6- and 12-o'clock positions; peripheral iridectomy was made, and the platinum clip was bent back against the superior haptic to secure the lens against dislocation. **C,** Original iris-fixated lens designed by Fyodorov, as made in the United States; 2 looped haptics were placed posterior to the iris, and the optic and 2 opposing loops were placed anterior to the iris. *(Courtesy of Robert C. Drews, MD.)*

that had closed loops and modified it by opening the loops and inserting the haptics into the capsular bag for posterior chamber placement. Subsequent modifications of this lens by Pierce, Sinskey, and Shearing allowed ECCE with posterior chamber lens implantation to become the standard for modern cataract surgery. The discovery that viscous sodium hyaluronate could protect the endothelium from critical damage during IOL implantation was a turning point in the acceptance of IOLs.

IOL optic geometry has evolved from the earlier plano-convex models to the newer biconvex design. Numerous changes in the shape of the posterior IOL surface and edge design were advanced to reduce late opacification of the posterior lens capsule and to facilitate laser capsulotomy. Other lens modifications include the incorporation of ultraviolet (UV)-absorbing chromophores into the IOL material to protect the retina from UV radiation. Special-purpose lenses, such as those designed specifically for suture fixation in the ciliary sulcus, were also developed. These lenses have eyelets molded into the inside curve of the haptics to facilitate suture attachment. Other types of special-use IOLs include lenses designed with opaque flanges to decrease glare in clinical conditions such as aniridia and iris coloboma.

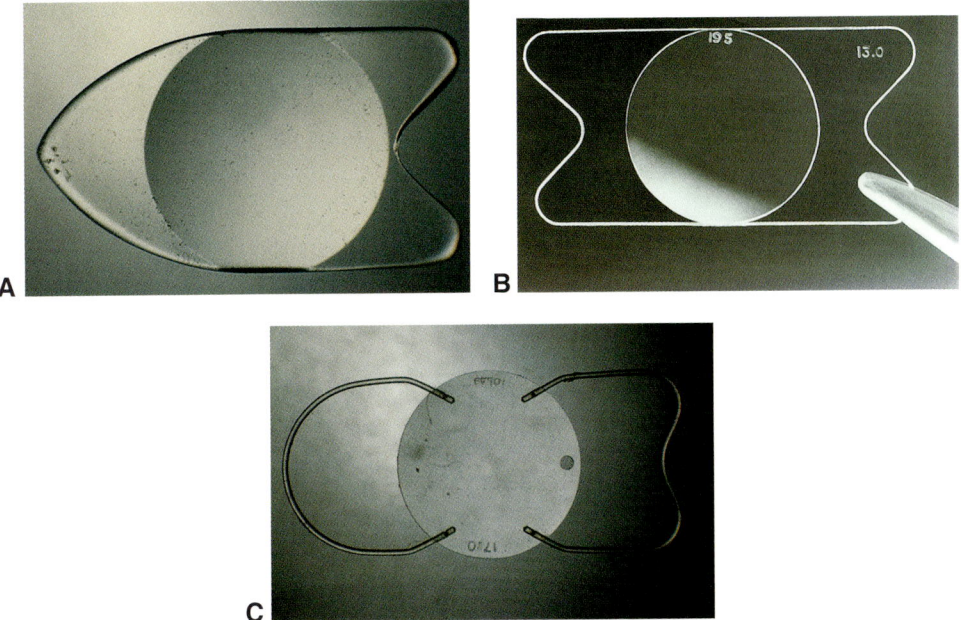

Figure 7-35 Early anterior chamber lens designs. **A,** Angle-supported lens designed by Strampelli; used from 1950 to 1955. **B,** Mark VIII lens designed by Choyce; rigid lens was implanted in anterior chamber angle either as a secondary lens implant or primarily after intracapsular cataract surgery. **C,** Azar 91Z lens; designed to be placed with rounded haptic in inferior chamber angle and notched haptic in superior chamber angle, with lens vaulted anteriorly. *(Courtesy of Robert C. Drews, MD.)*

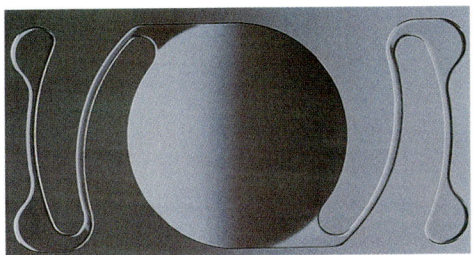

Figure 7-36 Kelman ACIOL with flexible 4-point fixation. *(Courtesy of Robert C. Drews, MD.)*

Mazzocco is generally given credit for developing a foldable IOL. His plate-style lens design (Fig 7-37) is still used for the correction of astigmatism at the time of cataract surgery, and it influenced the design of phakic refractive IOLs (see BCSC Section 13, *Refractive Surgery*). Foldable versions of the Shearing-style lens (Fig 7-38) soon followed. The obvious advantage of the foldable lens design is that it allows implantation of the IOL through a small incision. The availability of a small-incision lens was the factor that influenced the majority of ECCE surgeons to convert to using phacoemulsification. Although various materials have been evaluated, most foldable lenses are currently manufactured from either silicone or acrylic materials.

Although either silicone or acrylic materials are suitable for most patients, problems have been reported with silicone IOLs in patients who undergo vitrectomy with silicone oil injection. When cataract surgery is to be performed in a patient who is likely to require

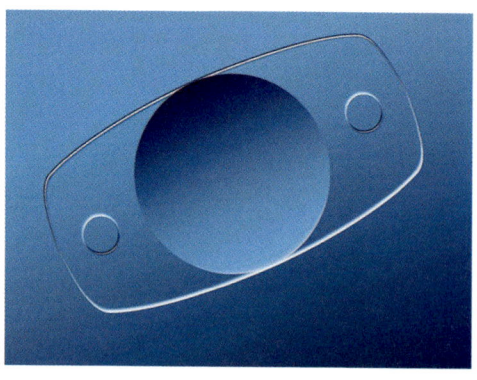

Figure 7-37 Mazzocco plate lens. *(Courtesy of STAAR Surgical.)*

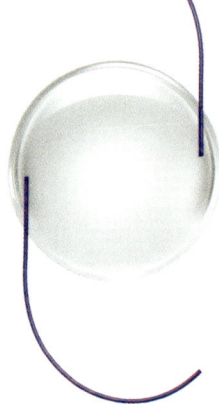

Figure 7-38 Modern 3-piece PCIOL. *(Courtesy of Bausch & Lomb Surgical.)*

vitreoretinal surgery in the future (eg, a patient with high myopia, proliferative diabetic retinopathy, retinal detachment in the fellow eye, uveitis, or any disease process that may lead to vitreous hemorrhage), an IOL material other than silicone is preferred.

> Hollick EJ, Spalton DJ, Ursell PG, et al. The effect of polymethylmethacrylate, silicone, and polyacrylic intraocular lenses on posterior capsular opacification 3 years after cataract surgery. *Ophthalmology.* 1999;106(1):49–54.

Multifocal Lenses

The original multifocal IOL concept was based on the principle that the pupil tends to constrict for near tasks, so the central portion of the lens was designed for near vision and the outer portion for distance vision. The disadvantage is that distance correction is not available when bright lights constrict the pupil. Present designs address this problem by having alternating zones for distance correction and for near. Other designs are supposed to move anteriorly with accommodative effort to allow near focusing. A combination of geometric optics and diffraction optics can also achieve a multifocal effect. The long-term effects of multifocal lenses are under investigation. Multiple multifocal lenses are available in the United States.

The advantages of these lenses include an increased range of vision with reduced dependence on spectacles. The drawbacks of multifocal IOLs include reductions in contrast sensitivity and best-corrected visual acuity and the presence of glare and halos (see also BCSC Section 3, *Clinical Optics*). The cataract surgeon should spend more "chair time" counseling these patients about intended postoperative visual outcome and limitations. Multifocal IOLs require accurate biometry and IOL power calculations, and they may work best when implanted bilaterally in patients with minimal astigmatism. Patients with hyperopia may be less bothered by some visual aberrations than are patients with myopia. It is strongly recommended that a special-consent process be used with this technology. The surgeon should have a strategy in place for managing postoperative residual refractive errors, including refractive surgery, spectacle or contact lens correction, and possible IOL exchange, performed preferably before capsular fibrosis increases the difficulty of explantation.

Pseudoaccommodative Lenses

A new classification of IOLs was introduced in 1996, the accommodative or pseudoaccommodative IOLs. These lenses work by various mechanisms designed to move the IOL during accommodative effort through either a single or dual optic mechanism. Whether these lenses work predominantly by IOL movement or by another mechanism has been an area of debate.

> Cionni RJ, Osher RH, Snyder ME, Nordlund ML. Visual outcome comparison of unilateral versus bilateral implantation of apodized diffractive multifocal intraocular lenses after cataract extraction: prospective 6-month study. *J Cataract Refract Surg.* 2009;35(6): 1033–1039.
>
> Cochener B, Lafuma A, Khoshnood B, Courouve L, Berdeaux G. Comparison of outcomes with multifocal intraocular lenses: a meta-analysis. *Clin Ophthalmol.* 2011;5:45–56.
>
> Menapace R, Findl O, Kriechbaum K, Leydolt-Koeppl C. Accommodating intraocular lenses: a critical review of present and future concepts. *Graefes Arch Clin Exp Ophthalmol.* 2007;245(4):473–489. Epub 2006 Aug 30.
>
> Rocha KM, Chalita MR, Souza CE, et al. Postoperative wavefront analysis and contrast sensitivity of a multifocal apodized diffractive IOL (ReSTOR) and three monofocal IOLs. *J Refract Surg.* 2005;21(6):S808–S812.
>
> Zhang F, Sugar A, Jacobsen G, Collins M. Visual function and patient satisfaction: Comparison between bilateral diffractive multifocal intraocular lenses and monovision pseudophakia. *J Cataract Refract Surg.* 2011;37(3):446–453.

Other Designs

Some IOLs have been designed, theoretically, to limit higher-order aberrations and to improve the quality of vision in low-contrast settings. Following are some examples of these IOLs: TECNIS (AMO, Santa Ana, CA), AcrySof IQ (Alcon, Ft Worth, TX), and SofPort Advanced Optics (AO) Model LI61 (Bausch & Lomb, Rochester, NY).

Although lenses with UV chromophores have been standard for several decades, a blue blocker has been added to Alcon's series of acrylic posterior chamber lenses. Blue-blocking IOLs attenuate blue-wavelength light (400–460 nm). Proponents say that these IOLs protect the patient from blue-light exposure to the macula. However, physicians critical of these lenses claim that there is no evidence of benefit from blue-blocking IOLs, and they are concerned that these lenses might create problems with scotopic vision.

A light-adjustable silicone IOL has been developed that allows noninvasive postoperative adjustment of refractive power. This IOL is currently under investigation.

> Chayet A, Sandstedt C, Chang S, et al. Use of the light-adjustable lens to correct astigmatism after cataract surgery. *Br J Ophthalmol.* 2010;94(6):690–692.
>
> Mainster MA, Turner PL. Blue-blocking IOLs decrease photoreception without providing significant photoprotection. *Surv Ophthalmol.* 2010;55(3):272–289.
>
> Schwartz DM. Light-adjustable lens. *Trans Am Ophthalmol Soc.* 2003;101:417–436.

IOL Power Determination

See Chapter 6 in this volume and BCSC Section 13, *Refractive Surgery.*

Techniques of Lens Implantation

PMMA IOLs may be safely handled with standard fine smooth forceps for insertion. Insertion forceps often have longer tips than do tying forceps to help in positioning the lens across the anterior chamber.

Silicone and acrylic IOLs must be handled more gently than PMMA IOLs. Surgeons implanting a foldable lens use a variety of instruments to hold the IOL in its folded position during insertion. These instruments are of 2 general designs:

- an injection tube that fits into the small incision and injects the IOL through the tube to unfold in the eye
- molded forceps that hold the folded IOL as it slides through the small incision

Procedure

The microscope should be adjusted to give a full-field view of the eye. The globe is positioned so that the cataract surgeon can insert the lens and ensure optimal access to and visibility of the anterior chamber, lens capsule, and incision.

The incision size must be large enough to accommodate the IOL. Larger incisions for intracapsular or extracapsular surgery are generally closed with sutures so that the appropriate opening size is obtained, whereas smaller incisions from phaco surgery may need to be enlarged if the surgeon plans to implant an IOL that is not folded. An OVD or air is used to stabilize the anterior chamber depth and to protect the corneal endothelium from contact with the IOL.

Posterior chamber IOL implantation

PMMA posterior chamber IOLs may be secured within the capsular bag or in front of the capsule within the ciliary sulcus. An OVD is injected either between the anterior and posterior capsules to open the capsular bag or between the iris and anterior capsular remnant for ciliary sulcus support. The IOL is advanced through the incision, with the leading haptic placed into position first. The IOL optic is then brought into the pupil, and the trailing haptic is flexed and placed into position or *dialed* (rotated clockwise with slight posterior pressure, so that the second haptic slides under the anterior capsule or into the ciliary sulcus following the edge of the optic). With other types of capsule openings, such as a can-opener capsulotomy, visualizing the anterior capsule for precise placement of the trailing haptic may be more difficult.

Foldable IOLs with haptics are inserted into the capsular bag with insertion forceps or an injector, after OVD injection, and then allowed to open in situ. For those foldable lenses with haptics, the leading haptic is slowly pushed under the edge of the anterior capsular rim into position within the capsular bag. The optic follows and the trailing haptic is placed, with forceps or with dialing, under the rim of the anterior capsule. Similar steps are used to place the lens in the ciliary sulcus, although lenses designed for insertion into the capsule may be inappropriate for placement in the ciliary sulcus. *Plate-haptic IOLs* must be inserted into a capsular bag protected by a CCC. The IOL position can be adjusted with a hook, and the lens may be rotated carefully to achieve adequate centration. Slight indentation of the sclera just posterior to the limbus should flex the plate without significantly altering centration. The surgeon then aspirates the OVD to minimize the risk of a rise in postoperative IOP. The anterior chamber depth is adjusted with balanced salt solution.

Several techniques have been described for securing a PCIOL behind the iris with sutures when capsular support is inadequate. Polypropylene sutures should be used instead of nylon sutures because nylon degrades over time and lens dislocation may result. Transscleral polypropylene sutures may be used to secure the IOL haptics in the ciliary sulcus (see Chapter 8 for a discussion of dislocation). Polypropylene sutures may also be used to attach PCIOL haptics to the overlying iris.

Sutured PCIOLs are most valuable as an alternative to ACIOL implantation in situations where an angle-supported lens might be considered problematic, such as with an angle compromised by peripheral anterior synechiae. Suture fixation techniques are more difficult than standard implantation and are associated with a greater risk of complications (such as vitreous hemorrhage, dislocation, lens tilt, or late endophthalmitis).

> Donaldson KE, Gorscak JJ, Budenz DL, Feuer WJ, Benz MS, Forster RK. Anterior chamber and sutured posterior chamber intraocular lenses in eyes with poor capsular support. *J Cataract Refract Surg.* 2005;31(5):903–909.
> Osher RH, Snyder ME, Cionni RJ. Modification of the Siepser slip-knot technique. *J Cataract Refract Surg.* 2005;31(6):1098–1100.

Anterior chamber IOL implantation

Primary anterior chamber IOL implantation Anterior chamber IOLs are supported by the chamber angle and are generally flexible. Modern 4-point-fixation flexible ACIOLs are acceptable for use when posterior chamber implantation is not feasible. It is common practice to use 1 mm plus the horizontal diameter of the limbus, as measured externally with a caliper (white to white) or with an automated IOL calculation device, to determine the appropriate length for the ACIOL.

A typical phaco incision must be enlarged with the keratome or with corneal scissors to allow ACIOL insertion. The pupil is generally constricted pharmacologically prior to IOL implantation. At least 1, and often 2, peripheral iridectomies are performed to avoid pupillary block. The anterior chamber depth is stabilized, and the corneal endothelium is protected with OVD or air. A lens glide may be inserted across the anterior chamber into the distal angle to isolate the iris from the advancing IOL haptic. The surgeon then inserts the IOL, placing its leading haptic into the angle while observing the iris for any indication of distortion. As the IOL is held against the distal angle stabilized with forceps, the glide is withdrawn. The posterior lip of the incision is gently retracted to allow placement of the trailing haptic in the angle. Visual inspection should confirm the proper insertion of the trailing haptic. The surgeon can adjust IOL position by using a hook to flex the optic toward either angle for repositioning.

The pupil will peak toward any area of iris "tuck," and the IOL should be repositioned until the pupil is round and the optic is centered. Light indentation of the sclera axial to the lens position should flex the IOL haptic without significant decentration of the optic, movement of the pupil, or rotation of the lens. The OVD is aspirated, and the chamber depth adjusted with balanced salt solution. The incision is carefully closed with nylon sutures.

Secondary anterior chamber IOL implantation When spectacles or contact lenses are unsatisfactory for correction of aphakia, secondary ACIOL implantation is indicated. The type of cataract surgery performed and the general condition of the anterior segment determine the appropriate style and technique of lens implantation. The cornea, angle, iris, and vitreous should be studied carefully before secondary ACIOL implantation. Pachymetry, gonioscopy, and endothelial cell counts may be considered before surgery.

Factors that influence selection of an incision site (superior versus temporal) include preexisting astigmatism, iris anatomy, conjunctival scarring, and corneal vascularization. If an anterior vitrectomy may be needed to remove any vitreous incarcerated in the wound or adherent to the iris, the pupil should be dilated; otherwise, the pupil may be constricted with a topical miotic prior to surgery. After vitrectomy, intraoperative acetylcholine or carbachol may be infused to constrict the pupil for lens implantation. Anterior and posterior synechiae that would interfere with the positioning of the IOL may be dissected. A lens glide may be useful during insertion of anterior IOLs, and the anterior chamber depth needs to be stabilized with an OVD. The positioning of secondary IOLs is similar to that described for primary lenses but may be more difficult because of scarring from the cataract surgery.

Relative Contraindications to Lens Implantation

The surgeon must determine whether the support structures within the eye are adequate to maintain centration and stability of the IOL for the type of lens fixation anticipated. If the angle is not open and available for ACIOL implantation, a sutured PCIOL is necessary. Although proliferative diabetic retinopathy and other retinal disorders were formerly considered relative contraindications, prospective studies have shown that these conditions are not adversely affected by PCIOL implantation that maintains an intact posterior capsule.

Corneas with Fuchs dystrophy can be further assessed with endothelial cell counts and pachymetry. If the values are near normal, phacoemulsification with a dispersive OVD, intraocular irrigating solution (with added glucose, glutathione, phosphate, and bicarbonate), and PCIOL implantation are strategies for minimizing further endothelial loss with surgery.

However, patients with increased central corneal thickness or other evidence of endothelial dysfunction such as stromal or epithelial edema may require a different procedure. One alternative is Descemet membrane–stripping automated endothelial keratoplasty (DSAEK) and phacoemulsification with IOL insertion (known as a "triple procedure") or penetrating keratoplasty and phacoemulsification with IOL insertion. Alternatively, cataract surgery may be followed by endothelial replacement procedures such as DSAEK. (See also BCSC Section 8, *External Disease and Cornea*.)

> Ford JG, Karp CL. *Cataract Surgery and Intraocular Lenses: A 21st-Century Perspective*. 2nd ed. Ophthalmology Monograph 7. San Francisco: American Academy of Ophthalmology; 2001.

Outcomes of Cataract Surgery

Contemporary cataract surgery has an excellent success rate in both improving visual acuity and enhancing subjective visual function. More than 90% of otherwise healthy eyes achieve a best-corrected postoperative visual acuity of 20/40 or better. The rate of achieving a postoperative acuity of 20/40 or better for all eyes has been reported to be 85% to 89% when eyes with comorbid conditions such as diabetic retinopathy, glaucoma, and age-related macular degeneration are included.

Visual acuity is but one measure of the functional success of cataract surgery. Research tools have been developed to assess how cataract progression and cataract surgery affect visual function (see Chapter 6).

Prospective studies using these tools show that patients who undergo cataract surgery have significant improvement in many quality-of-life parameters, including community and home activities, mental health, driving, and life satisfaction. Among patients with bilateral cataracts, the quality of life improves after cataract surgery on the first eye as well as the second eye. A reduction in falls and hip fractures has been documented in patients after cataract surgery.

> Brenner MH, Curbow B, Javitt JC, Legro MW, Sommer A. Vision change and quality of life in the elderly: response to cataract surgery and treatment of other chronic ocular conditions. *Arch Ophthalmol*. 1993;111(5):680–685.
>
> Harwood RH, Foss AJ, Osborn F, Gregson RM, Zaman A, Masud T. Falls and health status in elderly women following first eye cataract surgery: a randomized controlled trial. *British J Ophthalmol*. 2005;89(1):53–59.
>
> Javitt JC, Brenner MH, Curbow B, Legro MW, Street DA. Outcomes of cataract surgery: improvement in visual acuity and subjective visual function after surgery in the first, second, and both eyes. *Arch Ophthalmol*. 1993;111(5):686–691.

Mangione CM, Phillips RS, Lawrence MG, Seddon JM, Orav EJ, Goldman L. Improved visual function and attenuation of declines in health-related quality of life after cataract extraction. *Arch Ophthalmol.* 1994;112(11):1419–1425.

Powe NR, Schein OD, Gieser SC, et al. Synthesis of the literature on visual acuity and complications following cataract extraction with intraocular lens implantation: Cataract Patient Outcome Research Team. *Arch Ophthalmol.* 1994;112(2):239–252.

Steinberg EP, Tielsch JM, Schein OD, et al. National study of cataract surgery outcomes: variation in 4-month postoperative outcomes as reflected in multiple outcome measures. *Ophthalmology.* 1994;101(6):1131–1141.

CHAPTER 8

Complications of Cataract Surgery

Complications of cataract surgery vary in timing as well as scope. Undesirable consequences of surgery may occur intraoperatively or later in the postoperative period. Many large-scale peer-reviewed studies of cataract surgery complications contain data from larger-incision extracapsular surgery or from earlier phacoemulsification (phaco) technology than is available today. But a recent review of Medicare beneficiaries showed that the rate of severe adverse events after cataract surgery, including endophthalmitis, suprachoroidal hemorrhage, and retinal detachment, declined from 1994 to 2006.

Fortunately, complications resulting in permanent loss of vision are rare with modern surgical techniques and technology in the hands of experienced cataract surgeons. In a recent review, the most common intraoperative complication of phacoemulsification is posterior capsule rupture in 1.5% to 3.5% of cases. Common postoperative complications include posterior capsule opacification, corneal edema (in 0.03% to 5.18% of cases), clinically apparent cystoid macular edema (in 1.2% to 3.5% of cases), and retained lens fragments (in 0.45% to 1.70% of cases). The prevalence of retinal detachment ranges from 0.14% to 0.90%; that of endophthalmitis, 0.10% to 0.20%; and that of IOL dislocation, 0.19% to 1.10%. For further details, see Table 8-1.

> American Academy of Ophthalmology Cataract and Anterior Segment Panel. Preferred Practice Pattern Guidelines. *Cataract in the Adult Eye.* San Francisco: American Academy of Ophthalmology; 2011. Available at: www.aao.org/ppp.
> Greenberg PB, Tseng VL, Wu WC, et al. Prevalence and predictors of ocular complications associated with cataract surgery in United States veterans. *Ophthalmology.* 2011;118(3): 507–514.
> Jaffe NS, Jaffe MS, Jaffe GF. *Cataract Surgery and Its Complications.* 6th ed. St Louis: Mosby; 1997.
> Schmier JK, Halpern MT, Covert DW, Lau EC, Robin AL. Evaluation of Medicare costs of endophthalmitis among patients after cataract surgery. *Ophthalmology.* 2007;114(6): 1094–1099.
> Stein JD, Grossman DS, Mundy KM, Sugar A, Sloan FA. Severe adverse events after cataract surgery among Medicare beneficiaries. *Ophthalmology.* 2011;118(9):1716–1723. Epub 2011 Jun 2.
> Steinert RF, ed. *Cataract Surgery.* 3rd ed. Philadelphia: Saunders; 2010.

Table 8-1 Complication Rates From Selected Studies of Cataract Surgery

	Cataract PORT, 1994*	Schein et al, 1994†	NEON, 2000‡	Zaidi et al, 2007§	Jaycock et al, 2009‖	Greenberg et al, 2011#	Clark et al, 2011**
Number of cases	††	717	2603	1000	55,567	45,082	65,060
Percent phacoemulsification	65	65	92	100	99.7	95 (approx)‡‡	100
Intraoperative (%)							
Posterior capsular or zonular rupture	3.1	1.95	1.6	1.5	1.92§§	3.5‖‖	NA
Vitreous loss/anterior vitrectomy or aspiration	0.8	1.39	1.1	1.1	NA	NA	NA
Iris/ciliary body injury	0.7	0.84	0	1.2	0.55	0.1	NA
Loss of nuclear material into vitreous	NA	0.28	<1	0.1	0.18	0.2	0.16
Suprachoroidal hemorrhage	NA	0.14	0	0	0.07	0	NA
Retrobulbar hemorrhage	NA	0	0	0.1	NA	0	NA
Postoperative (%)					(n=16,731)##		
CME	3.5	3.21	NA	1.2	1.62	3.3	NA
Iris abnormalities	1.3	2.51	NA	NA	0.16	NA	NA
Corneal edema	NA	1.95	<1	0.7	5.18	NA	0.03
Wound leak or rupture	NA	0.84	<1	1.1	0.14	NA	0.06
IOL dislocation, removal, or exchange	1.1	0.28	<1	NA	0.22	0.9	0.19
Endophthalmitis	0.13	0.14	<1	0.1	NA	0.2	0.17
Retinal tear, break, or detachment	0.7	0.14	<1	0.2	NA	0.9	0.37
Visually significant CME	NA	NA	<1	NA	NA	NA	NA
Persistent iritis	NA	NA	1.1	1.1	NA	NA	NA

CME = cystoid macular edema; IOL = intraocular lens; NA = not available; NEON = National Eyecare Outcomes Network; PORT = Cataract Patient Outcomes Research Team.

* Powe NR, Schein OD, Gieser SC, et al; Cataract Patient Outcome Research Team. Synthesis of the literature on visual acuity and complications following cataract extraction with intraocular lens implantation. *Arch Ophthalmol.* 1994;112:239–252.
† Schein OD, Steinberg EP, Javitt JC, et al. Variation in cataract surgery practice and clinical outcomes. *Ophthalmology.* 1994;101:1142–1152.
‡ Lum F, Schein O, Schachat AP, et al. Initial two years of experience with the AAO National Eyecare Outcomes Network (NEON) cataract surgery database. *Ophthalmology.* 2000;107:691–697.
§ Zaidi FH, Corbett MC, Burton BJ, Bloom PA. Raising the benchmark for the 21st century—the 1000 cataract operations audit and survey: outcomes, consultant-supervised training and sourcing NHS choice. *Br J Ophthalmol.* 2007;91:731–736.
‖ Jaycock P, Johnston RL, Taylor H, et al. The Cataract National Dataset electronic multi-centre audit of 55,567 operations: updating benchmark standards of care in the United Kingdom and internationally. *Eye (Lond).* 2009;23:38–49.
Greenberg PB, Tseng VL, Wu WC, et al. Prevalence and predictors of ocular complications associated with cataract surgery in United States veterans. *Ophthalmology.* 2011;118:507–514.
** Clark A, Morlet N, Ng JQ, et al. Whole population trends in complications of cataract surgery over 22 years in Western Australia. *Ophthalmology.* 2011;118:1055–1061.
†† Number of cases varies depending on the studies included for each complication.
‡‡ The study used Current Procedural Terminology codes to identify cases, which do not specify whether cataract surgeries are performed by phacoemulsification or manual extracapsular cataract extraction. A survey*** of Veterans Health Administration facilities found that phacoemulsification was performed in approximately 95% of extracapsular cataract surgeries.
§§ This is a composite figure that includes posterior capsule rupture without vitreous loss, posterior capsule rupture with vitreous loss, and zonule rupture with vitreous loss.
‖‖ This is a composite figure that includes diagnostic codes for posterior capsule tear and procedural codes for anterior vitrectomy.
Postoperative information was not available for all study patients.
*** Chen CK, Tseng VL, Wu WC, Greenberg PB. A survey of the current role of manual extracapsular cataract extraction. *J Cataract Refract Surg.* 2010;36:692–693.

Modified from American Academy of Ophthalmology Cataract and Anterior Segment Panel. Preferred Practice Pattern Guidelines. *Cataract in the Adult Eye.* San Francisco: American Academy of Ophthalmology; 2011:26. Available at: www.aao.org/ppp.

Corneal Complications

Corneal Edema

Stromal and/or epithelial edema may occur in the immediate postoperative period. The incidence is higher in eyes with preexisting corneal endothelial dysfunction such as Fuchs dystrophy. Edema is most often caused by a combination of mechanical trauma, prolonged surgery, chemical injury, inflammation, or elevated intraocular pressure (IOP), resulting in acute endothelial decompensation with an increase in corneal thickness (Table 8-2).

Table 8-2 Principal Causes of Corneal Edema After Cataract Surgery

Surgical trauma
  Mechanical energy from phacoemulsification
  Instruments
  Intraocular lens (IOL)
  Irrigating solutions
  Lens fragments
  Prior surgery
Corneal endothelial disease
  Fuchs dystrophy
  Low endothelial cell density
Chemical injury
  Preservatives in intraocular solutions
  Residual toxic chemicals on instruments (eg, detergents, dried solutions)
  Improper concentrations of intraocular solutions (eg, antibiotics, anesthetics, irrigating solutions)
    Osmotic damage
    Direct toxicity
IOL related
  IOL endothelial touch
  Uveitis-glaucoma-hyphema (UGH) syndrome
  Long-term toxicity (chronic inflammation?)
Endothelial contact
  Flat chamber
    Wound leak
    Ciliary block
    Suprachoroidal effusion or hemorrhage
  Iris bombé
    Pupillary block
  Vitreous touch
Detachment of Descemet membrane
Late trauma from retained foreign material
  Nuclear fragments
  Particulate matter
Elevated intraocular pressure (IOP)
Inflammation
Membranous ingrowth
  Epithelial downgrowth
  Fibrous ingrowth
  Endothelial proliferation
Brown-McLean syndrome

Adapted with permission from Steinert RF. *Cataract Surgery*. 3rd ed. Philadelphia: Saunders; 2010:596.

Toxic substances inadvertently introduced into the anterior chamber can also cause acute endothelial dysfunction with diffuse corneal edema referred to as *toxic anterior segment syndrome* (*TASS*; discussed later). Late postoperative focal corneal edema may occur because of small nuclear fragments retained in the anterior chamber angle. These may be noticed on initial postoperative examinations or may be noticed up to years later if they migrate into the anterior chamber from a secluded location in the posterior chamber.

Edema from surgical trauma generally resolves completely within 4 to 6 weeks of surgery. The eye must be examined thoroughly for contributing factors that could exacerbate the edema. If epithelial edema is present in the face of a compact stroma immediately after surgery, it is likely due to elevated IOP with an intact endothelium. Decreasing IOP medically or via aqueous release from the paracentesis site often results in rapid resolution of epithelial edema in these cases. As a rule, if the corneal periphery is clear, the corneal edema will resolve with time. Corneal edema that persists after 3 months usually does not clear. Significant chronic corneal edema from loss of endothelial cells results in bullous keratopathy (Fig 8-1), which is associated with reduced visual acuity, irritation, foreign-body sensation, epiphora, and occasional infectious keratitis.

In its early stages, corneal edema after cataract surgery can be controlled by the use of topical hyperosmotic agents, topical corticosteroids, and, occasionally, bandage (therapeutic) contact lenses. Over time, subepithelial scarring may develop, resulting in a decrease in bulla formation and discomfort. Decreased visual acuity, recurrent infectious keratitis, and symptoms of pain are possible indications for endothelial or penetrating keratoplasty. Posterior lamellar or endothelial keratoplasty has been very successful in restoring clear corneas and improving visual acuity. The likelihood of obtaining a clear graft is high, but coexisting cystoid macular edema (CME) may limit full recovery of vision. Bulla formation and pain associated with bullous keratopathy may be alleviated with phototherapeutic keratectomy or anterior stromal micropuncture, but they may recur. In the case of an eye with little or no visual potential, a Gundersen conjunctival flap or an

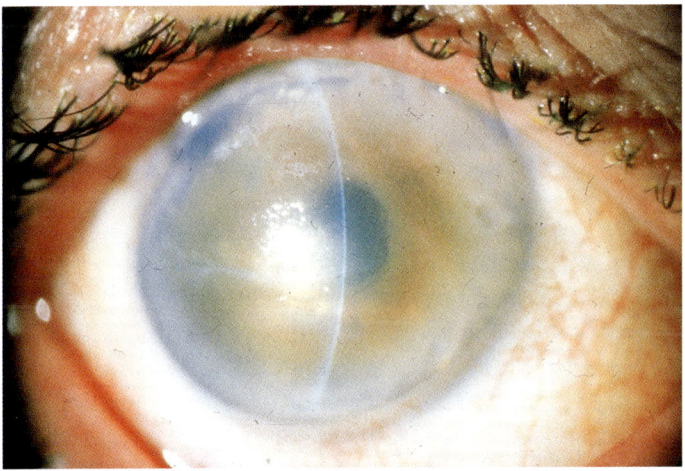

Figure 8-1 Pseudophakic bullous keratopathy. *(Courtesy of Karla J. Johns, MD.)*

amniotic membrane graft is an option that does not carry the greater risks of penetrating keratoplasty. (See also BCSC Section 8, *External Disease and Cornea*.)

Brown-McLean syndrome

Brown-McLean syndrome is a clinical condition that may occur after cataract surgery. It consists of peripheral corneal edema with a clear central cornea. This condition occurs most frequently following intracapsular cataract surgery, but it has also been reported following extracapsular surgery and phacoemulsification. The edema typically starts inferiorly and progresses circumferentially, but it spares the central 5–7-mm zone of the cornea. Central corneal guttae frequently appear, and punctate brown pigment often underlies the edematous areas. In rare cases, Brown-McLean syndrome progresses to clinically significant central corneal edema. The etiology of this syndrome is unknown.

Vitreocorneal adherence and persistent corneal edema

Vitreocorneal adherence and persistent corneal edema can occur early or late after uncomplicated intracapsular cataract extraction (ICCE), complicated extracapsular cataract extraction (ECCE), or phacoemulsification. An anterior vitrectomy may be indicated if corneal thickening or edema develops. In more advanced cases with prolonged corneal edema, penetrating or endothelial keratoplasty combined with vitrectomy may be indicated.

Incision and Wound Complications

Proper incision construction and closure are critical in reducing intraoperative and postoperative complications. Scleral, limbal, or corneal wound strength is only 10% of normal tissue at 1 week, increasing only to 40% by 8 weeks and 75% to 80% of its original strength by 2 years. There is concern that the increased use of nonsutured clear corneal incisions may be responsible for an increased incidence of postoperative wound leakage with influx into the anterior chamber and possible increased risk for endophthalmitis.

Clinical signs of wound leakage include decreased vision, hypotony, corneal striae, shallow anterior chamber, hyphema, choroidal folds, choroidal effusion, macular edema, and optic nerve edema. A Seidel test, gonioscopy, ultrasound biomicroscopy, or anterior segment optical coherence tomography (OCT) may help diagnose or confirm subtle cases. Management of wound leaks depends on etiology, timing, and severity. Small leaks during the first few days after surgery may be asymptomatic and self-limited. Medical treatment to enhance healing includes prophylactic topical antibiotics, cycloplegia, aqueous inhibitors, patching, decreasing or stopping corticosteroid therapy, or applying a collagen shield or bandage soft contact lens. In more serious or persistent cases with shallowing of the anterior chamber, iris prolapse, hypotony, or choroidal or macular edema, surgical repair is indicated. Suturing the wound is usually sufficient, but an amniotic membrane graft or tissue adhesives such as cyanoacrylate may be used. A wound leak under a conjunctival flap may lead to an inadvertent filtering bleb. Over time, the fistula may epithelialize and become resistant to medical management and require surgical intervention. Efforts to induce inflammation to promote wound healing and cicatrization of the bleb include cryotherapy, diathermy, chemical cauterization with trichloroacetic acid, or injection of an autologous blood patch. In chronic cases, it may be necessary to excise the bleb/conjunctiva and explore for a fistula, which should be scraped free of invading epithelium or excised and covered, if necessary, with a scleral patch graft with resuturing of the wound. Tenon capsule and conjunctiva should be used to cover the exposed sclera.

Thermal wound burns

Thermal injury to the incision may result in whitening of the corneal tissue, contraction, and wound gape. During phacoemulsification, heat may be transferred from the needle to the cornea because of inadequate cooling of the phaco tip. This can result from an insufficient inflow of coaxial irrigation fluid around the vibrating probe or from occlusion of outflow at the phaco tip or aspiration line by an ophthalmic viscosurgical device (OVD) or lens material.

Friction produces heat, which causes the corneal collagen to contract, with subsequent distortion of the incision. If the distortion is significant, wound gape may occur with associated leakage. These incisions are not usually self-sealing, and they require suturing or patch grafts for adequate closure. When the wound integrity is stable, induced astigmatism may be reversed by selective removal of sutures, based on keratometry readings or topography measurements.

Wound dehiscence or rupture

Postoperative wound dehiscence may be spontaneous or secondary to trauma. The incidence depends on the size and integrity of the wound and the degree of healing, which may be affected by the use of corticosteroids or the presence of systemic disease that alters collagen metabolism. The trend toward smaller incisions and minimally invasive surgery has decreased the occurrence of wound dehiscence. Traumatic wound rupture is often accompanied by extrusion of intraocular contents and almost always requires surgical repair.

Detachment of Descemet Membrane

Detachment of Descemet membrane results in stromal swelling and epithelial bullae localized in the area of detachment. This complication can occur when an instrument or IOL is introduced through the incision or when fluid is inadvertently injected between Descemet membrane and the corneal stroma. Small detachments may resolve spontaneously. Otherwise, they may be reattached with air or expansile gas (eg, sulfur hexafluoride [SF_6] or perfluoropropane [C_3F_8]) tamponade in the anterior chamber. Larger detachments can be sutured back into place. Gas may help position the detached area of Descemet membrane prior to suture placement. An OVD can facilitate chamber maintenance during the procedure, but the surgeon must take great care not to introduce the OVD between Descemet membrane and the corneal stroma. One or more 10-0 nylon or polypropylene sutures armed with long, curved cutting needles on both ends may be used. The needles are first passed through an incision in the peripheral cornea distant to the area of Descemet detachment. They are then passed from the anterior chamber through the detached area of Descemet membrane, stroma, and epithelium. The ends are tied on the external surface of the cornea, and the knots are buried.

Induced Astigmatism

Incisions in the cornea can alter the preexisting topography and astigmatism, as discussed in Chapter 7 and in BCSC Section 13, *Refractive Surgery*. Most well-constructed peripheral corneal, limbal, or scleral incisions less than 4 mm in length will induce less than 1 diopter (D) of astigmatism, usually flattening in the axis of the incision. Larger incisions closer to the corneal apex or those that require suture closure are more apt to induce additional astigmatism. Postoperative astigmatism may be caused by tight radial sutures, which steepen corneal curvature in the axis of the suture. The astigmatism induced by larger sutured incisions such as those used in ICCE, ECCE, or secondary IOL implantation may decrease by several diopters over time as the sutures dissolve or relax, possibly making suture removal unnecessary. Removing or cutting sutures 6 to 8 weeks postoperatively can reduce excessive astigmatism. If more than 1 suture is to be removed, it may be preferable to remove adjacent sutures in a series of visits rather than all at once. Removal of too many sutures too early in the postoperative course may result in either significant corneal flattening in the axis of the incision or a leaking incision. Postoperative astigmatism may also be induced by corneal burns from the phaco tip. Modification of preexisting astigmatism through incision architecture and location on the steeper axis combined with peripheral corneal relaxing incisions may be a desirable method to compensate for preoperative corneal astigmatism. (See Chapter 7.)

Corneal Melting

Keratolysis, or sterile melting of the cornea, may occur following cataract extraction. It is most frequently associated with preexisting tear-film abnormalities resulting from keratoconjunctivitis sicca, Sjögren syndrome, or autoimmune disease such as rheumatoid arthritis. Preoperative recognition of these predisposing factors is valuable because the frequent perioperative use of topical lubricants can lessen morbidity. Punctal plug placement or lateral tarsorrhaphy may also be performed at the time of surgery.

Severe stromal melting has been reported with the postoperative use of many topical nonsteroidal anti-inflammatory drugs (NSAIDs). The melting is due in part to the epithelial toxicity and hypoesthesia that these drugs can induce.

Persistent epithelial defects accompanied by stromal dissolution require intensive treatment with nonpreserved topical lubricants. Use of topical medications, particularly preserved medications, should be minimized to reduce epithelial toxicity. Additional treatment modalities to encourage epithelialization and to arrest stromal melting include punctal occlusion, bandage contact lenses, tarsorrhaphy, botulinum injections to induce ptosis, autologous serum eyedrops, and systemic tetracyclines. The prophylactic use of topical antibiotics must be monitored closely. After a week's application, many topical antibiotics begin to cause secondary toxic effects that may inhibit epithelial healing. If the disease continues to progress in spite of medical therapy, an amniotic membrane graft or lamellar or penetrating keratoplasty should be considered. Corneal melting may recur even with grafted tissue. For the treatment of any underlying autoimmune disease, systemic immunosuppressive therapy may be needed.

Other Anterior Segment Complications

Epithelial Downgrowth

Epithelial downgrowth is a rare complication of intraocular surgery. The condition is characterized by a sheet of epithelium growing intraocularly following trauma or a surgical incision and covering the corneal endothelium, trabecular meshwork, and/or iris surfaces. One possible explanation for this condition is that, if epithelial cells are introduced into the anterior chamber during surgery, they may adhere to intraocular structures and begin to proliferate as a cellular membrane. Another theory is that a sheet of epithelium from the ocular surface grows through the incision (possibly because the incision is not watertight) and then proliferates over the posterior corneal and iris surfaces.

The clinical signs of epithelial downgrowth include elevated IOP, clumps of cells floating in the anterior chamber, a visible retrocorneal membrane (usually with overlying corneal edema), an abnormal iris surface, and pupillary distortion. The mechanism for elevated IOP is outflow obstruction caused by the growth of the epithelial membrane over the trabecular meshwork or by epithelial cells clogging the meshwork. Diagnosis of epithelial downgrowth is confirmed with the argon laser; argon laser burns applied to the membrane or the iris surface will appear white if epithelial cells are present.

Many complex surgical procedures have been suggested for treating this condition. Local application of cryotherapy or of 5-fluorouracil has been reported to be effective. Neither of these interventions has been uniformly successful. In some patients, palliative surgery for comfort and glaucoma valve implants for IOP control are indicated.

Toxic Anterior Segment Syndrome

If a toxic substance enters the anterior chamber, it may produce severe intraocular inflammation and corneal edema. Toxic anterior segment syndrome (TASS) is an acute sterile postoperative inflammation. The symptoms and signs of TASS may mimic those of infectious endophthalmitis and include photophobia, severe reduction in visual acuity, corneal edema, and marked anterior chamber reaction, occasionally with hypopyon. TASS presents within hours of surgery, whereas acute infectious endophthalmitis typically develops 2 to 7 days after surgery. Other potentially distinguishing features of TASS include diffuse, limbus-to-limbus corneal edema; anterior chamber fibrinous exudate; a dilated, irregular, or nonreactive pupil; and elevated IOP. The pathologic changes are limited to the anterior chamber. Pain is typically much less than that experienced with an infection. If endophthalmitis is suspected, diagnostic and therapeutic interventions as described later in this chapter should be undertaken. Treatment of TASS consists of intensive topical corticosteroids until the inflammation subsides. A brief course of systemic corticosteroids may be beneficial. Frequent follow-up is necessary to monitor IOP and to reassess for signs of bacterial infection.

Subconjunctival antibiotic injections and ophthalmic ointments applied with patching have been reported to enter the anterior chamber through scleral tunnel incisions that act as 1-way valves. Skin cleansers containing chlorhexidine gluconate have been reported to cause irreversible corneal edema and opacification if they unintentionally come into contact with the endothelium. Other possible causes of TASS include substitution of sterile water for balanced salt solution or the intraocular use of inappropriate irrigating solutions, antibiotics, or anesthetics. All solutions used intracamerally should be free of preservatives, with physiologic osmolarity and pH. Clusters of TASS cases have occurred due to tainted balanced salt solution. The most common cause of sporadic cases of TASS may be the inadvertent intraocular introduction of residual toxic materials such as detergents, enzymatic cleaners, or denatured OVD from improperly cleaned instruments, especially reusable irrigation/aspiration (I/A) handpieces, cannulas, or irrigation tubing. The patient's risk of developing TASS is reduced by careful cleaning, rinsing, and air-drying of reusable cannulas; by use of disposable cannulas; and by avoidance of the intraocular use of any nonphysiologic or preserved solutions.

> Mamalis N. Toxic anterior segment syndrome (TASS). *Focal Points: Clinical Modules for Ophthalmologists.* San Francisco: American Academy of Ophthalmology; 2009, module 10.
> Mamalis N, Edelhauser HF, Dawson DG, Chew J, LeBoyer RM, Werner L. Toxic anterior segment syndrome. *J Cataract Refract Surg.* 2006;32(2):324–333.

Shallow or Flat Anterior Chamber

Intraoperative

During ECCE or phacoemulsification, the anterior chamber may become shallow because of inadequate infusion, leakage through an oversized incision, external pressure on the globe, positive vitreous pressure, fluid misdirection syndrome, suprachoroidal effusion, or suprachoroidal hemorrhage. If the reason for loss of normal chamber depth is not apparent, the surgeon should first reduce aspiration, raise the infusion bottle height, and check the incision. If the incision is too large and a significant volume of irrigation fluid flows out of the anterior chamber, the surgeon can place a suture across the incision in order to reduce the incision size and ultimately help keep the chamber formed. External pressure on the globe can be relieved by readjusting the surgical drapes or the eyelid speculum. "Positive vitreous pressure" or forward displacement of the lens–iris diaphragm occurs more commonly in obese, thick-necked patients, in patients with pulmonary disease such as chronic obstructive pulmonary disease (COPD), and in anxious patients or those with full bladders who perform a Valsalva maneuver. Placing obese patients in a reverse Trendelenburg position may be useful. Intravenous mannitol can be used to reduce the vitreous volume and allow the case to continue uneventfully.

If the reason for the loss of anterior chamber depth or elevated IOP is still unknown, the surgeon should check the red reflex to evaluate the possibility of a suprachoroidal hemorrhage or effusion. In these situations, the eye typically becomes very firm and the patient becomes agitated and complains of pain. To confirm this diagnosis, the surgeon should examine the fundus with an indirect ophthalmoscope. If a hemorrhage or effusion is significant, the incisions should be closed and the case postponed until the pressure has decreased.

Posterior fluid misdirection Fluid infused into the anterior chamber may be misdirected into the vitreous cavity through intact zonular fibers or through a zonular or capsular tear, causing an increase in the vitreous volume, with subsequent forward displacement of the lens and shallowing of the anterior chamber. The fluid may accumulate in the retrolental space or dissect posteriorly along the vitreoretinal interface. If gentle posterior pressure on the lens or reinflation of the capsular bag with OVD does not alleviate the situation, infusing intravenous mannitol and waiting at least 20 minutes may allow the anterior chamber to deepen. If suprachoroidal effusion/hemorrhage has been ruled out, the surgeon can insert a 20- to 23-gauge needle through the pars plana into the retrolental space by direct visualization, gently aspirate fluid vitreous, and deepen the anterior chamber with irrigation fluid or OVD. The surgeon must exercise care in placing the needle in order to avoid a retinal tear or detachment. Alternatively, vitreous aspiration may be performed with a cutting/aspirating pars plana vitrectomy tip inserted through a sclerotomy 3.5 mm behind the limbus, combined with balanced salt solution infusion or additional OVD placed into the anterior chamber.

Postoperative

A flat anterior chamber during the postoperative period may cause permanent damage to ocular structures. Prolonged apposition of the iris to angle structures can cause peripheral anterior synechiae and chronic angle-closure glaucoma. Following either ICCE or ECCE, iridovitreal or iridocapsular synechiae can also lead to pupillary block. Corneal contact with vitreous or an IOL can result in endothelial cell loss and chronic corneal edema.

Postoperative shallow or flat anterior chambers can be classified according to their etiology and level of IOP. Causes include leaking incision, choroidal detachment, pupillary block, ciliary block, and suprachoroidal hemorrhage.

Cases associated with ocular hypotension (IOP below 10 mm Hg) are usually secondary to leakage of aqueous at the incision site or to choroidal detachment. Patients may be asymptomatic, especially if a leaking incision is plugged by iris incarceration, allowing re-formation of the anterior chamber. Even without iris incarceration, slow or intermittent leaks may coexist with a formed anterior chamber. Carefully comparing the chamber depth of the surgical eye with that of the fellow eye may help the surgeon identify these cases.

For a discussion of evaluation and management of an incisional leak, see the section Incision and Wound Complications. The methods noted are appropriate both for the management of minor incision leaks and as temporary measures until more secure incision closure can be accomplished surgically. Patients may develop an associated ciliochoroidal detachment that resolves spontaneously after incision closure. Surgical exploration with re-formation of the anterior chamber and repair of the incision is indicated in any of the following cases: if no improvement occurs within 24 to 48 hours, if obvious wound gape is present, if the iris is prolapsed out of the incision, or if intraocular structures such as the IOL are in contact with the corneal endothelium.

Late hypotony without obvious leakage from the incision is uncommon after cataract surgery. It may result from retinal detachment, cyclodialysis, filtering bleb formation, or persistent uveitis.

Cases of a shallow anterior chamber with normal or high IOP are usually the result of pupillary block, ciliary block, or suprachoroidal hemorrhage. Pupillary block that occurs in the early postoperative period may follow a resolved incision leak. Postoperative uveitis with iridovitreal or iridocapsular synechiae may cause relatively late pupillary block.

Failure to perform a peripheral iridectomy after placement of an anterior chamber IOL may also be associated with early or late postoperative pupillary block. If initial attempts at pupillary dilation fail to deepen the anterior chamber and lower the pressure, a laser peripheral iridotomy is usually effective. Ciliary block glaucoma and suprachoroidal hemorrhage are discussed later in this chapter.

Elevated Intraocular Pressure

A rise in IOP is common following cataract surgery. It is generally mild and self-limited and does not require prolonged antihypertensive therapy. However, a significant and sustained rise in IOP after surgery may require timely and specific management.

OVD retained in the eye after cataract surgery is frequently responsible for postoperative IOP elevation. These large molecules can impair aqueous outflow through the trabecular meshwork. Even when all apparent OVD is removed from the anterior chamber at the conclusion of surgery, residual OVD can lodge in the posterior chamber or behind the lens implant, especially dispersive OVD. All types of OVDs, but in particular the higher-viscosity agents, may cause the pressure to rise. The IOP tends to peak 4 to 6 hours after surgery. IOP elevation usually does not last more than a few days and is amenable to medical treatment. The clinician may quickly manage marked IOP elevation in the early postoperative period by applying gentle pressure on the posterior lip of a preexisting paracentesis to release a small amount of aqueous humor. Topical and/or systemic pressure-lowering agents should also be administered, as pressure reduction after aqueous release is short-lived, with the IOP likely to rise again within 1 to 2 hours of the decompression.

Causes of elevated IOP without angle closure after cataract surgery include hyphema, TASS, endophthalmitis, retained lens material (phacolytic or phacoanaphylactic reactions), uveitis, iris pigment release, preexisting glaucoma, corticosteroid usage, vitreous in the anterior chamber, ghost cell glaucoma, or α-chymotrypsin. Angle-closure glaucoma may be due to pupillary block, ciliary block, epithelial ingrowth, neovascular glaucoma, or peripheral anterior synechiae. Treating the underlying cause of the IOP elevation should be curative.

Uncomplicated phacoemulsification may actually lower the long-term IOP by 10% to 34% in many eyes by an amount proportional to the preoperative pressure.

> Poley BJ, Lindstrom RL, Samuelson TW, Schulze R Jr. Intraocular pressure reduction after phacoemulsification with intraocular lens implantation in glaucomatous and nonglaucomatous eyes: evaluation of a causal relationship between the natural lens and open-angle glaucoma. *J Cataract Refract Surg.* 2009;35(11):1946–1955.

Intraoperative Floppy Iris Syndrome

Intraoperative floppy iris syndrome (IFIS) is the intraoperative triad of iris billowing and floppiness, iris prolapse into the incisions, and progressive pupillary miosis. Studies have shown that IFIS, especially when unexpected, will result in a higher rate of surgical complications, including iris trauma, posterior capsule rupture, and vitreous loss. It was originally associated with either the current or prior use of the adrenergic antagonist tamsulosin, a selective α_{1a}-adrenergic antagonist. Since then, IFIS has been reported with the use of other selective and nonselective α-adrenergic antagonists such as doxazosin, terazosin, alfuzosin, and silodosin, and following the use of some antipsychotic agents such as chlorpromazine or other drugs and supplements with α-adrenergic antagonist activity. Drugs that are selective $α_{1a}$-adrenergic antagonists seem to have greater effect on the iris dilator muscle than do nonselective drugs. Tamsulosin is most commonly used to treat lower urinary tract symptoms associated with benign prostatic hypertrophy. It is also used to treat renal stones and occasionally to treat women with urinary retention. Doxazosin, terazosin, prazosin, and labetalol (an α-adrenergic antagonist and a β-adrenergic antagonist) are used to treat hypertension. IFIS may be present in patients who have no apparent exposure to α-adrenergic antagonists; other associated causes remain undefined. IFIS has a wide range of clinical severity with approximately equal numbers of mild, moderate, or severe involvement in patients taking tamsulosin. There is no correlation with adrenergic antagonist dosage or duration of therapy, and discontinuing the medication preoperatively seems to have no effect on the degree of IFIS.

All preoperative patients should be questioned about their use of α-adrenergic antagonists and the degree of dilation noted. Since 2005, the Food and Drug Administration (FDA) has required that $α_{1a}$-adrenergic antagonists be labeled with a precautionary statement about IFIS and cataract surgery.

The following interventions have been proposed to reduce the intraoperative effects of IFIS: preoperative atropine; intracameral injection of α-agonists such as preservative-free phenylephrine or epinephrine; careful attention to incision location and construction to reduce wound leak; bimanual microincision surgical techniques; employment of highly retentive OVDs to "viscodilate" the pupil and maintain a concave iris near the incisions; discontinuation of fluid inflow prior to withdrawal of instruments to prevent fluid and iris egress; and the use of low-flow settings and lens removal techniques that minimize anterior chamber turbulence and eliminate a higher pressure gradient posterior to the iris. Intracameral irrigation of 0.5 to 1.0 mL of buffered, preservative-free 0.75% lidocaine mixed with preservative/bisulfate-free epinephrine 1:4000, when combined with surgical strategies noted earlier, has been successful in minimizing complications for many surgeons.

Despite these interventions, some patients still have significant miosis and/or iris prolapse intraoperatively. In these cases, use of iris retractors or pupil expansion rings (Fig 8-2) can maintain adequate dilation and iris stability to complete the procedure safely. These are best inserted prior to capsulorrhexis in order to avoid capture of the anterior capsule rim. Mechanical pupil-stretching techniques are ineffective in treating IFIS.

Bell CM, Hatch WV, Fischer HD, et al. Association between tamsulosin and serious ophthalmic adverse events in older men following cataract surgery. *JAMA*. 2009;301(19): 1991–1996.

Chang DF. Intraoperative floppy iris syndrome. *Focal Points: Clinical Modules for Ophthalmologists*. San Francisco: American Academy of Ophthalmology; 2010, module 11.

Chang DF, Braga-Mele R, Mamalis N, et al; ASCRS Cataract Clinical Committee. ASCRS white paper: clinical review of intraoperative floppy-iris syndrome. *J Cataract Refract Surg.* 2008;34(12):2153–2162.

Chang DF, Campbell JR. Intraoperative floppy iris syndrome associated with tamsulosin. *J Cataract Refract Surg.* 2005;31(4):664–673.

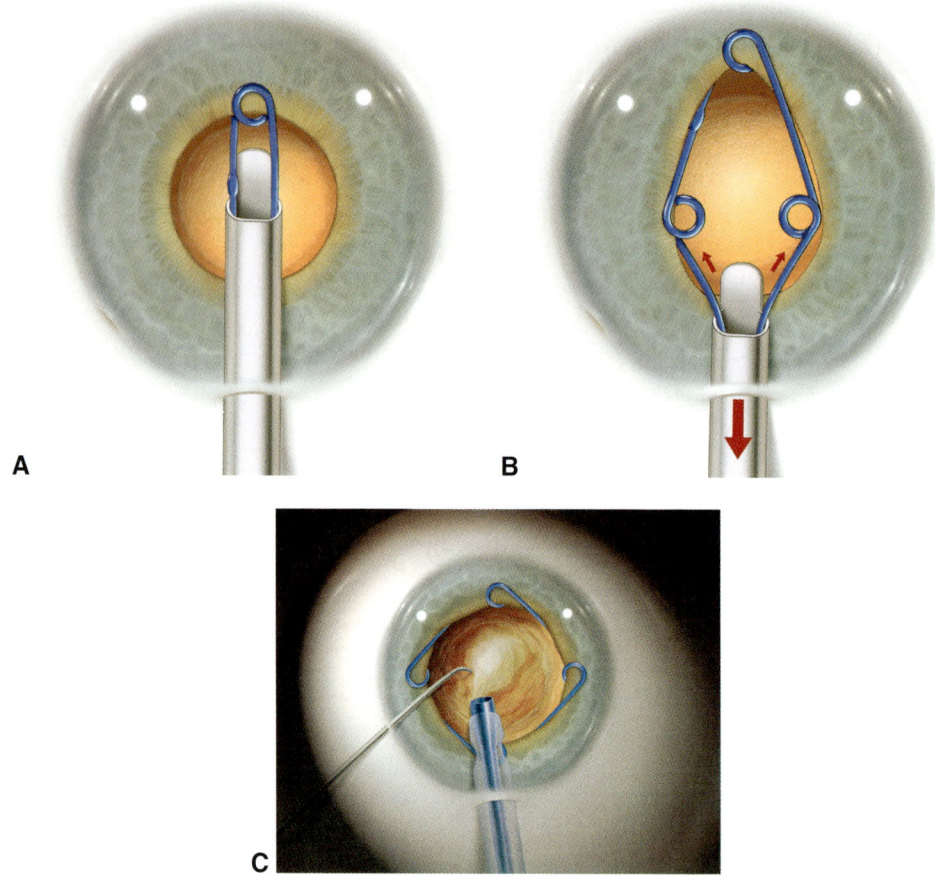

Figure 8-2 Malyugin Ring (MicroSurgical Technology). **A,** Pupil expansion ring introduced with a disposable injector. **B,** After the distal pupillary margin is engaged with the leading ring, the 2 lateral rings are introduced, followed by the trailing ring, which must be positioned with a lens hook. **C,** Insertion of the ring results in a rounded 6-mm pupil and allows easy access to the posterior chamber. *(Courtesy of MST [MicroSurgical Technology].)*

Lens–Iris Diaphragm Retropulsion Syndrome

Lens–iris diaphragm retropulsion syndrome (LIDRS) during cataract extraction is characterized by posterior displacement of the lens–iris diaphragm with a marked deepening of the anterior chamber, posterior iris bowing, and pupil dilation. It is due to a high level of infusion pressure in the anterior chamber with a reverse pupillary block and may result in stress on the zonular apparatus, considerable patient discomfort under topical anesthesia, and more-difficult surgery due to the excessively deep chamber. Lifting the iris off the anterior capsule is usually sufficient to break the pupillary block and restore the normal anterior chamber depth.

> Cionni RJ, Barros MG, Osher RH. Management of lens-iris diaphragm retropulsion syndrome during phacoemulsification. *J Cataract Refract Surg.* 2004;30(5):953–956.

Iridodialysis and Iris Trauma

Iridodialysis, the tearing of the iris at its root or insertion, may occur intraoperatively as a result of the manipulation of intraocular tissues. Insertion of the phaco tip or IOL can sometimes damage the iris. Traction on the iris root due to aspiration of iris tissue during phacoemulsification can cause a tear and a subsequent hyphema. If the iridodialysis is small or insignificant, it can be left alone. More extensive iridodialysis that could cause optical problems or that could be cosmetically significant may require surgical reattachment of the iris root to the wall of the eye with a permanent monofilament suture.

Chronic mydriasis or iris damage from surgery or trauma may cause excessive glare, particularly if the pupillary light response is inadequate or if the edge of the IOL is uncovered by the iris. Suturing an iris defect, pupillary circlage, or implanting artificial iris devices may alleviate symptoms or improve a patient's cosmetic concerns. An iris-colored contact lens may be considered as a nonsurgical alternative.

Cyclodialysis

Cyclodialysis, the separation of the ciliary body from its insertion at the scleral spur, also may occur as a result of trauma or of surgical manipulation of intraocular tissue. Gonioscopic observation shows a deep-angle recess with a gap between the sclera and the ciliary body. Repair of a cyclodialysis cleft is often indicated to relieve prolonged hypotony. Closure may be achieved by applying argon laser photocoagulation to the cleft. If this is ineffective, it may be necessary to reattach the ciliary body with sutures.

Ciliary Block Glaucoma

Ciliary block glaucoma, also known as *malignant glaucoma*, results from the posterior misdirection of aqueous into the vitreous body. This misdirection displaces the lens–iris diaphragm anteriorly, causing the central and peripheral portions of the anterior chamber to become very shallow. This leads to a secondary elevation of IOP as a consequence of angle obstruction. Ciliary block glaucoma occurs most commonly after intraocular surgery in eyes with prior angle-closure glaucoma, but it can also occur after cataract or glaucoma surgery or various laser procedures in eyes with open angles. It must be differentiated from pupillary block glaucoma, suprachoroidal hemorrhage, or choroidal detachment.

The posterior diversion of aqueous into the vitreous cavity can elevate the IOP despite the presence of a patent iridectomy or iridotomy. Thus, ciliary block glaucoma, unlike pupillary block, is not relieved by iridectomy but requires either intense medical therapy or more aggressive surgical therapy.

Medical treatment consists of cycloplegia and mydriasis with drugs such as atropine 1% and phenylephrine 10% 4 times a day to attempt to relieve the obstruction and allow aqueous to enter the anterior chamber, thereby moving the lens–iris diaphragm posteriorly. This therapy is coupled with the use of aqueous suppressants (such as β-blockers, α-agonists, and/or oral carbonic anhydrase inhibitors) and hyperosmotic agents (such as oral glycerin or intravenous mannitol) to reduce aqueous production and vitreous volume and thus lower the IOP. Miotics should be avoided because they make ciliary block glaucoma worse by exacerbating the anterior displacement of the lens–iris diaphragm. Medical therapy is successful in 50% of these cases.

Surgical intervention consists of maneuvers to disrupt the anterior vitreous face and vitreous/ciliary body interface in order to reestablish a channel for aqueous to circulate into the anterior chamber. Techniques include mechanical disruption with a knife, use of the Nd:YAG laser, or pars plana vitrectomy. (See also BCSC Section 10, *Glaucoma.*)

> Lundy DM. Ciliary block glaucoma. *Focal Points: Clinical Modules for Ophthalmologists.* San Francisco: American Academy of Ophthalmology; 1999, module 3.

Chronic Uveitis

With uncomplicated surgery and the use of postoperative topical corticosteroids or NSAIDs, most eyes should be free of inflammation by 3 to 4 weeks after surgery. Complicated cases requiring manipulation of intraocular tissues (eg, iris sphincterotomy, iridectomy, or iris prolapse), vitreous loss, or sulcus fixation of an IOL may have a more prolonged recovery. Increased inflammation can be seen in children, in patients with diabetes, and in eyes with previous surgery, exfoliation syndrome, pigment dispersion syndrome, or long-term miotic use. The presence of hypopyon or vitritis should prompt intervention to determine the source of the inflammation. Low-grade inflammation lasting more than 4 weeks should raise the possibility of chronic infection, retained lens fragments, or other causes of chronic inflammation. The clinician should investigate the possibility of microbial endophthalmitis in patients who have persistent uveitis without a previous inflammatory history.

Chronic uveitis following cataract surgery has been reported in association with low-grade bacterial pathogens, including *Propionibacterium acnes* and *Staphylococcus epidermidis.* Patients with this condition may have an unremarkable early postoperative course and lack the classic findings of acute endophthalmitis. Weeks or months after surgery, however, they develop chronic uveitis that is variably responsive to topical corticosteroids. This condition is usually associated with granulomatous keratic precipitates and less commonly with hypopyon. A localized focus of infection sequestered within the capsular bag may occasionally be observed, most often within the remaining lens capsule. Diagnosis requires a high level of clinical suspicion, coupled with examination and cultures of appropriate specimens of aqueous, vitreous, and, where applicable, retained lens material that may harbor a nidus of infection. Appropriate intravitreal antibiotic therapy is indicated. If this treatment fails, the clinician may need to search for and remove any visible focus of potentially infectious material in order to sterilize the eye. In some cases, total removal of the residual capsule and IOL is necessary.

Patients with preexisting uveitis may have excessive postoperative inflammation but generally do well with small-incision cataract surgery and IOL implants. Debate continues as to whether different IOL materials incite more or less inflammatory response. Some surgeons favor acrylic IOL material over silicone in patients with preexisting uveitis or a risk for chronic inflammation. IOL malposition is a more important cause of chronic inflammation if the IOL contacts the iris, ciliary body, or angle structures. Vitreous prolapse or vitreous incarceration in the wound may be a cause of prolonged inflammation.

Retained lens material is occasionally an insidious cause of chronic low-grade inflammation or corneal edema (see the following section, Retained Lens Material).

Management of chronic uveitis is directed toward the cause. Surgery corrects mechanical issues with IOL malposition, vitreous incarceration, or retained lens fragments. The clinician must rule out infectious etiologies. If no obvious causes are found, prolonged use of topical or subconjunctival steroids is indicated, with efforts to identify potential systemic causes of uveitis.

> Van Gelder RN, Leveque TK. Cataract surgery in the setting of uveitis. *Curr Opin Ophthalmol.* 2009;20(1):42–45.

Retained Lens Material

During cataract extraction, lens fragments may remain in the anterior chamber angle or in the posterior chamber behind the iris, or they may migrate into the vitreous cavity if zonular dehiscence or posterior capsule rupture occurs. Retained lens material is thought to be more frequent with phacoemulsification than with ECCE, with a reported postoperative prevalence of 0.45% to 1.7%. (For a discussion of the surgical management of this intraoperative complication, see the Capsular Rupture section later in this chapter.)

Patients with retained lens fragments present with varying degrees of inflammation depending on the size of the lens fragment, the type of lens material, the amount of time elapsed since surgery, and the patient's individual response. The clinical signs of retained lens material may include uveitis, elevated IOP, corneal edema, and vitreous opacities.

Retained cortical lens material does not necessarily require surgical intervention. In general, cortical material is better tolerated and more likely to reabsorb over time than is nuclear material, which, even in small amounts, persists longer and is more likely to incite a significant inflammatory reaction and elevated IOP. Smaller fragments of lens material are better tolerated than larger pieces for the same reasons.

Observation is warranted for patients with small amounts of retained cortical lens material in the hope that this material will be reabsorbed. Inflammation should be controlled with corticosteroid and nonsteroidal anti-inflammatory drops and cycloplegics. IOP can be controlled with topical agents and with carbonic anhydrase inhibitors given systemically. Surgical intervention may be necessary to remove residual lens material in the following situations:

- presence of a large or visually significant amount of lens material
- increased inflammation not readily controlled with topical medications
- medically unresponsive elevated IOP resulting from inflammation
- corneal edema
- associated retinal detachment or retinal tears
- associated endophthalmitis

If the posterior capsule is intact, simple aspiration of residual lens material through an anterior incision may be carried out with the use of an I/A instrument. If lens material has migrated into the vitreous cavity through a defect in the zonular fibers or posterior capsule, pars plana vitrectomy and removal of lens material are indicated. When such major intervention is necessary, a surgeon skilled in pars plana vitrectomy techniques should remove the retained lens material from the vitreous. The vitreoretinal surgeon can delay intervention up to 7 to 14 days following the initial cataract surgery without jeopardizing the successful outcome. Chronic glaucoma and CME may be more likely when intervention is delayed more than 3 weeks after the cataract surgery.

> Monshizadeh R, Samiy N, Haimovici R. Management of retained intravitreal lens fragments after cataract surgery. *Surv Ophthalmol.* 1999;43(5):397–404.
>
> Vilar NF, Flynn HW Jr, Smiddy WE, Murray TG, Davis JL, Rubsamen PE. Removal of retained lens fragments after phacoemulsification reverses secondary glaucoma and restores visual acuity. *Ophthalmology.* 1997;104(5):787–792.

Capsular Rupture

If capsular rupture occurs during phacoemulsification, lens fragments may enter the posterior segment. At the time of posterior capsule rupture, the surgeon should reduce the high fluid flow and stabilize the anterior segment. Evaluation of the location and size of the tear will determine the appropriate surgical response. A radial tear in an anterior capsulorrhexis may extend through the capsular fornix into the posterior capsule. A small rupture in the posterior capsule during emulsification of the nucleus can be managed by alteration of the surgical technique. If the majority of the nucleus remains and the capsular tear is large, further attempts at phacoemulsification should be abandoned. To extract the remaining nuclear fragments mechanically, the surgeon should enlarge the incision and remove the nucleus with a lens loop or spoon in a manner that minimizes vitreous traction and further damage to the capsule.

If only a small portion of the nucleus remains to be aspirated or if the rent in the capsule is small, the surgeon, by compartmentalizing the vitreous with OVD and using low-flow–low-vacuum settings, may be able to use the phaco tip to remove the remaining nuclear material. Full occlusion of the aspiration port and minimal phaco power will reduce the risk of further damage to the capsule or aspiration of vitreous. Insertion of a second instrument or lens glide behind the nuclear remnant may help prevent the remnant from being dislocated into the vitreous. Alternatively, OVD can be introduced posterior to the fragment in an effort to float it anteriorly. If the nuclear material drops posteriorly but is still visible and if the surgeon is familiar with pars plana techniques, a posterior assisted-levitation maneuver may be attempted. A spatula or OVD cannula is placed through a stab incision in the pars plana and used to elevate the nuclear fragment into the anterior segment. Retrieval of nuclear fragments from the deep vitreous is not recommended.

If the nuclear fragment is not visible or if the surgeon is not experienced with pars plana vitrectomy techniques, a biaxial anterior vitrectomy can be performed with an aspirating guillotine cutter to remove prolapsed vitreous and the peripheral cortical material. A 2-port anterior vitrectomy, separating infusion from the aspiration/cutting instrument, facilitates the removal of vitreous from the anterior segment of the eye. For better visualization, the vitreous may be stained with unpreserved or washed triamcinolone. Preferably, the aspiration/cutting instrument should be placed through a pars plana incision and directly visualized in the posterior segment through the pupil while irrigation is continued through the limbus or cornea. This directs flow posteriorly and reduces the amount of vitreous that migrates into the anterior segment. Alternatively, both the irrigation instrument and the aspiration/cutting instrument may be placed through 2 separate limbal or corneal incisions.

If posterior capsule support for an intracapsular placement of the IOL is inadequate, an attempt to preserve the anterior capsulorrhexis should be made to allow for capture of the IOL optic in the capsular bag with the haptics placed in the ciliary sulcus. A 3-piece IOL with a total diameter greater than 12.5 mm may be inserted into the ciliary sulcus after confirmation of the anterior capsule's integrity. A single-piece uniplanar acrylic IOL is not suitable for the ciliary sulcus. If capsular integrity is insufficient, the surgeon may substitute an anterior chamber lens of appropriate power and size. A posterior chamber IOL may also be used in the absence of capsular support by suturing the haptics to the iris or to the wall of the eye through the ciliary sulcus. If posteriorly dislocated nuclear material remains, it should be approached within 1 to 2 weeks by a vitreoretinal surgeon via a pars plana vitrectomy route (see BCSC Section 12, *Retina and Vitreous*). Retained lens material, especially nuclear material, is often associated with elevated IOP, significant inflammation, and corneal edema. Following are some guidelines for the anterior segment surgeon faced with managing posteriorly dislocated lens fragments:

- Attempt retrieval of the fragments only if they are visible and easily accessible.
- Perform an anterior vitrectomy until no vitreous is seen anterior to the capsule.
- Insert an IOL only when safe and indicated, preferably a posterior chamber lens in the ciliary sulcus or an anterior chamber lens with prophylactic peripheral iridotomy. Adjust the lens power appropriately for the position and type of IOL used.
- Perform a watertight incision closure and remove the OVD.
- Prescribe frequent postoperative topical corticosteroids, NSAIDs, and IOP-lowering agents as necessary.
- Arrange a referral for prompt vitreoretinal consultation.
- Disclose and discuss all surgical complications with the patient.

If a small rent appears in the posterior capsule during aspiration of the cortex and the vitreous face remains intact, the surgeon should attempt to remove the residual cortex without expanding the tear. After stabilizing the anterior chamber with the use of an OVD, capsulorrhexis forceps may be used to convert the tear into a round posterior capsulorrhexis that will not spread equatorially. Use of a low flow of I/A helps the surgeon avoid disrupting the vitreous face, and the residual cortex is then removed from the peripheral lens capsule. Some surgeons prefer a manual dry-aspiration technique, using a cannula attached to a handheld syringe to remove the residual cortex after a capsular rupture, thereby avoiding any pressure from irrigation.

If larger posterior capsule tears occur or when the anterior vitreous face is broken, a vitrectomy is recommended to facilitate the removal of residual cortex and the subsequent placement of an IOL. In addition, a vitrectomy can prevent the development of vitreomacular traction from the IOL or the incision. Vitreous loss during cataract surgery is associated with an increased risk of retinal detachment, CME, and endophthalmitis.

Arbisser LB. Anterior vitrectomy for the anterior segment surgeon. *Focal Points: Clinical Modules for Ophthalmologists.* San Francisco: American Academy of Ophthalmology; 2009, module 2.

Arbisser LB, Charles S, Howcroft M, Werner L. Management of vitreous loss and dropped nucleus during cataract surgery. *Ophthalmol Clin North Am.* 2006;19(4):495–506.

Chang DF, Packard RB. Posterior assisted levitation for nucleus retrieval using Viscoat after posterior capsule rupture. *J Cataract Refract Surg.* 2003;29(10):1860–1865.

Fishkind WJ. The torn posterior capsule: prevention, recognition, and management. *Focal Points: Clinical Modules for Ophthalmologists.* San Francisco: American Academy of Ophthalmology; 1999, module 4.

Kaynak S, Celik L, Kocak N, Oner FH, Kaynak T, Cingil G. Staining of vitreous with triamcinolone acetonide. *J Cataract Refract Surg.* 2006;32(1):56–59.

Monshizadeh R, Samiy N, Haimovici R. Management of retained intravitreal lens fragments after cataract surgery. *Surv Ophthalmol.* 1999;43(5):397–404.

Vitreous Prolapse in the Anterior Chamber

In cases with vitreous prolapse during any intraocular surgery, the surgeon should attempt to remove all of the vitreous in the anterior chamber to reduce the chance of long-term complications. Vitreous in the anterior chamber may lead to chronic intraocular inflammation with or without associated CME. The incidence of corneal edema and glaucoma increases. The pupil may be distorted by vitreous adherent to the incisions or iris. Inflammation or symptoms of glare due to exposing the edge of the IOL as well as the cosmetic appearance of the iris may prompt surgical intervention. In symptomatic patients, Nd:YAG laser vitreolysis or anterior vitrectomy may be considered if response to topical anti-inflammatory therapy is inadequate. Severing vitreous strands to incisions may reduce CME, originally described in the era of intracapsular surgery as the Irvine-Gass syndrome. If the vitreous extends through the incision to the ocular surface, a vitrectomy should be performed. The exposed vitreous may act like a wick, enabling bacteria to gain entrance into the eye and increasing the risk of endophthalmitis (vitreous wick syndrome). In cases showing considerable corneal compromise, a posterior vitrectomy approach may be preferable to an anterior approach to reduce surgical trauma to the cornea.

Complications of IOL Implantation

Decentration and Dislocation

A 0.19% to 3.00% incidence of subluxation or dislocation of an IOL has been reported after uncomplicated surgery. The position of the dislocated IOL, either within the capsule (intracapsular) or outside of it (extracapsular), determines the best means for correction (Fig 8-3). The most common cause of extracapsular dislocation is sulcus placement of the IOL in situations in which the IOL is inadequately sized for this location or in which a decentered or oversized capsulorrhexis, localized zonular defects, haptic damage, and/or haptic memory loss have occurred. Asymmetric bag/sulcus haptic positions aggravated by capsular fibrosis and contraction may tilt or decenter an IOL. The most common cause

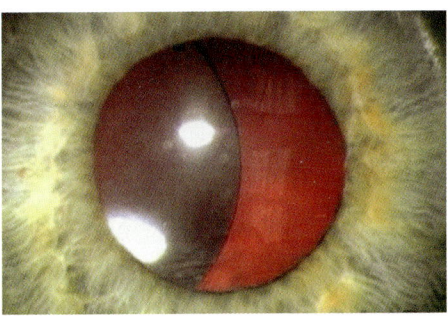 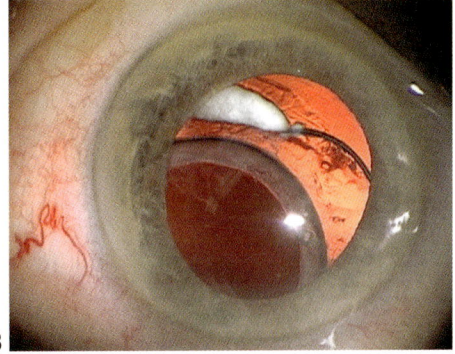

Figure 8-3 Intraocular lens (IOL) dislocation. **A,** Out-of-the-bag dislocation. **B,** In-the-bag dislocation. *(Part A from Dorey MW, Condon GP. Management of dislocated intraocular lenses.* Focal Points: Clinical Modules for Ophthalmologists. *San Francisco: American Academy of Ophthalmology; 2009, module 9:2. Part B reprinted from Gimbel HV, Condon GP, Kohnen T, Olson RJ, Halkiadakis I. Late in-the-bag intraocular lens dislocation: incidence, prevention, and management.* J Cataract Refract Surg, *pages 2193–2204, Volume 31, copyright 2005, with permission from Elsevier.)*

for intracapsular IOL dislocation is zonular degradation associated with exfoliation syndrome. Insufficient zonular support may also be due to trauma, previous vitreoretinal surgery, capsular contraction, retinitis pigmentosa, high myopia, uveitis, or other congenital conditions that affect zonular integrity.

Decentration can produce unwanted glare and reflections or multiple images if the edge of the lens is within the pupillary space. Decentration of an aspheric, multifocal, or accommodating lens diminishes the lens's desired effect. Aspheric lenses with negative spherical aberration used to counteract the positive spherical aberration of the aging cornea may cause increased higher orders of aberration than would spherical lenses if decentered. Decentration of any posterior chamber IOL may lead to pupillary capture or any component of the uveitis-glaucoma-hyphema syndrome due to contact with uveal tissue. Minor, asymptomatic cases call for observation. They may be treated with miotics to constrict the pupil over the IOL optic or with cycloplegics to reduce iris/IOL chafing in the cases of pigment dispersion or recurrent hyphema. More-severe cases of IOL decentration are managed by IOL repositioning, stabilization with sutures, or exchange.

An IOL that is designed for intracapsular fixation is prone to decentration or dislocation when one or both haptics are placed in the sulcus. At times, a lens decentered in the sulcus or in the bag with a posterior capsule rent may be stabilized by prolapsing the optic through an intact capsulorrhexis. An extracapsular decentered IOL may be rotated and repositioned into a stable axis if clinical evidence shows sufficient capsule and zonular fibers to support the implant. Many extracapsular and selected intracapsular 3-piece IOL dislocations can be managed with peripheral iris suture fixation using a McCannel suture or Siepser slipknot technique with nonabsorbable monofilament suture such as 9-0 or 10-0 polypropylene (Fig 8-4). Microinstruments for intraocular grasping and cutting through small incisions may facilitate repositioning the IOL and tying sutures. Current single-piece uniplanar acrylic IOLs are not suitable for sulcus or iris fixation. Iris fixation has some advantages over scleral fixation with a decreased chance of late suture erosion

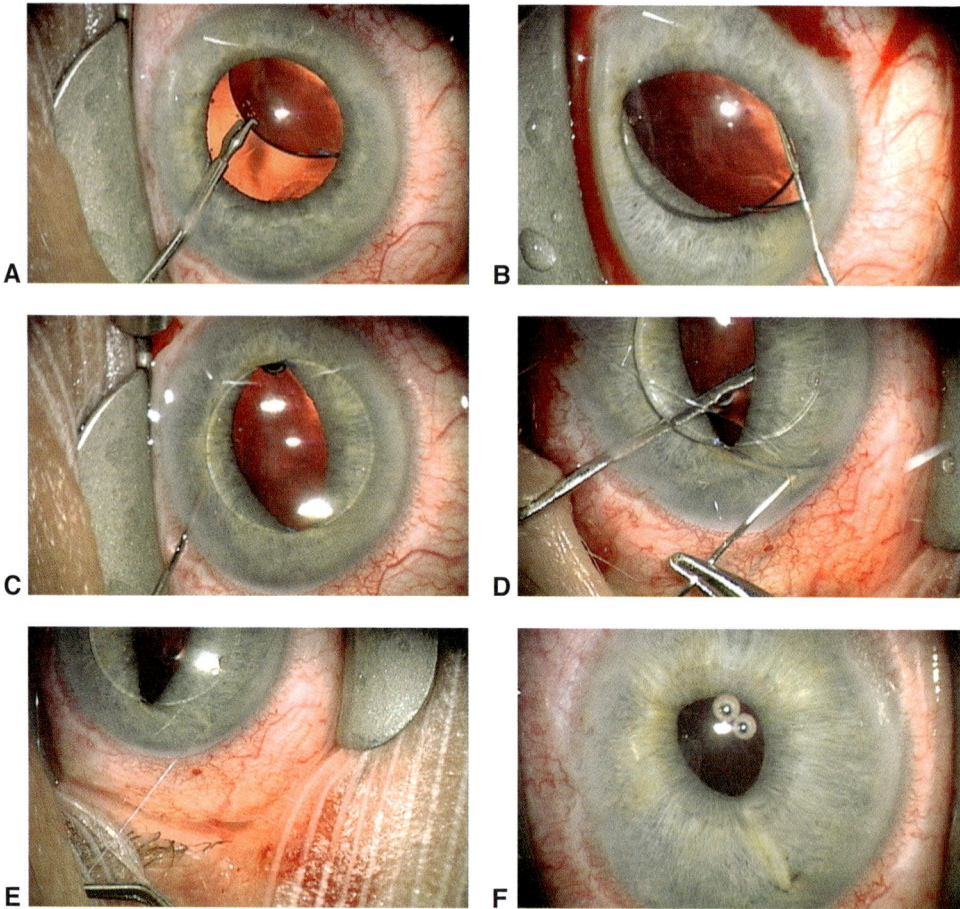

Figure 8-4 Peripheral iris fixation technique for out-of-the-bag IOL dislocation. **A,** Grasping and rotation IOL with microsurgical forceps. **B,** Iris hooks used to bring optic above the iris plane. **C,** Optic capture by the pupil is completed by adding acetylcholine to induce miosis. **D,** Needle has been passed through a paracentesis, then through iris and behind the haptic, and then back out through iris and distal clear cornea. **E,** A Siepser sliding knot is used to secure the haptic to the peripheral iris. **F,** After both haptics are secured, the optic is prolapsed back into the posterior chamber, and the sutures are minimally visible at the 5- and 10-o'clock positions. *(Reprinted with permission from Condon GP. Following a posterior capsular rent, the sulcus-fixated intraocular lens has become decentered. How should I proceed? In: Chang DF, ed. Curbside Consultation in Cataract Surgery. Thorofare, NJ: Slack; 2007:227–232.)*

or breakage, IOL tilting, intraocular hemorrhage, and endophthalmitis. Disadvantages include posterior iris pigment chafing, distortion of the pupil, possible pseudophakodonesis, and hyphema.

Irregular capsule fibrosis may gradually decenter an in-the-bag IOL. Deformation of the haptics may render simple rotation insufficient to center the IOL properly. It may become necessary in these cases to move the IOL haptics into the ciliary sulcus or replace the capsule-fixated IOL with a posterior chamber sulcus-fixated IOL.

Severe pseudophakodonesis or intracapsular (in-the-bag) dislocation of an IOL due to zonular loss may be managed with suture fixation to the sclera. Many different *ab externo* and *ab interno* approaches and suture configurations have been described (Fig 8-5). A concurrent anterior vitrectomy is often necessary. Iris retractors may be used for better visualization or to stabilize the haptics during suturing. Sutures through the scleral wall should be covered by a flap to prevent erosion through the conjunctiva. If dislocation of the IOL is complete, pars plana vitrectomy techniques are required to retrieve the lens or lens/capsule complex and elevate it safely into the anterior segment, where it can then be stabilized until suture fixation to the iris or sclera is accomplished from an anterior approach. Alternatively, the implant may be removed altogether and replaced with either an anterior chamber IOL or a transscleral or iris-sutured posterior chamber IOL. Suture breakage and subluxation of scleral-fixated sutured IOLs has been reported 3 to 9 years after implantation with 10-0 polypropylene fixation sutures. Double-fixation techniques and thicker 9-0 polypropylene or 9-0 Gore-Tex sutures are currently recommended for scleral fixation of IOLs. Other complications of sutured IOLs include vitreous or suprachoroidal hemorrhage, lens tilting, CME, retinal tears or detachment, suture erosion, and infection. (See BCSC Section 12, *Retina and Vitreous*.)

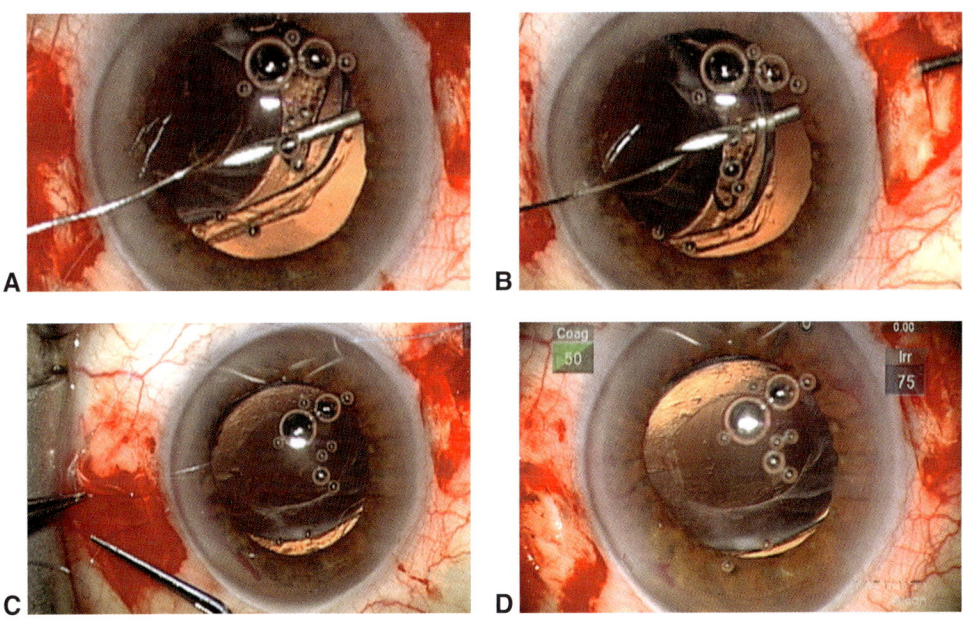

Figure 8-5 *Ab externo* scleral fixation technique. **A,** A partial-thickness scleral groove is made 1.0–1.5 mm posterior to the limbus. A hollow 26-gauge needle is inserted through the scleral groove behind the iris plane and over the haptic into the pupillary zone. A preplaced 9-0 polypropylene suture on a long needle is placed through a corneal paracentesis tract in the opposite direction. This needle can fit into the hollow 26-gauge needle and can then be retrieved back through the original scleral groove site. **B,** The 26-gauge needle is inserted again into the scleral groove about 1 mm away from the original pass site; it is then inserted behind the iris plane beneath the haptic/capsule complex and up again into the pupillary zone. A similarly preplaced 9-0 polypropylene suture on a long needle is placed, and the suture retrieved in an identical fashion through the original scleral groove site. **C,** The knot is tied but not yet locked. **D,** The other haptic is secured in a similar process. The optic is centered, and the knots are locked and then buried in the scleral grooves. *(Reprinted from Masket S. Cataract surgical problem: February consultation #1. J Cataract Refract Surg. Volume 34, issue 2, copyright February 2008, with permission from Elsevier.)*

Decentration, iris tucking, or pseudophakodonesis of an anterior chamber IOL is treated if necessary by repositioning the properly sized flexible IOL or by exchanging that lens with either a correctly sized anterior chamber IOL or a sutured 3-piece posterior chamber IOL. Dislocated iris-supported lenses are rare in clinical practice today, but they should be surgically exchanged; in cases in which more extensive surgery is contraindicated, simple repositioning may be successful.

> Chang DF. Siepser slipknot for McCannel iris-suture fixation of subluxated intraocular lenses. *J Cataract Refract Surg.* 2004;30(6):1170–1176.
>
> Dorey MW, Condon GP. Management of dislocated intraocular lenses. *Focal Points: Clinical Modules for Ophthalmologists.* San Francisco: American Academy of Ophthalmology; 2009, module 9.
>
> Gimbel HV, Condon GP, Kohnen T, Olson RJ, Halkiadakis I. Late in-the-bag intraocular lens dislocation: incidence, prevention, and management. *J Cataract Refract Surg.* 2005;31(11): 2193–2204.
>
> Hannush SB. Sutured posterior chamber intraocular lenses. *Focal Points: Clinical Modules for Ophthalmologists.* San Francisco: American Academy of Ophthalmology; 2006, module 9.

Pupillary Capture

Postoperative pupillary capture of the IOL optic can occur for a variety of reasons, including formation of synechiae between the iris and underlying posterior capsule, improper placement of the IOL haptics, shallowing of the anterior chamber, or anterior displacement of the posterior chamber IOL optic. The latter is associated with placement of nonangulated IOLs in the ciliary sulcus, upside-down placement of an angulated IOL so that the IOL vaults anteriorly, excessive Soemmering ring formation, or asymmetric capsule contraction. Placement of a posteriorly angulated posterior chamber IOL in the capsular bag decreases the likelihood of pupillary capture.

Often, pupillary capture is only a cosmetic issue; the patient is otherwise asymptomatic and can be left untreated. Occasionally, pupillary capture can cause problems with glare, photophobia, chronic uveitis, unintended myopia, or even monocular diplopia. Mydriatics can sometimes be used successfully to free the iris through pharmacologic manipulation of the pupil. If conservative management fails, surgical intervention may be required to free the iris, lyse synechiae, manage capsule contraction or residual lens proliferation, and reposition the lens (Figs 8-6, 8-7).

Capsular Block Syndrome

Capsular block syndrome is an uncommon postoperative complication of capsular bag–fixated posterior chamber IOLs. Most cases occur in the immediate postoperative period, but some may be seen years later. Aqueous or OVD from surgery becomes trapped within the capsular bag between the posterior capsule and the posterior surface of the IOL. A myopic shift in the refractive error is due to a forward displacement of the lens optic. When an anterior displacement of the iris diaphragm and shallowing of the anterior chamber occur, posterior synechiae can form and elevate the IOP if left untreated. The fluid behind the IOL may have a turbid or milky appearance. Nd:YAG laser anterior or

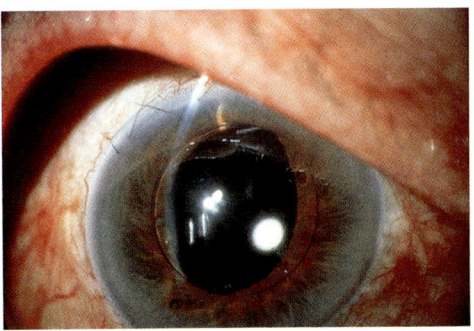

Figure 8-6 Pupillary capture. *(Courtesy of Karla J. Johns, MD.)*

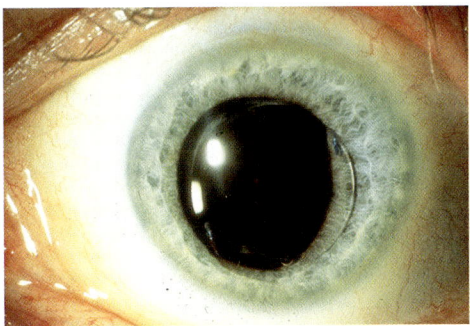

Figure 8-7 Pupillary capture by an angled posterior chamber IOL in a patient who was assaulted 2 months after surgery. *(Courtesy of Steven I. Rosenfeld, MD.)*

posterior capsulotomy results in release of the fluid, posterior movement of the IOL optic to its intended position, and resolution of the myopic shift.

Uveitis-Glaucoma-Hyphema Syndrome

Uveitis-glaucoma-hyphema (UGH) syndrome was first described in the context of rigid or closed-loop anterior chamber IOLs. UGH can also be seen in patients with posterior chamber lenses, owing to contact between lens haptics and uveal tissue in the posterior chamber. The classic triad or individual elements may occur as a result of inappropriate IOL sizing, contact between the implant and vascular structures or the corneal endothelium, or defects in implant manufacturing. Uveitis, glaucoma, and/or hyphema may respond to treatment with cycloplegics and topical anti-inflammatory or antiglaucoma medications. If medical therapy does not sufficiently alleviate the symptoms or if inflammation threatens either retinal or corneal function, IOL removal must be considered. This procedure may be very complicated because of inflammatory scars, particularly in the chamber angle or posterior to the iris. If such scarring is present, the surgeon may need to amputate the haptics from the optic and remove the lens piecemeal, rotating the haptic material out of the synechial tunnels to minimize trauma to the eye. In some cases, it is safer to leave portions of the haptics in place. Early lens explantation may reduce the risk of corneal decompensation and CME.

Pseudophakic Bullous Keratopathy

Certain IOL designs, particularly iris-clip lenses (iris-fixated lenses with the optic anterior to the iris) and closed-loop flexible anterior chamber lenses, are associated with increased risk of corneal decompensation. Iris-clip lenses have been shown to contact the corneal endothelium during eye movement. Endothelial cell loss associated with closed-loop anterior chamber IOLs is thought to be due to chronic inflammation and contact between the lens and peripheral corneal endothelial cells. Thus, these two lens types are no longer in clinical use. Patients with underlying corneal endothelial dysfunction such as Fuchs corneal dystrophy are at greater risk for developing postoperative corneal edema.

Unexpected Refractive Results

Unintended postoperative refractive errors are usually the result of a preoperative error in measurement of axial length or in keratometry readings. Choosing the correct IOL power is more difficult in patients who are undergoing simultaneous penetrating keratoplasty, in patients with silicone oil in the vitreous cavity, and in patients who have had prior refractive surgery (see Chapter 6). The surgeon or staff member's failure to confirm the proper IOL at the time of surgery may result in implantation of the incorrect lens. Unexpected postoperative refractive results may occur because of inverting an angulated IOL or placing the lens in the sulcus when it was calculated for in-the-bag placement, either of which results in anterior displacement and changes the effective power of the IOL. The clinician should rule out or treat other causes of an anterior or posterior shift in the IOL position, such as posterior capsule rupture, capsular block, or ciliary block. Mislabeling or manufacturing defects are rarely the cause. Incorrect lens power should be suspected early in the postoperative course when the uncorrected visual acuity is less than expected and is confirmed by refraction. Medical record documentation of the source of the error and full disclosure to the patient are necessary.

If the magnitude of the postoperative refractive error produces symptomatic ametropia, anisometropia, or dissatisfaction on the part of the patient, the surgeon can consider several options: overrefraction, contact-lens wear, IOL exchange with a lens of the appropriate power, insertion of a piggyback IOL, or a secondary keratorefractive procedure.

IOL Glare, Dysphotopsia, and Opacification

In addition to lens decentration and capsular opacification, glare can result when the diameter of the IOL optic is smaller than the diameter of the scotopic pupil. Optics with a square-edge design and multifocal IOLs are more prone to produce glare and halos. Spherical aberration may produce some degree of distortion or glare under scotopic conditions when the pupil is dilated, even if the iris covers the edge of the lens optic. Aspheric IOLs may reduce some of these phenomena and improve contrast sensitivity. Spherical aberration of the cornea changes with age and corneal refractive surgery, and various aspheric IOLs can be matched to the degree of corneal asphericity.

Positive dysphotopsias, described as glare, streaks, flashes, arcs, or halos of light, are more common with truncated square-edge IOLs and those manufactured from higher-index materials. Some patients with apparently ideal placement of an IOL in the capsular bag see *negative dysphotopsias,* described as an arcuate dark or dim region usually in the temporal visual field. The cause is unknown, but the dysphotopsia may be due to the overlap of the optic by the anterior capsulorrhexis edge. Symptoms abate in some cases with surgical repositioning of the optic anterior to the capsulorrhexis, implantation of a piggyback IOL, or an anterior capsulectomy. Most patients who experience dysphotopsias improve with time. Initially, observation is advised.

A number of IOLs have developed opacities or discoloration immediately after implantation or progressively over years. Many different causes have been identified and vary with the IOL manufacturer, material, and storage, as well as surgical adjuvants and associated patient conditions. Five general processes of IOL opacification have been identified.

- deposits or precipitates on the surface of or in the IOL optic (such as calcium deposits on silicone IOLs in asteroid hyalosis)
- influx of water in hydrophobic optic material (glistenings)
- staining of the IOL by capsular dyes or medications
- IOL coating by substances such as ophthalmic ointment or silicone oil
- progressive degradation of the IOL material (such as snowflake degeneration in polymethylmethacrylate [PMMA] IOLs)

Glistenings are observed with all types of IOLs but are primarily associated with hydrophobic acrylic IOLs. Although their appearance may be striking on slit-lamp examination, they have not been shown to affect corrected distance visual acuity. Whether they have an effect on contrast sensitivity or glare is a matter of controversy, and IOL explantation is rarely reported. Calcium deposition within or on the surface of hydrophilic acrylic lenses has produced significant visual symptoms, leading in some cases to lens explantation. Interlenticular opacifications have been noted between piggybacked posterior chamber IOLs, particularly if both are made of hydrophobic acrylic material and placed in the capsular bag. Enlarging the capsulorrhexis, using 2 different materials, and placing 1 lens in the bag and 1 in the sulcus may reduce the incidence.

Patients who have had diffractive or refractive multifocal IOLs implanted are more prone to experience glare, decreased contrast sensitivity, or loss of desired multifocality with minor IOL decentration or posterior capsule opacity. Extra care in IOL centration and management of capsular opacity or contraction is advised. An accommodating lens such as Crystalens (Bausch & Lomb, Rochester, NY) may vault anteriorly (Z syndrome) due to misplaced haptics or asymmetric capsular contraction and must be surgically repositioned. Toric IOLs must be located at a precise axis for maximal astigmatic correction and may need to be repositioned if they have rotated away from the intended axis. Repositioning should be accomplished before the haptics are fibrosed into the capsule.

Jin H, Limberger IJ, Ehmer A, Guo H, Auffarth GU. Impact of axis misalignment of toric intraocular lenses on refractive outcomes after cataract surgery. *J Cataract Refract Surg.* 2010;36(12):2061–2072.

Werner L. Causes of intraocular lens opacification or discoloration. *J Cataract Refract Surg.* 2007;33(4):713–726.

Werner L. Glistenings and surface light scattering in intraocular lenses. *J Cataract Refract Surg.* 2010;36(8):1398–1420.

Capsular Opacification and Contraction

Posterior Capsule Opacification

The most common late complication of cataract surgery by means of ECCE or phacoemulsification is posterior capsule opacification (PCO). In addition, contracture of a continuous curvilinear capsulorrhexis may occlude the visual axis because of anterior capsule phimosis and fibrosis. Fortunately, posterior or anterior capsule opacification is amenable to treatment by means of Nd:YAG laser capsulotomy.

Capsular opacification stems from the continued viability of lens epithelial cells that remain after removal of the nucleus and cortex. Opaque secondary membranes are formed by proliferating lens epithelial cells, fibroblastic metaplasia, and collagen deposition. Lens epithelial cells proliferate in several patterns. Sequestration of nucleated bladder cells (Wedl cells) in a closed space between the adherent edges of the anterior and posterior capsule results in a doughnut-shaped configuration, referred to as a *Soemmering ring*. If the epithelial cells migrate out of the capsular bag, translucent globular masses resembling fish eggs *(Elschnig pearls)* form on the edge of the capsular opening. These pearls can fill the pupil or remain hidden behind the iris. Histologic examination shows that each "fish egg" is a nucleated bladder cell, identical to those proliferating within the capsule of a Soemmering ring but usually lacking a basement membrane. If the epithelial cells migrate across the anterior or posterior capsule, they may cause capsular wrinkling and opacification. Significantly, the lens epithelial cells are capable of undergoing metaplasia with conversion to myofibroblasts. These cells can produce a matrix of fibrous and basement membrane collagen. Contraction of this collagen matrix will cause wrinkles in the posterior capsule, with resultant distortion of vision and glare.

The reported incidence of posterior capsule opacification varies widely and seems to be diminishing with current IOL design and placement. Analysis of pooled multiple reports prior to 1995 found the overall rate of visually significant posterior capsule opacification to be approximately 28% at 5 years. Factors thought to influence this rate include the age of the patient, history of intraocular inflammation, presence of exfoliation syndrome, size of the capsulorrhexis, quality of the cortical cleanup, capsular fixation of the implant, design of the lens implant (specifically a reduction in incidence with posterior convex or a truncated square-edge optic design), modification of the lens surface, and time elapsed since surgery. There seems to be no difference in PCO rates with prolonged use of postoperative topical corticosteroids or NSAIDs. Mitotic inhibitors instilled in the capsular bag reduce capsular opacification but are rarely used clinically. The presence of intraocular silicone oil may dramatically speed the progression of opacity.

The IOL material has a modest effect on opacification rates: hydrogel IOLs have the highest rate, followed by PMMA, then silicone and hydrophobic acrylic material with the lowest rate. However, the IOL design is now considered the dominant factor in inhibiting the posterior migration of lens epithelial cells and influencing the rate of PCO. Truncated-edge design is associated with lower rates of PCO in both silicone and acrylic IOLs, although these lenses may increase the incidence of undesirable optical reflections and positive dysphotopsias.

Apple DJ, Peng Q, Visessook N, et al. Eradication of posterior capsule opacification: documentation of a marked decrease in Nd:YAG laser posterior capsulotomy rates noted in an analysis of 5416 pseudophakic human eyes obtained postmortem. *Ophthalmology.* 2001;108(3):505–518.

Apple DJ, Solomon KD, Tetz MR, et al. Posterior capsule opacification. *Surv Ophthalmol.* 1992;37(2):73–116.

Daynes T, Spencer TS, Doan K, Mamalis N, Olson RJ. Three-year clinical comparison of 3-piece AcrySof and SI-40 silicone intraocular lenses. *J Cataract Refract Surg.* 2002; 28(7):1124–1129.

Dewey S. Posterior capsule opacification. *Curr Opin Ophthalmol.* 2006;17(1):45–53.

Hollick EJ, Spalton DJ, Ursell PG, et al. The effect of polymethylmethacrylate, silicone, and polyacrylic intraocular lenses on posterior capsular opacification 3 years after cataract surgery. *Ophthalmology*. 1999;106(1):49–55.

Rönbeck M, Zetterström C, Wejde G, Kugelberg M. Comparison of posterior capsule opacification development with 3 intraocular lens types: five-year prospective study. *J Cataract Refract Surg*. 2009;35(11):1935–1940.

Schaumberg DA, Dana MR, Christen WG, Glynn RJ. A systematic overview of the incidence of posterior capsule opacification. *Ophthalmology*. 1998;105(7):1213–1221.

Anterior Capsule Fibrosis and Phimosis

Capsular fibrosis is associated with clouding of the anterior capsule. If a substantial portion of the IOL optic is covered by the opaque anterior capsule, including portions exposed through the undilated pupil, the patient may become symptomatic. Symptoms may include glare, especially at night owing to physiologic mydriasis in darkness, or the sensation of a peripheral cloud or haze.

The term *capsular phimosis* is used to describe the postoperative contraction of the anterior capsule opening as a result of fibrosis. Phimosis produces symptoms similar to and often more pronounced than those of fibrosis itself and may cause stress on the zonular fibers or decentration of an IOL optic. Anterior capsule contraction and fibrosis occur more frequently with smaller capsulorrhexis openings, in patients with underlying exfoliation syndrome, in other situations with abnormal or asymmetric zonular support (eg, penetrating or blunt trauma, Marfan syndrome, or surgical trauma), and with silicone rather than acrylic IOL material. Anterior capsule contraction may lead to or hasten late pseudophakodonesis or in-the-bag IOL subluxation due to stress on the zonular apparatus.

Capsular phimosis can be treated with several radial Nd:YAG-laser anterior capsulotomies to release the annular contraction, reduce the traction on the zonular fibers, and enlarge the anterior capsule opening (Fig 8-8). This procedure is performed in a fashion similar to a Nd:YAG-laser posterior capsulotomy, with care taken not to defocus too far posteriorly and damage the underlying IOL with laser pitting. In general, the anterior capsule tissue or a fibrotic ring is tougher and requires more laser power than does the posterior capsule.

Nd:YAG Laser Capsulotomy

Use of the Nd:YAG laser is now a standard procedure for the treatment of secondary opacification of the posterior capsule or contraction of the anterior capsule. However, a discission knife can be used through an *ab externo* corneal incision to open an opacified capsule in special cases.

Indications

The following are indications for Nd:YAG capsulotomy:

- best-corrected visual acuity symptomatically decreased as a result of a hazy posterior capsule
- a hazy posterior capsule preventing the clear view of the ocular fundus required for diagnostic or therapeutic purposes

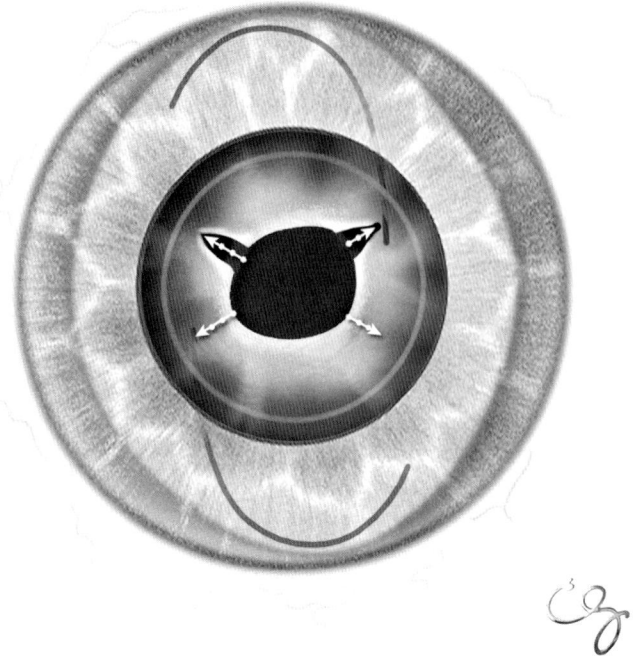

Figure 8-8 Nd:YAG laser anterior capsulotomy. Multiple radial anterior capsulotomies can relieve anterior capsule phimosis and traction on the zonular fibers. *(Illustration by Christine Gralapp.)*

- monocular diplopia, a Maddox rod–like effect, or glare caused by wrinkling of the posterior capsule or by encroachment of a partially opened posterior capsule into the visual axis
- contraction of anterior capsulotomy (capsular phimosis), causing encroachment on the visual axis, excessive traction on the zonular fibers, or alteration of the lens optic position

Contraindications

The following are contraindications to Nd:YAG laser capsulotomy:

- inadequate visualization of the posterior capsule
- an uncooperative patient who is unable to remain still or hold fixation during the procedure (use of a contact lens or retrobulbar anesthesia may enhance the feasibility of a capsulotomy in some of these patients)
- active intraocular inflammation, uncontrolled glaucoma, high risk for retinal detachment, suspected CME, and so forth (relative contraindications)

Procedure

Observation of the posterior capsule through an undilated pupil can help the surgeon pinpoint the location of the visual axis. The center of the visual axis is the desired site for the opening, which is usually adequate at 3–4 mm in diameter. In some circumstances, larger-diameter openings may be required for more complete visualization of the fundus. Dilation is not always necessary for the procedure, but it may be helpful in producing a larger opening in the posterior capsule. When viewing the posterior capsule, the surgeon should note *before* dilation any specific landmarks near the visual axis, because the location of the visual axis may not be obvious through the dilated pupil.

A high-plus-power anterior segment laser lens, used with topical anesthesia, improves ocular stability and enlarges the cone angle of the beam, reducing the depth of focus. The smaller-focus diameter facilitates the laser pulse puncture of the capsule, and structures in front of and behind the point of focus are less likely to be damaged.

Capsulotomy can be performed in a spiral (Fig 8-9A), cruciate (Fig 8-9B), or inverted D-shaped pattern, beginning in the periphery to reduce the chance of pitting the central optic until ideal energy levels and focus have been established. Occasional reports of IOL dislocation into the vitreous following capsulotomy have been of concern, particularly with silicone plate-haptic lenses. Constructing the capsulotomy in a spiraling circular pattern, rather than in a cruciate pattern, creates an opening less likely to extend radially and reduces the risk of dislocation.

If the energy output applied is minimal, the anterior vitreous face may remain intact. A ruptured anterior vitreous face will usually be kept in check by the presence of a posterior chamber IOL, although vitreous strands occasionally migrate around the lens and through the pupil.

Any posterior chamber IOL can be damaged by laser energy, but the threshold for lens damage appears to be lower for silicone than for other materials. The laser pulse should be focused just behind the posterior capsule, although pulses too far behind the IOL will be ineffective. The safest approach is to focus the laser beam slightly behind the posterior surface of the capsule for the initial application and then move subsequent applications anteriorly until the desired puncture is achieved.

In cases of anterior capsule contraction, multiple relaxing incisions of the fibrotic ring are applied to relieve the contracting force and create a larger optical opening (see Fig 8-8). Cycloplegic drugs are not routinely necessary. Some surgeons prescribe preoperative and postoperative antiglaucoma medications; others prescribe NSAIDs to reduce the risk of postprocedure CME.

The success rate of Nd:YAG laser capsulotomy appears to exceed 95%. Occasionally, opacification that is exceptionally thick and dense is not affected by the Nd:YAG laser; these patients may require an invasive surgical procedure using a discission knife or scissors.

In addition to capsulotomy, the Nd:YAG laser can also be used for vitreolysis, synechialysis, iris cystotomy, coreoplasty, iridotomy, rupture of the hyaloid face for ciliary block, removal of precipitates and membranes from an IOL surface, and liquefaction of retained cortical material.

Complications

Complications of Nd:YAG laser capsulotomy include transient or long-term increased IOP, retinal detachment, CME, hyphema, damage to the IOL, dislocation of the IOL, corneal edema, and corneal abrasions (from the focusing contact lens for the laser surgery). Transient elevation of IOP can appear in a significant number of patients and may be treated prophylactically with a topical aqueous suppressant. Pressure levels peak within 2 to 3 hours. This elevation appears to be a consequence of obstruction of the outflow

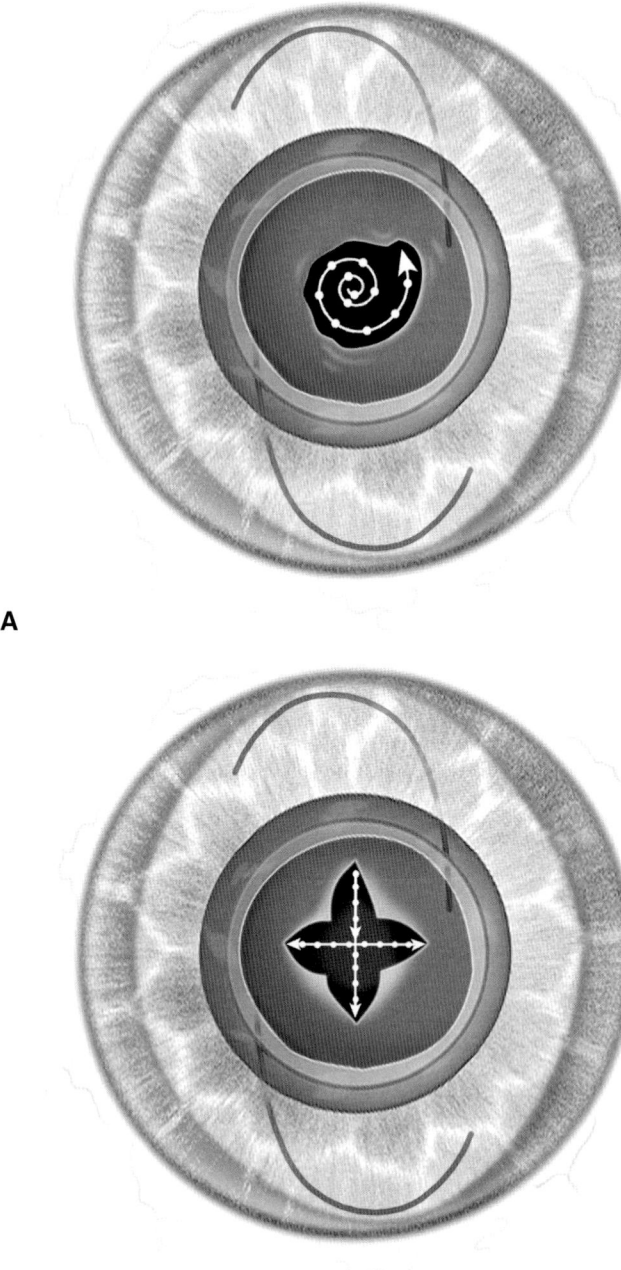

Figure 8-9 Nd:YAG laser posterior capsulotomy. A spiral pattern **(A)** may reduce the risk of radial tears, but a cruciate pattern **(B)** or an inverted D pattern (not shown) with an inferior flap hinge allows for initial punctures in the periphery and may help reduce the risk of central IOL laser damage. *(Illustration by Christine Gralapp.)*

pathways by debris or macromolecules scattered by the laser treatment; it is more common in eyes with vitreous prolapse, without in-the-bag fixation of the IOL, or with preexisting glaucoma. Elevations respond quickly to topical glaucoma medications, which can be continued for 3 to 5 days following the procedure.

Nd:YAG laser capsulotomy may increase the risk of retinal detachment, with a reported incidence of 0.1% to 3.6%. Approximately half of the retinal detachments following cataract extraction occur within 1 year of capsulotomy, often associated with a posterior vitreous detachment (PVD). In many cases, it is difficult to ascertain whether the retinal detachment is related to the capsulotomy or to the cataract surgery itself or is just a consequence of a naturally occurring PVD. High myopia, vitreous trauma, a family history of retinal detachment, and preexisting pathology are factors that increase the risk of retinal detachment following Nd:YAG capsulotomy. Routine dilated fundoscopy is unlikely to detect retinal pathology that requires surgery in the absence of symptoms, but all patients at increased risk for retinal detachment should be instructed to report promptly any new symptoms suggesting a PVD or retinal tear.

CME can occur following Nd:YAG capsulotomy. In patients with a history of CME, or in high-risk patients such as those with diabetic retinopathy, the use of topical steroids and nonsteroidal anti-inflammatory agents (before and after treatment) may be beneficial. Nd:YAG capsulotomy should be delayed at least 3 months postoperatively when a silicone plate-haptic lens is present to increase the likelihood of capsular fixation and decrease the chance of posterior dislocation.

> American Academy of Ophthalmology Cataract and Anterior Segment Panel. Preferred Practice Pattern Guidelines. *Cataract in the Adult Eye*. San Francisco: American Academy of Ophthalmology; 2011. Available at: www.aao.org/ppp.
>
> Jahn CE, Richter J, Jahn AH, Kremer G, Kron M. Pseudophakic retinal detachment after uneventful phacoemulsification and subsequent neodymium: YAG capsulotomy for capsule opacification. *J Cataract Refract Surg.* 2003;29(5):925–929.
>
> Javitt JC, Tielsch JM, Canner JK, Kolb MM, Sommer A, Steinberg EP. National outcomes of cataract extraction: increased risk of retinal complications associated with Nd:YAG laser capsulotomy: the Cataract Patient Outcomes Research Team. *Ophthalmology.* 1992;99(10):1497–1498.
>
> Olsen G, Olson RJ. Update on a long-term, prospective study of capsulotomy and retinal detachment rates after cataract surgery. *J Cataract Refract Surg.* 2000;26(7):1017–1021.
>
> Tuft SJ, Minassian D, Sullivan P. Risk factors for retinal detachment after cataract surgery: a case-control study. *Ophthalmology.* 2006;113(4):650–656.

Hemorrhage

Systemic Anticoagulation

A large prospective cohort study did not show an increased risk of hemorrhagic complications in patients on anticoagulant or antiplatelet therapy during cataract surgery. In addition, no increase in the risk of medical complications was observed when such therapy was temporarily discontinued for surgery. This result is in contrast to earlier reports, which suggested that anticoagulation increases the risk of suprachoroidal effusion and suprachoroidal hemorrhage, and to more recent reports that cessation of anticoagulation therapy carries significant risks of thromboembolic complications. In general, patients undergoing cataract surgery with topical or sub-Tenon anesthesia do not require cessation of anticoagulant therapy. If the surgeon is considering discontinuation of anticoagulants, consultation with the patient's primary care physician is recommended.

> Katz J, Feldman MA, Bass EB, et al; Study of Medical Testing for Cataract Surgery Team. Risks and benefits of anticoagulant and antiplatelet medication use before cataract surgery. *Ophthalmology.* 2003;110(9):1784–1788.
>
> Kobayashi H. Evaluation of the need to discontinue antiplatelet and anticoagulant medications before cataract surgery. *J Cataract Refract Surg.* 2010;36(7):1115–1119.

Retrobulbar Hemorrhage

Retrobulbar hemorrhages are more common with retrobulbar anesthetic injections than with peribulbar injections, and they may vary in intensity. Reports estimate the incidence of significant retrobulbar hemorrhage to be 0.44% to 0.74%.

Venous retrobulbar hemorrhages are usually self-limited and tend to spread slowly. They often do not require treatment.

Arterial retrobulbar hemorrhages occur more rapidly and are associated with taut orbital swelling, marked proptosis, elevated IOP, reduced mobility of the globe, inability to separate the eyelids, and massive ecchymosis of the eyelids and conjunctiva. This type of retrobulbar hemorrhage causes an increase in orbital volume and associated orbital pressure, which can restrict the vascular supply to the globe. Large orbital vessels may be occluded. Tamponade of the smaller nutrient vessels in the optic nerve may occur, resulting in severe vision loss from anterior ischemic optic neuropathy and subsequent optic atrophy, despite the absence of obvious retinal vascular occlusion.

Ophthalmologists can often make the diagnosis of retrobulbar hemorrhage by observing the rapid onset of eyelid and conjunctival ecchymosis and tightening of the orbit. The diagnosis can be confirmed by tonometry revealing elevated IOP. Direct ophthalmoscopy may reveal pulsation or occlusion of the central retinal artery in severe cases.

Treatment of acute retrobulbar hemorrhage consists of maneuvers to lower the orbital and intraocular pressure as quickly as possible. These may include digital massage, intravenous osmotic agents, aqueous suppressants, lateral canthotomy and cantholysis, localized conjunctival peritomy (to allow egress of blood), and, occasionally, anterior chamber paracentesis. Serial tonometry demonstrating a reduction in IOP will help confirm the success of the treatment. Without demonstration of normalization of IOP and mobility of the globe, surgery should be postponed. In general, cataract surgery should not be performed when a serious retrobulbar hemorrhage occurs, as the risk of iris prolapse or even an expulsive choroidal hemorrhage is far greater than usual. The surgery can be rescheduled for several days later. To reduce the risk of a recurrent retrobulbar hemorrhage, many surgeons would consider using peribulbar, sub-Tenon, topical, or general anesthesia for the second attempt at surgery.

In addition to retrobulbar hemorrhage, there have been reports of central retinal artery occlusion, ischemic optic neuropathy, toxic neuropathy or myopathy, and inadvertent subdural injections after retrobulbar anesthesia (see BCSC Section 1, *Update on General Medicine,* and BCSC Section 6, *Pediatric Ophthalmology and Strabismus*).

> Davis DB II, Mandel MR. Efficacy and complication rate of 16,224 consecutive peribulbar blocks: a prospective multicenter study. *J Cataract Refract Surg.* 1994;20(3):327–337.
>
> Dutton JJ, Hasan SA, Edelhauser HF, Kim T, Springs CL, Broocker G. Anesthesia for intraocular surgery. *Surv Ophthalmol.* 2001;46(2):172–184.
>
> Feibel RM. Current concepts in retrobulbar anesthesia. *Surv Ophthalmol.* 1985;30(2):102–110.
>
> Morgan CM, Schatz H, Vine AK, et al. Ocular complications associated with retrobulbar injections. *Ophthalmology.* 1988;95(5):660–665.

Hyphema

Hyphema in the immediate postoperative period usually originates from the incision or the iris; it is commonly mild and resolves spontaneously. The risk of hyphema is greater in patients with exfoliation syndrome. Resolution may take longer if vitreous is mixed with the blood. The 2 major complications from prolonged hyphema are elevated IOP and corneal blood staining. IOP should be monitored closely and treated medically at first, although it may be difficult to control if the blood is mixed with the OVD used during the procedure.

Hyphema that occurs months to years after surgery usually comes from incision vascularization or erosion of vascular tissue by an IOL. Argon laser photocoagulation of the bleeding vessel, often performed through a goniolens, may stop the bleeding or prevent rebleeding. To reduce the risk of continued or recurrent bleeding, antiplatelet or anticoagulation therapy may be withheld, if medically possible, until the hyphema resolves. Occasionally, it is necessary to reposition or exchange an IOL that comes in contact with iris or angle structures and results in recurrent intraocular hemorrhage or chronic inflammation.

Suprachoroidal Effusion or Hemorrhage

Suprachoroidal effusion with or without suprachoroidal hemorrhage usually occurs intraoperatively but may also occur later. Secure incision closure to prevent hypotony can significantly reduce the postoperative risk of this complication. Typically, a forward prolapse of posterior ocular structures including iris and vitreous occurs, generally accompanied by a change in the red reflex. Clinically, suprachoroidal effusion may be difficult to differentiate from suprachoroidal hemorrhage. Patient agitation and pain followed by an extremely firm globe suggest suprachoroidal hemorrhage. Both complications are more common in the presence of associated hypertension, arteriosclerotic cardiovascular disease, tachycardia, obesity, high myopia, glaucoma, advanced age, nanophthalmos, choroidal hemangioma associated with Sturge-Weber syndrome, or chronic ocular inflammation. Fortunately, both suprachoroidal effusion and suprachoroidal hemorrhage are much less likely with phacoemulsification because the relatively closed system formed by the architecture of the small, self-sealing incisions and the relatively tight fit of the phaco tip in the incision avoids prolonged hypotony and reduces intraoperative fluctuations in IOP.

Suprachoroidal effusion may be a precursor to suprachoroidal hemorrhage. Exudation of fluid from choroidal vasculature ultimately stretches veins or arteries that supply the choroid after coursing through the sclera. If suprachoroidal hemorrhage occurs in this situation, it is presumably a result of disruption of one or more of these taut blood vessels. Alternatively, suprachoroidal hemorrhage may represent a spontaneous rupture of choroidal vasculature, particularly in patients with underlying systemic vascular disease. (See BCSC Section 12, *Retina and Vitreous*.)

Expulsive Suprachoroidal Hemorrhage

Expulsive suprachoroidal hemorrhage, a rare but serious problem, generally occurs intraoperatively. It requires immediate action. This condition usually presents as a sudden increase in IOP accompanied by acute onset of pain and the following:

- darkening of the red reflex
- incision gape
- iris prolapse
- expulsion of the lens, vitreous, and bright red blood

The instant this condition is recognized, the surgeon must close the incision with sutures or digital pressure. Prolapsed vitreous should be removed, and uveal tissue reposited. After secure wound closure, posterior sclerotomies may be considered to allow the escape of suprachoroidal blood to decompress the globe, allow the repositioning of prolapsed intraocular tissue, and facilitate permanent closure of the cataract incision. Drainage of suprachoroidal blood may be achieved by performing sclerotomies in one or more quadrants, 5–7 mm posterior to the limbus. Elevated IOP serves both to stop bleeding and to expel suprachoroidal blood. Once there is optimal clearance of blood from the suprachoroidal space, the sclerotomies may be left open to allow further drainage postoperatively. It may be necessary to repeat the drainage procedure 7 days or more after an expulsive hemorrhage in cases of residual suprachoroidal blood that threatens ocular integrity or visual acuity. These procedures may lower dangerously elevated IOPs and restore appropriate anatomical relationships within the eye, but they carry some risk that bleeding will recur.

If the incision can be closed without posterior sclerotomies, more-rapid tamponade of the bleeding vessel can be achieved. Most surgeons would then terminate the operation and observe for 7 to 14 days to allow clotting and liquefaction of the hemorrhage, while managing elevated IOP medically. Referral to a vitreoretinal surgeon for management and subsequent drainage of choroidal hemorrhage should be considered. The patient needs to be informed of the extremely guarded prognosis for restoration of vision.

Delayed Suprachoroidal Hemorrhage

Less commonly, suprachoroidal hemorrhage may occur in the early postoperative period, presenting with sudden onset of pain, loss of vision, and shallowing of the anterior chamber. Predisposing factors for postoperative choroidal hemorrhage or effusion include hypotony, wound leak, unrecognized scleral perforation, trauma, uveitis, cyclodialysis, excessive filtration, or following laser photocoagulation or cryotherapy. If the incision remains intact and the IOP can be controlled medically, limited suprachoroidal hemorrhage may be observed and frequently will resolve spontaneously. If the incision is not intact, surgical revision alone may be sufficient to allow the hemorrhage to resolve. Surgical drainage of the suprachoroidal space is indicated if a flat anterior chamber, medically uncontrolled glaucoma, adherent (kissing) choroidals, or a choroidal detachment persists. Medical management consists of systemic corticosteroids, topical and oral ocular hypotensive agents for elevated IOP, topical cycloplegia, and close observation.

Endophthalmitis

Endophthalmitis is a rare but dreaded complication of cataract surgery that may lead to severe loss of vision or loss of the eye. Early diagnosis and prompt treatment are essential for achieving a satisfactory outcome. Large retrospective studies of the incidence of endophthalmitis after cataract surgery reveal rates between 0.04% and 0.22%. A comprehensive review of 440,000 consecutive cataract surgeries performed in Canada from 2002 to 2006 revealed an incidence of 0.14%. Factors that increase the risk of infection include diabetes mellitus, complicated or prolonged surgery, vitreous loss, posterior capsule rupture, and wound leaks.

Infectious endophthalmitis may present in an acute form or in a more indolent or chronic form; the latter is associated with organisms of lower pathogenicity. The symptoms of endophthalmitis include mild to severe ocular pain, vision loss, floaters, and photophobia. The hallmark of endophthalmitis is vitreous inflammation, but other signs include eyelid or periorbital edema, ciliary injection, chemosis, anterior chamber reaction, hypopyon, decreased visual acuity, corneal edema, and retinal hemorrhages (Fig 8-10). The majority of cases present within 3 to 10 days after surgery, with a median of 6 days in the Endophthalmitis Vitrectomy Study. A significant percentage (22%) presented 2 to

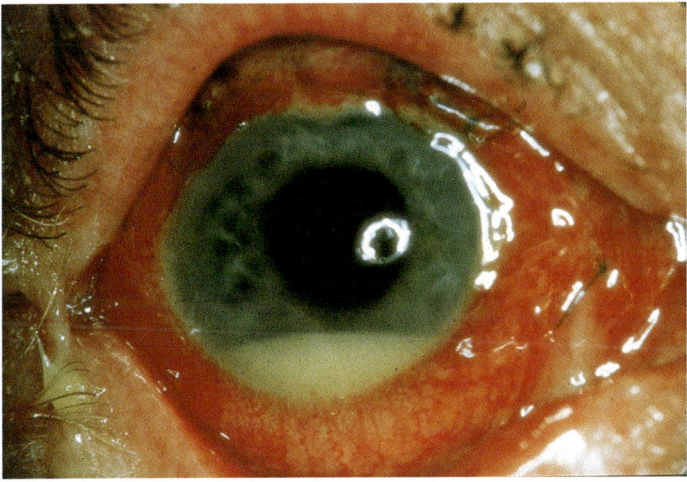

Figure 8-10 Endophthalmitis. *(Courtesy of Karla J. Johns, MD.)*

6 weeks after surgery. The most common bacterial causes in that study were gram-positive coagulase-negative *Staphylococcus epidermidis* (70%), *Staphylococcus aureus* (9.9%), *Streptococcus* (9.0%), other gram-positive (3.1%), *Enterococcus* (2.2%), and gram-negative (5.9%). Most infections are due to organisms similar to the patients' own periocular bacterial flora. Drug-resistant strains are becoming more common.

Meticulous attention to watertight incision closure is an important element of endophthalmitis prevention, particularly when clear corneal incisions are employed. The effectiveness of antibiotics in the prevention of endophthalmitis has been controversial. Topical therapy for 1 to 3 days prior to surgery can reduce bacterial counts but has not been shown to reduce the incidence of infection. In 2006, the Endophthalmitis Study Group of the European Society of Cataract and Refractive Surgeons reported a decrease in endophthalmitis rates from 0.34% to 0.07% in patients given intracameral cefuroxime 1 mg at the conclusion of surgery compared to those given topical levofloxacin drops alone. The high incidence of infection in the control group has confounded the results. Although the practice is not universally accepted, many surgeons routinely use intracameral antibiotics such as vancomycin, moxifloxacin, or a broad-spectrum cephalosporin. Given the difficulty of obtaining commercially available preservative-free antibiotics in doses appropriate for intracameral prophylaxis, surgeons must weigh these results against the risk of TASS from dilutional errors or preservative toxicity.

Diagnosis

Acute endophthalmitis typically develops 3 to 7 days postoperatively and runs a fulminant course. Decreasing vision and increasing pain and inflammation are hallmarks. Early diagnosis is extremely important, as delay of treatment can substantially alter the visual prognosis.

Chronic endophthalmitis, in contrast, may have its onset weeks or months after surgery. It may be characterized by chronic iridocyclitis or granulomatous uveitis and is often associated with decreased visual acuity, little or no pain, and the presence of a nidus of the infectious agent within the eye. The most common causes are *Propionibacterium acnes, S epidermidis,* and fungi. (See also BCSC Section 9, *Intraocular Inflammation and Uveitis,* and BCSC Section 12, *Retina and Vitreous.*)

Acute infectious endophthalmitis must be differentiated from TASS (discussed previously). The clinical presentation is often diagnostic but, at times, the clinician may only diagnose sterile endophthalmitis by excluding possible infectious causes by means of appropriate aqueous and vitreous cultures.

Treatment

The recommended approach to the diagnosis and management of postoperative endophthalmitis is based on the results of the Endophthalmitis Vitrectomy Study. As soon as a clinical diagnosis of endophthalmitis is suspected, assessment of visual acuity will help direct management decisions. Needle biopsy for anterior chamber and vitreous samples for culture and gram stain will help determine the appropriate antibiotic selection. Fortified topical antibiotics may be started if doing so does not delay referral to a vitreoretinal specialist. Immediate pars plana vitrectomy and antibiotic injections are indicated when the patient's visual acuity has been reduced to light perception.

When the visual acuity is hand motions or better, a less-invasive anterior chamber and vitreous biopsy for cultures with subsequent intravitreal injection of antibiotics may be sufficient. To expedite the delivery of antibiotics, this procedure can be performed in the office if sterile conditions can be achieved. Because clinical features do not distinguish between gram-positive and gram-negative organisms, the mainstay of treatment for both remains broad-spectrum intravitreal antibiotics. Currently, vancomycin 1 mg and ceftazidime 2.25 mg or amikacin 0.4 mg are preferred. Fortified topical and subconjunctival antibiotics are administered in the period following intravitreal antibiotic injection while waiting for culture results. Topical cycloplegic and frequent corticosteroid drops are advised. Intravenous or oral antibiotics have shown little benefit, although bactericidal aqueous and intravitreal concentrations of parenteral fourth-generation fluoroquinolones have been documented. Although intravitreal corticosteroids are frequently used because of their theoretical role in reducing inflammation and scarring, their benefit has yet to be demonstrated in a controlled study.

Chronic or delayed-onset endophthalmitis is also best treated with vitreous biopsy and intraocular antibiotics. However, due to sequestration of infectious material in the capsular bag or vitreous, a vitrectomy and posterior capsulectomy or even IOL exchange is often necessary to remove the nidus of infection.

See BCSC Section 12, *Retina and Vitreous*, for additional discussion.

> Doft BH. Managing infectious endophthalmitis: results of the Endophthalmitis Vitrectomy Study. *Focal Points: Clinical Modules for Ophthalmologists*. San Francisco: American Academy of Ophthalmology; 1997, module 3.
>
> Endophthalmitis Study Group, European Society of Cataract and Refractive Surgeons (ESCRS). Prophylaxis of postoperative endophthalmitis following cataract surgery: results of the ESCRS multicenter study and identification of risk factors. *J Cataract Refract Surg.* 2007;33(6):978–988.
>
> Hatch WV, Cernat G, Wong D, Devenyi R, Bell CM. Risk factors for acute endophthalmitis after cataract surgery: a population-based study. *Ophthalmology*. 2009;116(3):425–430.
>
> Ness T, Kern WV, Frank U, Reinhard T. Postoperative nosocomial endophthalmitis: is perioperative antibiotic prophylaxis advisable? A single centre's experience. *J Hosp Infect.* 2011;78(2):138–142.
>
> Packer M, Chang DF, Dewey SH, et al. Prevention, diagnosis, and management of acute postoperative bacterial endophthalmitis. *J Cataract Refract Surg.* 2011;37(9):1699–1714.

Retinal Complications

Cystoid Macular Edema

Cystoid macular edema (CME) is a common cause of decreased vision after cataract surgery (originally known as *Irvine-Gass syndrome*). Although the pathogenesis of CME is unknown, the final common pathway appears to be increased perifoveal capillary permeability with accumulation of fluid in the inner nuclear and outer plexiform layers. CME is often associated with intraocular inflammation and may be mediated through the release of prostaglandins and leukotrienes. Associated intraoperative risk factors include vitreomacular traction, excessive exposure to ultraviolet (UV) light, posterior capsule rupture, vitreous loss, iris prolapse, and transient or prolonged hypotony.

CME can be recognized by an otherwise unexplained reduction in visual acuity, by the characteristic petaloid appearance of cystic spaces in the macula on ophthalmoscopy or fluorescein angiography (Fig 8-11A), or by cystic areas of low reflectivity and retinal thickening on spectral domain optical coherence tomography (SD-OCT; Fig 8-11B). Angiographic CME occurs in 40% to 70% of eyes following ICCE and in approximately 1% to 19% of eyes following ECCE via nuclear expression or phacoemulsification. Most of the affected patients are visually asymptomatic. CME after cataract surgery may be associated with some loss of contrast sensitivity even in the absence of reduced Snellen acuity.

If the diagnosis of clinical CME is based on vision loss to the 20/40 level or worse, the incidence is 2% to 10% following intracapsular surgery and 1% to 2% following extracapsular surgery with an intact posterior capsule. The risk of clinical CME after phacoemulsification with an intact posterior capsule is believed to be even lower. However, patients with angiographic CME after phacoemulsification score significantly lower in logMAR (logarithm of minimum angle of resolution) visual acuity than do patients with no CME, even though their Snellen visual acuities remain better than 20/40.

The peak incidence of both angiographic and clinical CME occurs 6 to 10 weeks after surgery. Spontaneous resolution occurs in approximately 95% of uncomplicated cases, usually within 6 months. In rare cases, CME may develop many years after ICCE, especially in association with delayed postoperative rupture of the anterior vitreous face. CME has also been associated with the use of epinephrine and dipivefrin topically for the treatment of aphakic glaucoma. Prostaglandin analogues have been associated with reversible CME in eyes that have undergone recent intraocular surgery, although a cause-and-effect relationship has not been established. The risk is believed to be greater in the absence of an intact posterior capsule. Although glaucoma medications may be associated with CME, at times the need to prevent elevation of IOP outweighs the risk of CME. Other risk

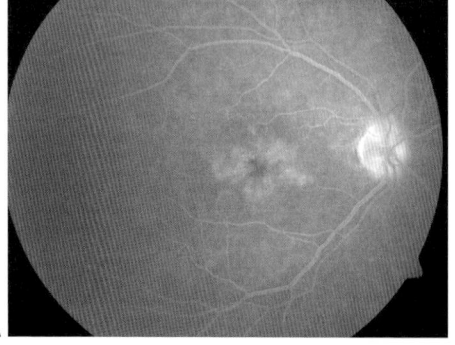 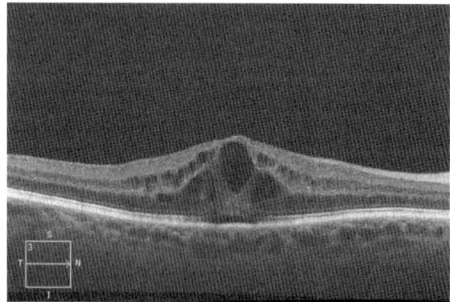

Figure 8-11 Cystoid macular edema. **A,** Fluorescein angiogram demonstrates late pooling of dye in a petaloid pattern in the macula and staining of the optic disc. **B,** Spectral domain optical coherence tomography (SD-OCT) scan shows diffuse retinal thickening with cystic areas of low reflectivity predominantly in the inner nuclear and outer plexiform layers. A nonreflective cavity beneath the neurosensory retina can also be seen. *(Courtesy of Thomas L. Beardsley, MD.)*

factors for CME include poorly controlled postoperative inflammation, coexisting uveitis, preexisting epiretinal membrane, diabetes and diabetic retinopathy, previous retinal vein occlusion, retinitis pigmentosa, and a previous occurrence of CME.

Eyes with improperly sized or malpositioned IOLs in contact with uveal tissue, cornea, or angle structures may have a higher incidence of CME. The presence of a well-positioned posterior chamber IOL in the capsular bag or of a flexible, open-loop anterior chamber IOL does not appear to increase the risk of CME. CME with vision loss occurs more commonly in eyes with prolonged surgery or surgical complications such as posterior capsule rupture and vitreous prolapse, and in eyes with vitreous adhering to the incision, the iris, or the IOL. The risk of CME may be reduced with preoperative and postoperative prophylactic use of topical ketorolac or other NSAID eyedrops. Because most cases of postoperative CME resolve spontaneously, it is difficult to assess the effect of these therapeutic agents. In a prospective randomized controlled clinical trial, topical ketorolac 0.5% or prednisolone acetate 1.0% was demonstrated to be effective therapy for chronic CME, but greater improvement in acuity was obtained with a combination of ketorolac and prednisolone 4 times a day than with either medication alone. If topical medications fail, sub-Tenon or intravitreal injections of corticosteroids may be effective.

Surgical therapy may be indicated when an inciting source of chronic CME can be defined and the edema fails to respond to medical therapy. Any retained lens fragments should be removed. Nd:YAG laser vitreolysis or vitrectomy can be used to remove vitreous adhering to the cataract incision in order to relieve iris deformity or vitreomacular traction. If the IOL is malpositioned and contributing to chronic uveitis, repositioning or exchange may be helpful. For further discussion of CME, see BCSC Section 12, *Retina and Vitreous*.

> Conway MD, Canakis C, Livir-Rallatos C, Peyman GA. Intravitreal triamcinolone acetonide for refractory chronic pseudophakic cystoid macular edema. *J Cataract Refract Surg.* 2003;29(1):27–33.
>
> Donnenfeld ED, Perry HD, Wittpenn JR, Solomon R, Nattis A, Chou T. Preoperative ketorolac tromethamine 0.4% in phacoemulsification outcomes: pharmacokinetic-response curve. *J Cataract Refract Surg.* 2006;32(9):1474–1482.
>
> Heier JS, Topping TM, Baumann W, Dirks MS, Chern S. Ketorolac versus prednisolone versus combination therapy in the treatment of acute pseudophakic cystoid macular edema. *Ophthalmology.* 2000;107(11):2034–2038.
>
> Ursell PG, Spalton DJ, Whitcup SM, Nussenblatt RB. Cystoid macular edema after phacoemulsification: relationship to blood–aqueous barrier damage and visual acuity. *J Cataract Refract Surg.* 1999;25(11):1492–1497.
>
> Wand M, Shields BM. Cystoid macular edema in the era of ocular hypotensive lipids. *Am J Ophthalmol.* 2002;133(3):393–397.

Retinal Light Toxicity

Prolonged exposure to the illuminating filament of the operating microscope can result in an increased risk of CME or a burn to the retinal pigment epithelium (RPE). The risk of an RPE burn is particularly high during cataract surgery, when the filtering effects of the natural lens (cataract) are removed, exposing the vulnerable RPE to unfiltered blue light and near-UV radiation. If the burn occurs in the fovea, visual acuity may be reduced. If the burn is extrafoveal, the patient may complain of a paracentral scotoma. Minimizing retinal exposure to the operating microscope light is the key to avoiding this complication.

Actions to reduce the risk of retinal photic injury include the following:

- Use the minimum light intensity needed to perform the procedure safely.
- Replace lamps with manufacturer-approved products.
- Add a filter to exclude light below 515 nm.
- Use oblique lighting, when possible.
- Use pupillary shields, either built into the microscope or placed on the cornea.
- Minimize direct exposure of the fovea.

Retinal Photic Injuries From Operating Microscopes During Cataract Surgery: FDA Public Health Advisory. Rockville, MD: US Dept of Health and Human Services; 1995.

Retinal Detachment

Rhegmatogenous retinal detachment (RRD) occurs in 2.0% to 3.0% of eyes following ICCE, in 0.5% to 2.0% of eyes following ECCE, and in less than 1.0% of eyes following phacoemulsification. RRD occurs most frequently within 1 year of cataract surgery or 6 months following posterior capsulotomy.

Most acute RRDs are subsequent to a posterior vitreous detachment (PVD). Uncomplicated cataract surgery and laser posterior capsulotomy are risk factors for RRD primarily because these procedures are risk factors for earlier onset of PVD. Pseudophakic eyes do not appear to be at increased risk for retinal tears from PVD compared to age-matched and axial length–matched phakic eyes.

Predisposing and nonmodifiable risk factors for RRD include axial myopia (>25 mm), younger age, male sex, lattice degeneration of the retina, a previous retinal tear or detachment in the surgical eye, a history of retinal detachment in the fellow eye, or a family history of retinal detachment. The presence of any of these factors should make the surgeon more vigilant in examining the peripheral fundus in these patients before and after surgery. The risk factors should also be considered in the decision to treat asymptomatic retinal breaks preoperatively.

The presence of an intact posterior capsule reduces the incidence of RRD. Conversely, complicated cataract surgery with a broken posterior capsule and vitreous loss increases the risk of postoperative RRD. Nd:YAG laser posterior capsulotomy may increase the risk for RRD. The incidence following capsulotomy is estimated to be between 0.1% and 3.6%. Neither the size of the capsulotomy nor the total energy delivered is thought to increase risk. Although no prospective randomized controlled studies confirm this belief, delaying capsulotomy for at least 3 to 6 months after cataract surgery may allow for posterior vitreous separation and be less disruptive to the vitreoretinal interface.

The successful repair of retinal detachment is not influenced by the presence or absence of either an anterior chamber or a posterior chamber IOL. Pars plana vitrectomy with or without a scleral buckle is the preferred procedure for repair of RRD, with approximately 85% success with one operation and ultimately a 98% reattachment rate with multiple procedures. (See also BCSC Section 12, *Retina and Vitreous*.)

> Arya AV, Emerson JW, Engelbert M, Hagedorn CL, Adelman RA. Surgical management of pseudophakic retinal detachments: a meta-analysis. *Ophthalmology.* 2006;113(10): 1724–1733.
>
> Boberg-Ans G, Henning V, Villumsen J, la Cour M. Long-term incidence of rhegmatogenous retinal detachment and survival in a defined population undergoing standardized phacoemulsification surgery. *Acta Ophthalmol Scand.* 2006;84(5):613–618.
>
> Haller JA. Retinal detachment. *Focal Points: Clinical Modules for Ophthalmologists.* San Francisco: American Academy of Ophthalmology; 1998, module 5.
>
> Steinert RF, Puliafito CA, Kumar SR, Dudak SD, Patel S. Cystoid macular edema, retinal detachment, and glaucoma after Nd:YAG laser posterior capsulotomy. *Am J Ophthalmol.* 1991;112(4):373–380.
>
> Tuft SJ, Minassian D, Sullivan P. Risk factors for retinal detachment after cataract surgery: a case-control study. *Ophthalmology.* 2006;113(4):650–656.

Needle Penetration of the Globe

Inadvertent penetration of the globe during ocular anesthesia or periocular injections is more common after retrobulbar injection but may occur with any periocular needle insertion. Factors predisposing to needle penetration of the globe include the following:

- axial myopia
- posterior staphyloma
- previous surgery for scleral buckling
- uncooperative patient
- inexperience in technique
- sharp needles
- retrobulbar location

Management of this complication varies with the severity of the intraocular damage. (See BCSC Section 12, *Retina and Vitreous*.)

> Rodriguez-Coleman H, Spaide R. Ocular complications of needle perforations during retrobulbar and peribulbar injections. *Ophthalmol Clin North Am.* 2001;14(4):573–579.

CHAPTER **9**

Preparing for Cataract Surgery in Special Situations

A complete discussion of the indications for and technique of cataract surgery in the pediatric age group is presented in BCSC Section 6, *Pediatric Ophthalmology and Strabismus*.

Psychosocial Considerations

Claustrophobia

Patients find it helpful to be told about the operating room and sterile-draping requirement prior to their surgery. The medical team can make accommodations for the patient who becomes anxious and extremely uncomfortable when confined to a small space or when the patient's head is covered by a surgical drape. The anesthetist can optimize intravenous sedation and hold the patient's hand to provide comfort and reassurance during surgery. When feasible, the surgeon can supplement topical or local ocular anesthesia with a "vocal local," providing soothing support to the patient. Placing a suction catheter under the drape or tenting open the side of the drape avoids accumulation of carbon dioxide, which can cause even a cooperative patient to become anxious or restless. General anesthesia is chosen when a patient cannot tolerate the aforementioned measures to address claustrophobia.

Dementia or Other Mental Disabilities

When dementia or other central nervous system impairment interferes with a patient's ability to communicate symptoms of cataract, the patient's functional deficit must be evaluated by other methods, such as degradation of the retinoscopic reflex, slit-lamp findings, and view of the retina. The patient's caregiver or family member may provide helpful information about the patient's capacity to carry out activities of daily living. The power to tolerate sedation and draping throughout surgery must be appraised, and general anesthesia should be considered for patients who cannot lie still for surgery. Improving the view into the fundus to monitor and treat retinal disease as well as the potential for vision rehabilitation and improved quality of life remain the foundation for the decision to proceed with cataract extraction in this situation.

Patient Communication During Eye Surgery

Reviewing the mechanics of the surgical experience is beneficial for all patients preoperatively and especially for those who have hearing loss or who do not speak the same language as the surgical team. Patients may wear their hearing aid in the ear opposite to the eye having surgery, both to permit communication and avoid water damage to the hearing aid ipsilateral to the surgical site. The surgeon, anesthesiologist, and patient should determine how best to communicate with each other in the operating room. For example, simple hand signals between the patient and anesthesiologist are effective. If the patient is too anxious and cannot communicate adequately, general anesthesia should be considered instead of topical or local anesthesia.

Systemic Considerations

Medical Status

Medical evaluation by the patient's primary care physician should always be part of the preoperative planning process. Hypertension and diabetes should be stabilized. Because patients are required to fast after midnight before surgery, insulin or oral hypoglycemic medication often requires adjustment in diabetic patients. Procedures on these patients should be performed as early in the day as possible to minimize large fluctuations in blood glucose levels. Pulmonary function in patients with lung disease should be optimized, and patients may be permitted to bring their inhalers into the operating room. Small-incision surgery offers a distinct advantage for wound security and reduced intraoperative complications related to coughing. Coughing during surgery may damage ocular structures and should be controlled judiciously with medication. The patient should be instructed to warn the surgeon of his or her need to cough. Patients with chronic obstructive pulmonary disease (COPD), bronchitis, congestive heart failure, or obesity will benefit from being placed in the reverse Trendelenburg position to reduce venous congestion to the head and neck and lessen the risk of vitreous loss and choroidal hemorrhage. Ocular inflammation such as scleritis and uveitis associated with connective tissue or inflammatory diseases should be controlled to minimize the chance of scleral or corneal necrosis. The ophthalmologist can work in conjunction with the other physicians involved in the patient's care to gauge therapy with systemic corticosteroid and immunosuppressive agents. For a more complete discussion of ocular surgery in patients with systemic disease, see BCSC Section 1, *Update on General Medicine*.

It is more difficult for a patient with severe arthritis to lie comfortably during surgery. Usually, the surgical table can be adjusted and pillows added to provide sufficient patient comfort without interfering with surgical access to the eye. A patient who has ankylosing spondylitis with cervical immobility presents an extreme challenge in surgical positioning (Fig 9-1). If no systemic medical contraindications exist and if adequate access cannot be attained otherwise, the surgeon should consider general anesthesia.

> Katz J, Feldman MA, Bass EB, et al. Injectable versus topical anesthesia for cataract surgery: patient perceptions of pain and side effects. *Ophthalmology*. 2000;107(11):2054–2060.
> Sainz de la Maza M, Vitale AT. Scleritis and episcleritis. *Focal Points: Clinical Modules for Ophthalmologists*. San Francisco: American Academy of Ophthalmology; 2009, module 1.

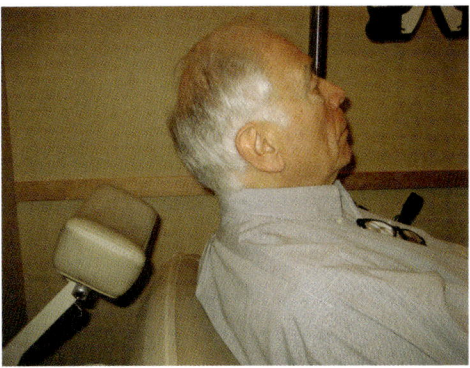 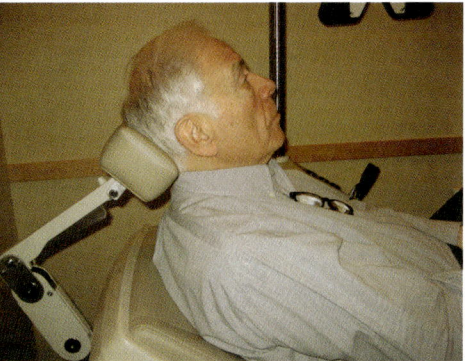

Figure 9-1 Inflammatory systemic disease. Persons with ankylosing spondylitis, such as the patient shown in these photos, often have cervical immobility. Evaluating patients in the office examination chair allows the surgeon to anticipate accommodations necessary for carrying out surgery safely and comfortably for both patient and surgeon in the operating room. This patient requires adjustment of the headrest to provide adequate support of his head and neck. *(Courtesy of Lisa Rosenberg, MD.)*

Anticoagulation Therapy or Bleeding Disorders

When managing patients on chronic anticoagulation therapy, the surgeon and primary care physician should carefully consider the role of this therapy in preventing systemic adverse events such as transient ischemic attack, cerebrovascular accident, myocardial infarction, pulmonary embolus, and failure of vascular bypass grafts—weighing this role against the risk of ocular complications such as suprachoroidal hemorrhage, retrobulbar hemorrhage, and hyphema from use of blood thinners. Retrospective studies have shown that maintenance of anticoagulation is relatively safe in intracapsular cataract extraction (ICCE), extracapsular cataract extraction (ECCE), and small-incision phacoemulsification (phaco). Cataract surgery in patients receiving anticoagulation therapy is not associated with an increased incidence of sight-threatening intraoperative or perioperative ocular bleeding. However, systemic blood thinners can increase the amount of bleeding should it occur. In the setting of anticoagulation, the rate of retrobulbar hemorrhage is 3 times higher when this technique of anesthetic is administered. Choroidal hemorrhage is rare. Minor forms of ocular hemorrhage, such as subconjunctival bleeding, eyelid ecchymosis, or hyphema, are transient and will resolve without additional therapy.

When the decision is made to discontinue anticoagulation therapy or, as an alternative, to bridge warfarin with heparin or low-molecular-weight heparin before surgery, the prescribing physician should decide and carry out the timing and management. Discontinuation of anticoagulation is strongly recommended in patients who have previously experienced a suprachoroidal hemorrhage because these patients are predisposed to recurrent bleeding. The clinician should note that restoring normal coagulation usually requires 3–5 days after stopping warfarin and that restoring platelet function requires at least 10–21 days after stopping antiplatelet therapy. Patients should be questioned about the use of all medications, including nonprescription items such as aspirin and those containing vitamins E and K that could affect coagulation status. Assessment of a coagulation profile prior to surgery should be considered for systemic conditions that might alter clotting ability, such as chronic liver disease, bone marrow suppression, deficiencies in clotting factors, and malabsorption syndrome. For further discussion of ocular hemorrhage, see the section titled "Hemorrhage" in Chapter 8.

> Jonas JB, Pakdaman B, Sauder G. Cataract surgery under systemic anticoagulant therapy with Coumadin. *Eur J Ophthalmol.* 2006;16(1):30–32.
>
> Katz J, Feldman MA, Bass EB, et al; Study of Medical Testing for Cataract Surgery Team. Risks and benefits of anticoagulant and antiplatelet medication use before cataract surgery. *Ophthalmology.* 2003;110(9):1784–1788.
>
> Morris A, Elder MJ. Warfarin therapy and cataract surgery. *Clin Experiment Ophthalmol.* 2000;28(6):419–422.

External Ocular Abnormalities

Blepharitis and Acne Rosacea

Blepharitis should be controlled before surgery in order to reduce the risk of endophthalmitis. Uncontrolled blepharitis causing irritation and an unhealthy tear film may adversely impact the quality of vision after cataract surgery. Signs of anterior blepharitis include crusting and flaking of the eyelid margins and collarettes at the base of the eyelashes. Treatment includes hot compresses and eyelid scrubs with baby shampoo. Nonprescription supportive preparations are available. Posterior blepharitis is manifested by plugging of the meibomian gland and by foaminess and vascularization of the eyelid margin. Systemic tetracycline saponifies inspissated meibomian secretions and is the mainstay of therapy for posterior blepharitis. Although topical ointments poorly penetrate meibomian orifices, newer topical eyedrops such as azithromycin aim to reduce bacterial flora at the surface of the meibomian glands. Injection of the bulbar conjunctiva and hypersensitivity-induced corneal infiltration are consequences of acute or chronic eyelid disease. Patients with acne rosacea are prone to developing blepharitis.

> Novosad BD, Callegan MC. Severe bacterial endophthalmitis: towards improving clinical outcomes. *Expert Rev Ophthalmol.* 2010;5(5):689–698.
>
> Packer M, Chang DF, Dewey SH, et al. Prevention, diagnosis, and management of acute postoperative bacterial endophthalmitis. *J Cataract Refract Surg.* 2011;37(9):1699–1714.
>
> Wykoff CC, Parrott MB, Flynn HW Jr, Shi W, Miller D, Alfonso EC. Nosocomial acute-onset postoperative endophthalmitis at a university teaching hospital (2002–2009). *Am J Ophthalmol.* 2010;150(3):392–398.

Keratoconjunctivitis Sicca

Optimizing dry-eye therapy prior to cataract surgery improves visual outcomes. A variety of aqueous layer supportive treatments can be personalized for each surgical candidate, including topical preserved and nonpreserved liquid tear preparations, gels, and ointments; topical cyclosporine; and punctum plugs. (For a detailed discussion of dry-eye therapy, see BCSC Section 8, *External Disease and Cornea.*) During surgery, desiccation of the corneal epithelium can be prevented by frequently hydrating the area with irrigating solution or by coating the cornea with a topical viscoelastic agent. Visual recovery may be delayed by exacerbation of the patient's dry-eye condition.

Patients with dry eyes associated with collagen vascular disease, pemphigoid, rheumatoid arthritis, or Sjögren syndrome present a special challenge to the cataract surgeon. Close observation of these patients in the weeks following surgery is warranted to identify and treat toxic keratoconjunctivitis and corneal ulceration from collagenase activation by postoperative corticosteroid therapy. Topical nonsteroidal anti-inflammatory drugs (NSAIDs) should not be prescribed for these patients because they are associated with a high risk of corneal melting. In extreme cases, persistent epithelial defects with stromal loss may require a bandage (therapeutic) contact lens, tarsorrhaphy, or amniotic membrane transplant.

> Asai T, Nakagami T, Mochizuki M, Hata N, Tsuchiya T, Hotta Y. Three cases of corneal melting after instillation of a new nonsteroidal anti-inflammatory drug. *Cornea*. 2006;25(2):224–227.
>
> Guidera AC, Luchs JI, Udell IJ. Keratitis, ulceration, and perforation associated with topical nonsteroidal anti-inflammatory drugs. *Ophthalmology*. 2001;108(5):936–944.

Pemphigoid

Eyes with cicatricial pemphigoid suffer from severe dryness due to scarring of meibomian glands and accessory lacrimal glands and occlusion of lacrimal gland orifices. Corneal haze or opacification impairs the surgeon's view into the anterior segment during surgery. Extensive symblepharon or ankyloblepharon may limit positioning and exposure of the eye during surgery. The eyelid speculum must be positioned carefully to avoid traction and pressure on the globe.

Corneal Conditions

Corneal Disease

The cornea is the most important refracting element of the eye. The surgeon should identify corneal abnormalities that might contribute to visual impairment and affect the degree of improvement in visual acuity expected after cataract extraction. Conditions such as dry eye, blepharitis, and epithelial basement membrane dystrophy disrupt the anterior refractive surface of the cornea and may induce irregular astigmatism. An abnormal tear film should be addressed (see previous section, Keratoconjunctivitis Sicca). Trial of a gas-permeable contact lens can mask an irregular astigmatism and help the clinician determine the contribution that astigmatism has on visual impairment.

Corneal irregularities interfere with accurate keratometry and lead to erroneous lens power calculation. In the setting of epithelial basement membrane dystrophy, epithelial debridement may help produce a smoother corneal surface (Fig 9-2). After debridement, it is necessary to wait at least 6 to 8 weeks for the corneal surface to smooth and stabilize before repeating keratometry. Mild corneal stromal opacities in the presence of a pristine anterior refractive surface are unlikely to reduce visual acuity.

When both cataract and corneal opacity contribute to a patient's vision loss, the surgeon has the option of removing the cataract first, repairing the cornea first, or combining the procedures. Removing the cataract first requires adequate visualization of the anterior segment; it may be possible in these circumstances to remove the cataract and monitor

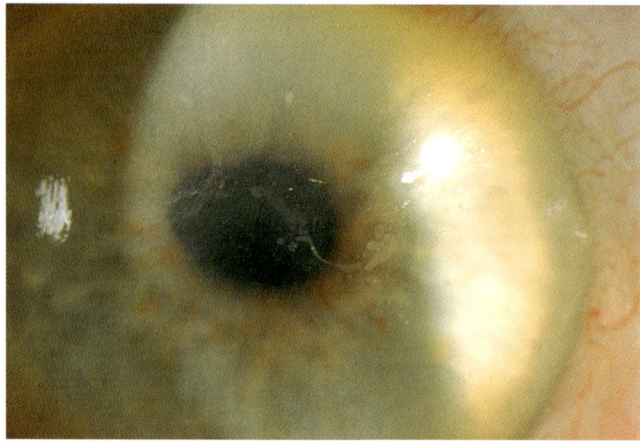

Figure 9-2 Epithelial basement membrane dystrophy. Irregular corneal astigmatism occurs in patients with epithelial basement membrane dystrophy. This corneal condition can further decrease vision in a patient with cataract-related visual impairment, in which case the visual improvement after cataract surgery might be less than expected. *(Courtesy of Christopher J. Rapuano, MD.)*

the patient for worsening corneal opacity. Eyes with endothelial corneal dystrophy are more likely to have diurnal visual fluctuations. If the cornea is clear in the morning, when edema is most likely to be greatest, then the cornea will probably heal following uncomplicated cataract surgery. Depending on the corneal pathology, a penetrating keratoplasty (PK) or an endothelial keratoplasty (EK) may be performed. The advantages of EK in those patients with primarily endothelial disease include faster rehabilitation and more dependable keratometry to calculate intraocular lens (IOL) power, although a hyperopic shift from 0.5 to 1.5 D may be encountered. Predicting correct IOL power after PK is less reliable.

If the cornea is too opaque for cataract surgery alone, then PK may be combined with cataract surgery in a triple procedure, or EK or PK may be performed first. The advantages of the triple procedure include a single visit to the operating room, which reduces the attendant perioperative surgical risks, and relatively rapid rehabilitation. Disadvantages include less-predictable IOL calculation and a period of "open sky," or exposure of intraocular contents prior to replacement of the corneal button.

The advantages of combining EK with cataract surgery include rapid corneal rehabilitation with greater likelihood of regular astigmatism, more-predictable calculation of subsequent IOL power, and relative ease of regrafting. Disadvantages include possible damage to grafted corneal endothelium when the additional entry into the anterior chamber is made and possible disruption of the graft. Corneal surgeons find EK easier to perform in the aphakic or pseudophakic eye than in the phakic eye.

If the cataract is not the primary source of visual impairment, it may still be advisable to remove the cataract at the time of corneal surgery because of the eventual need for cataract removal, the possible progression of cataract due to prolonged postoperative corticosteroid therapy, and the risk of additional damage to the corneal endothelium during secondary surgery.

Cataract Following Keratoplasty

Cataract formation soon after keratoplasty may be caused by lens trauma during the transplantation procedure or by prolonged corticosteroid use to prevent graft rejection. A corneal graft may not survive even routine cataract surgery. A scleral tunnel approach is farther from the corneal transplant and minimizes endothelial trauma during surgery. Before surgery, the surgeon should evaluate the corneal graft for thickening and anticipate reduced intraoperative clarity through the graft. Postoperative graft failure is minimized by protecting the endothelium with a viscoelastic agent during surgery and by treating postoperative inflammation.

Ideally, cataract surgery should be delayed until all PK sutures are removed, the corneal contour and surface are stable, and accurate keratometric readings can be obtained for IOL power selection. Symptomatic anisometropia is risked when IOL power is chosen before the cornea is fully healed. Posterior chamber lenses are preferred because they minimize contact between the optic and the corneal endothelium. If capsular support is inadequate for in-the-bag placement of an IOL, then a posterior chamber lens sutured to the sclera or iris may be placed. Alternatively, if the additional manipulation required for securing a sutured lens risks excessive endothelial trauma, insertion of a flexible anterior chamber IOL is an option. The probability of graft survival 5 years after cataract surgery is at least 80%.

Cataract Following Refractive Surgery

Patients who have undergone corneal refractive surgery and later develop a visually significant cataract present several unique challenges. First, IOL power calculation and visual outcome are less predictable in eyes that have had previous refractive surgery. Irregular astigmatism from a refractive surgical procedure may also compromise the ultimate visual result after cataract removal (Fig 9-3). Therefore, the clinician must thoroughly inform the patient about the limits of precision in lens power calculation and the possible requirement for postsurgical refractive correction to obtain the best visual acuity.

In general, postoperative hyperopia is more commonly encountered after cataract surgery in patients who have undergone previous refractive surgery. The corneal refractive

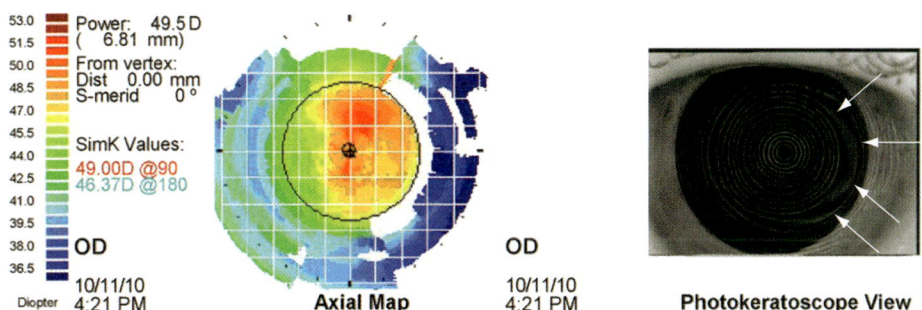

Figure 9-3 Irregular topography. Accurate lens implant power is difficult to determine when the corneal surface is abnormal, as shown here by an irregular corneal topographic map *(left)* and distorted corneal rings *(right, arrows)*. *(Courtesy of Lisa Rosenberg, MD.)*

incisions in radial keratotomy (RK) patients often swell after cataract surgery, thereby flattening the cornea and inducing hyperopia. Swelling may require more than 3 months to resolve. If a corneal cataract incision is chosen, it should be placed between RK incisions. Violating an old RK incision can destabilize the wound, causing it to pull apart. The presence of multiple deep RK incisions or unstable wounds increases the likelihood of anterior chamber shallowing during cataract surgery and makes final closure of the wound difficult. Alternatively, a scleral tunnel incision avoids previous keratotomy wounds. In eyes that have undergone laser in situ keratomileusis (LASIK), the surgeon should take care to avoid disrupting the flap while creating the clear corneal cataract incision. Corneal swelling may require more than 1 month to resolve. Photorefractive keratectomy (PRK) does not present the same technical problems. (For a detailed discussion of IOL power calculation, see Chapter 6 in this volume and BCSC Section 13, *Refractive Surgery*.)

Compromised Visualization of the Lens

Small Pupil

A small pupil minimally responsive to dilating agents may be widened intraoperatively using several different techniques. Bimanual pupil stretching with instruments such as Kuglen or Lester hooks or tethering the iris with hooks (Fig 9-4) or pupil-expansion devices (Fig 9-5) breaks posterior synechiae and releases the pupil sphincter muscle. However, excessive manipulation of the iris with these instruments risks greater postoperative inflammation. Also, the iris tends to be flaccid and floppy after manual stretching and release, and it is more likely to be damaged by the phaco tip. Viscodissection with a high-viscosity ophthalmic viscosurgical device (OVD) is another method to enlarge a pupil.

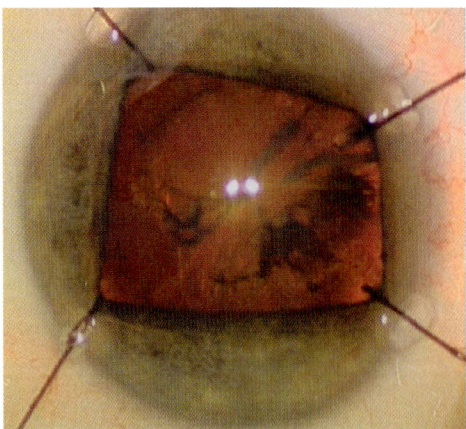 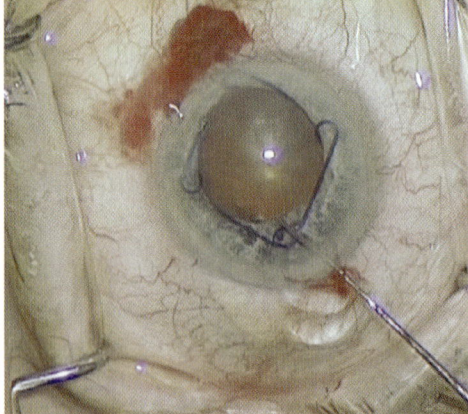

Figure 9-4 Iris hooks. A pupil that dilates insufficiently to permit access to the lens may be widened with iris hooks. Here, 4 hooks are placed to expose the lens for surgery. *(Courtesy of Lisa Rosenberg, MD.)*

Figure 9-5 Malyugin ring. A Malyugin ring is positioned at the pupil margin to open it circumferentially. *(Courtesy of Steven Vold, MD.)*

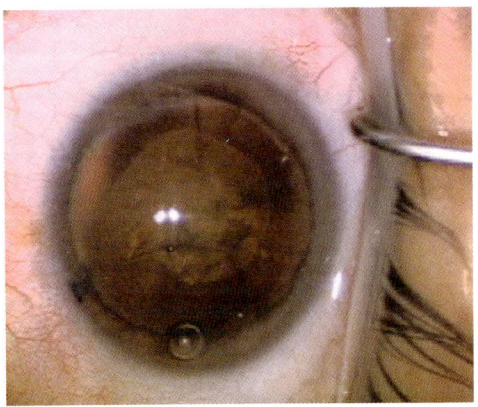

Figure 9-6 Trypan blue solution. The anterior capsule is stained lightly blue by trypan blue, thereby making the capsule easier to see during creation of a capsulorrhexis. This technique is very helpful in eyes with dense brunescent or cortical cataracts that interfere with the red reflex. *(Courtesy of Lisa Rosenberg, MD.)*

Poor Red Reflex

Conditions that cause an abnormal red reflex make it difficult to discriminate the capsular edge, thereby increasing the chance for incomplete or errant capsulorrhexis. The capsule becomes subject to radial tears with brunescent and dense cortical or capsular cataracts. Anterior pressure from hemorrhage or expansion of vitreous volume also affects the capsule. Corneal scars not only compromise the surgeon's view of the capsule but also make intraocular manipulation treacherous.

Trypan blue capsular dye makes visualization and manipulation of the capsule easier (Fig 9-6). Prior to capsulotomy, anterior chamber fluid can be replaced with air tamponaded with a small amount of OVD to occlude the paracentesis site. Trypan blue is then injected through a 27-gauge blunt cannula, starting as far away from the paracentesis as possible to deliver the dye directly to the capsule. The dye is then rinsed out of the anterior chamber with balanced salt solution and replaced with OVD, under which the stained anterior capsule is easily visible as the continuous curvilinear capsulorrhexis (CCC) is created.

Pandey SK, Werner L, Wilson ME Jr, Izak AM, Apple DJ. Anterior capsule staining: techniques, recommendations, and guidelines for surgeons. *Indian J Ophthalmol.* 2002;50(2):157–159.

Altered Lens and Zonular Anatomy

Advanced Cataract

In the case of very advanced, dense, and brunescent cataracts, surgical manipulation increases the chance for iris trauma, zonular tearing, capsular rupture, vitreous loss, and the dropping of lens fragments into the posterior segment. High-energy ultrasound causes corneal endothelial trauma and risks wound burn. It is helpful to create a larger capsulorrhexis to permit maneuvers required to minimize these complications. Thorough hydrodissection and hydrodelineation of the nucleus facilitate smooth rotation during phacoemulsification. When an initial groove is made in the hard nucleus, it is important that the surgeon make a deep and even pass so that the nucleus cracks without leaving interdigitations. These interdigitations would interfere with removal and would be more likely to lead to posterior capsule rupture. Viscodissection helps in separating sticky cortical attachments that impede rotation. A surgeon who uses excessive mechanical force on a nucleus that does not freely rotate risks creating a zonular dialysis from the transmittal of that force to the capsular bag. Mechanical segmentation of the nucleus decreases total ultrasound time, particularly when the lens is divided into very small pieces. Cataract-chopping techniques are effective in such cases.

If cataract surgery by phacoemulsification is no longer an appropriate technique for removing the lens, the clinician should consider converting to an extracapsular technique. The surgeon must decide whether to proceed through the temporal clear corneal incision by enlarging it to permit passage of the cataract and lens implant. Alternatively, the surgeon can close the temporal wound and move to the superior portion of the eye in order to work more comfortably through a new, larger corneoscleral incision, which may induce less astigmatism postoperatively compared to a large corneal wound.

Intumescent Cataract

This type of cataract has become swollen and enlarged with cortical material that often envelops a hard nucleus floating inside the capsular bag. Intumescent cataracts have weak zonular fibers and fragile capsules. Use of trypan blue has made creating the capsulorrhexis in this type of cataract much easier. Intumescence creates positive pressure in the capsular bag, so the initial capsular entry may extend outward toward the lens periphery. High-viscosity OVD exerts pressure on the anterior capsule and maintains chamber depth. OVD also limits the milky cortex from obscuring the surgeon's view of the capsule. Using a cystitome attached to the OVD syringe during creation of the capsular opening enables injection of additional OVD to clear the milky egress away from view while the surgeon works in the anterior chamber. After making the anterior capsule incision with the cystitome, the surgeon can reduce capsular pressure with immediate use of a 27-gauge cannula to aspirate cortical material from the capsular bag. Caution is advised during phacoemulsification because the freely mobile lens makes segmentation challenging.

Iris Coloboma and Corectopia

Zonular dehiscence or absence commonly occurs in the area of iris coloboma or a misshapen pupil (Fig 9-7A). Pharmacologic dilation reveals the extent of zonular abnormality. Iris hooks can be used intraoperatively to pull a flaccid iris out of the way. A capsular tension ring that incorporates a coloboma diaphragm (Fig 9-7B) not only helps stabilize the capsular bag but also serves as an artificial iris diaphragm. The surgeon also has the option to repair the coloboma with a suture at the conclusion of the case.

Posterior Polar Cataract

A weak or absent area of posterior lens capsule in the region of a posterior polar opacity places the eye at increased risk for capsular rupture during surgery. To minimize the likelihood of this complication, the surgeon should avoid creating excessive pressure within

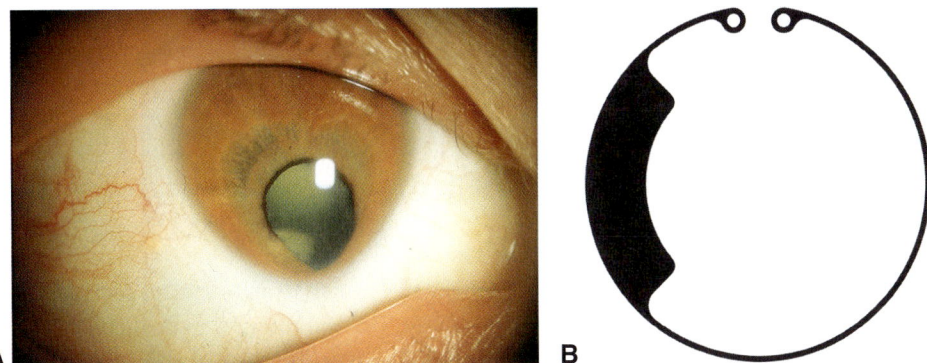

Figure 9-7 **A,** Coloboma of the iris with nuclear cataract. Absent or abnormal zonular fibers correlate with the area of the iris defect. Preoperative evaluation to identify associated posterior segment abnormalities is important in determining visual potential. **B,** A capsular tension ring with coloboma diaphragm. *(Part A courtesy of Robert S. Feder, MD; part B courtesy of Morcher GmbH, Stuttgart.)*

the bag or placing excessive pressure on the posterior capsule. Complete hydrodissection is avoided because of possible tearing of the capsule directly under the opacity. Instead, small volumes of fluid are directed around the cortex up to but not across the opacity. Next, gentle hydrodelineation is carried out, leaving a generous amount of epinuclear bowl in which to mobilize the nucleus and protect the capsule. Anterior chamber depth should be maintained and fluctuations in IOP controlled by low irrigation and aspiration. After the nucleus is removed, OVD is used to viscodissect the epinucleus from the bag. The posterior polar opacity is removed last. It, too, can be viscodissected. If the central portion of the posterior capsule is missing, filling the bag with OVD before removing the irrigating phaco handpiece from the eye stabilizes the chamber for lens insertion. Alternatively, if the posterior polar opacity is very adherent, it can be left in place and assessed for its visual impact postoperatively and treated by laser capsulotomy if indicated. After the surgeon places the IOL in the bag in uncomplicated surgery, care should be used to minimize capsular bag movement with slow and gentle OVD removal.

Zonular Dehiscence With Lens Subluxation or Dislocation

Common causes of zonular incompetence include exfoliation syndrome, ocular trauma, and high myopia (Fig 9-8). Marfan syndrome and inborn errors of metabolism are less-common sources of inadequate zonular support. Iridodonesis detected at the slit lamp may be the initial finding that signals zonular weakness or absence. If the entire lens becomes dislocated into the posterior segment, surgical removal of the lens may not be required unless uveitis develops. In some cases, the remaining zonular fibers may tether the lens within the anterior vitreous such that when the patient sits upright at the slit lamp the lens seems accessible for extraction. However, when the patient is supine during surgery, the lens may tilt backward and out of reach for the anterior segment surgeon. Thus, when iridodonesis or phacodonesis is detected preoperatively, it is helpful to confirm lens position with the patient supine during preoperative examination.

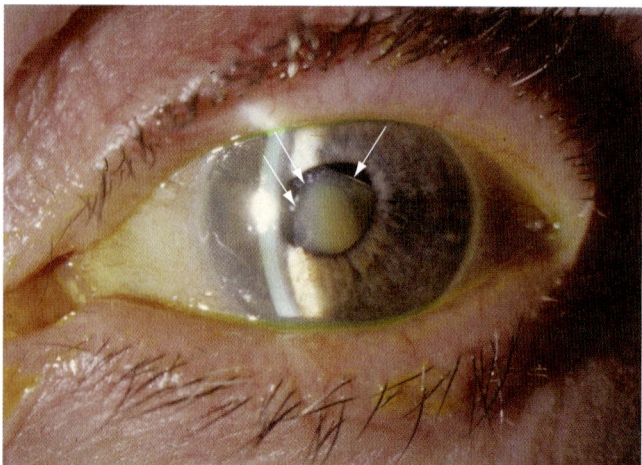

Figure 9-8 Subluxed lens. This lens with exfoliation is displaced inferiorly because zonular fibers at the inferior edge of the lens are stretched, damaged, or broken. *Arrows* indicate the superior edge of the inferiorly displaced lens. Working with a lens displaced out of the central visual axis demands meticulous preoperative planning to minimize surgical complications. *(Courtesy of Lisa Rosenberg, MD.)*

The clinician may determine zonular status by direct visualization of the lens equator through a widely dilated pupil or by use of a goniolens to visualize zonular fibers behind the dilated pupil. If zonular disruption encompasses more than 120° or if phacodonesis prevents CCC, the surgeon may consider removal of the cataract using an extracapsular or intracapsular technique (see Chapter 7). If the zonular weakness is less than 120°, the surgeon can use capsular hooks to stabilize a mobile capsular bag for phacoemulsification (Fig 9-9). In addition, capsular tension rings can be inserted into the capsular bag during surgery.

Zonular incompetence becomes apparent intraoperatively with phacodonesis, decentration of the capsular bag, and sometimes vitreous prolapse into the anterior chamber. Phacoemulsification could proceed safely with application of the same measures

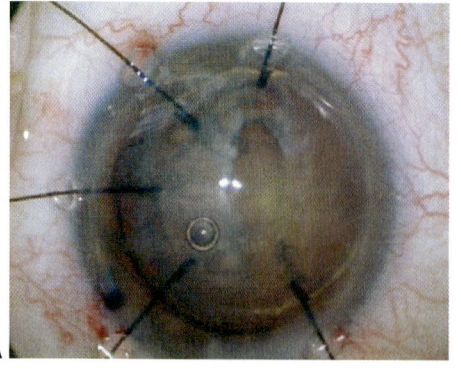
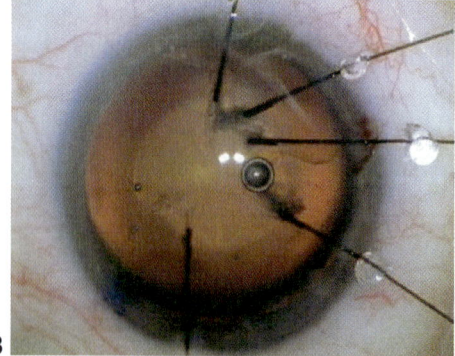

Figure 9-9 Capsular hooks. **A,** Hooks are placed around the anterior capsule edge to stabilize the capsular bag during phacoemulsification in this eye with a subluxed lens. **B,** Trypan blue solution has been used to aid visualization of the capsular edge. *(Courtesy of Lisa Rosenberg, MD.)*

recommended in the previous section on advanced cataract. Reducing the flow rate diminishes fluctuation and turbulence in anterior chamber depth and reduces the risk of vitreous prolapse through the area of zonular absence. A larger capsulorrhexis allows easier separation of lens components within the capsular bag. Thorough hydrodissection and hydrodelineation of the nucleus facilitate smooth rotation during phacoemulsification. Viscodissection helps separate cortical attachments that may impede rotation. Excessive mechanical maneuvers in the nucleus, cortical aspiration, or inadvertent aspiration of the anterior capsular edge contributes to further zonular compromise. Viscodissection of cortical remnants and IOL insertion prior to complete cortical removal are maneuvers that help maintain capsular integrity. Tangential, rather than radial, removal of cortex from the bag minimizes zonular stress.

If capsular support is insufficient for safe phacoemulsification, the surgeon can place iris or capsular hooks inside the capsulorrhexis edge to help stabilize the bag. Alternatively, a capsular tension ring (CTR) can be inserted into the capsular bag. This device provides support by exerting centrifugal force against the capsule equator to areas of absent or weakened zonular fibers. Because radial tension may further extend the capsular defect, placement of a CTR should be avoided if the anterior capsule is torn radially or if the capsulorrhexis is interrupted. The ring can be used in patients with posterior capsule defects as long as the anterior rhexis remains continuous. With a CTR in position, the surgeon can proceed to nuclear and cortical removal more safely and place an in-the-bag IOL. Insufficient zonular support can also be managed with a Cionni-modified CTR sutured to the scleral wall. If zonular support is insufficient for a 1-piece in-the-bag IOL, a 3-piece IOL with the haptics placed in the location of zonular weakness helps prevent postoperative capsular contraction. Otherwise, the surgeon must decide between using a 3-piece lens implant placed in the ciliary sulcus, a transcleral-fixated or iris-fixated posterior chamber IOL, or an anterior chamber lens.

> Rosenthal KJ. The capsular ring: indications and surgery. *Focal Points: Clinical Modules for Ophthalmologists.* San Francisco: American Academy of Ophthalmology; 2002, module 7.

Exfoliation Syndrome

Eyes with exfoliation are characterized by poor pupillary dilation and weakened zonular fibers. These findings increase the likelihood of intraoperative complications such as lens dislocation, capsular rupture, and vitreous loss. The techniques suggested for safe cataract surgery in these eyes are the same as those suggested for advanced cataract and zonular dehiscence in the previous sections.

Progressive capsular contraction, or capsular phimosis, is common in eyes with exfoliation. Possible dislocation of the implant into the vitreous is of concern. The surgeon should carefully consider the style of and placement for the chosen lens implant. Capsular contraction is less likely with a 3-piece lens placed inside the capsular bag. If capsular phimosis occurs, the Nd:YAG laser may be used to create radial incisions in the anterior capsule to release tension on the zonular fibers and maintain central lens position. Alternatively, a 3-piece lens may be placed in the ciliary sulcus if anterior capsular support is adequate, or an anterior chamber lens may be used at the conclusion of cataract removal.

Cataract in Aniridia

The lens capsule in patients with aniridia is thinner than that in patients with normal lenses, which makes it inherently more fragile and challenging when creating a capsulorrhexis. Ideally, the edge of a well-centered capsulorrhexis should overlap the optic edge by 1 mm. Corneal haze and neovascularization in these eyes are common because of stem-cell deficiency, so capsular staining may aid visualization through the cornea while creating an adequately sized capsular opening. High-viscosity OVD also optimizes visualization while stabilizing the capsular surface. The surgeon should avoid working inside the bag to eliminate potential tension on the capsular rim. Low infusion helps reduce turbulence and capsular fluctuation. The capsule in aniridic eyes acts as a pseudoiris when it opacifies.

Extremes in Axial Length

High Myopia

When the surgeon introduces the phaco tip into the anterior chamber of a highly myopic eye, the chamber may deepen dramatically, making nuclear sculpting difficult. To avoid extensive deepening of the anterior chamber and prevent difficulty with nuclear sculpting, the surgeon is advised to lower the irrigation bottle and increase the flow rate before entering the eye with the phaco tip. In spite of this maneuver, these eyes are susceptible to lens–iris diaphragm retropulsion syndrome, wherein 360° of iridocapsular contact occurs, causing reverse pupillary block, pupil dilation, and pain. A defect or laxity in the zonular fibers predisposes these eyes to this situation. Manual separation of the iris from the anterior capsule rim using a Sinskey hook or iris retractor corrects the situation.

Preoperative IOL power calculation in these eyes indicates whether a special-order IOL is required, such as a plano-powered or minus-powered implant. Whenever possible, the patient should receive an IOL because the lens implant serves as a barrier to the movement of the vitreous base and associated traction on the retina. Because myopic eyes are at increased risk for retinal detachment postoperatively, acrylic lens implants are favored when the patient's chance of undergoing future vitreoretinal surgery is significant. If the posterior capsule is open, silicone IOLs develop condensation that compromises the retinal surgeon's view into the eye. Silicone lenses have also been observed to migrate through the capsular opening into the vitreous.

> Cionni RJ, Barros MG, Osher RH. Management of lens-iris diaphragm retropulsion syndrome during phacoemulsification. *J Cataract Refract Surg.* 2004;30(5):953–956.
> Nahra Saad D, Castilla Cespedes M, Martinez Palmer A, Pazos Lopez M. Phacoemulsification and lens-iris diaphragm retropulsion syndrome. *Ophthalmic Surg Lasers Imaging.* 2005; 36(6):512–513.

High Hyperopia and Nanophthalmos

The eye of a cataract patient with high hyperopia often has a shallow anterior chamber and is prone to uveal prolapse, iris damage, and excessive corneal endothelial trauma. Anterior chamber deepening and intraocular tissue protection are achieved by using high-viscosity

OVD, a low aspiration rate, or elevation of the irrigation bottle prior to insertion of the phaco tip. Mannitol can be administered preoperatively to dehydrate vitreous volume in a patient with no systemic contraindications to use of this medication. Iris prolapse is avoided through an anterior corneal incision entry and by taking care not to overfill the eye with OVD. If all of these measures fail to provide sufficient anterior chamber volume for cataract removal, a small amount of liquid vitreous can be removed using a 25-gauge needle or vitrectomy handpiece through a pars plana puncture.

Nanophthalmos is a rare condition in which the eye is extremely short (<20.5 mm) and the ratio of lens volume to eye volume is larger than normal. These eyes have shallow anterior chambers, narrow angles, and thickened sclerae, with little room for the surgeon to maneuver. Small-incision bimanual surgery is an alternative technique to consider. Intraoperative or postoperative uveal effusion is a unique hazard in these small eyes. Maintaining positive pressure and a short procedure time aid in avoiding intraoperative effusion formation. Scleral windows should be considered as a prophylactic measure to treat uveal effusion. A sutured wound prevents hypotony from contributing to this complication postoperatively.

Hypotony

Chronic hypotony is often accompanied by posterior scleral flattening and shortened axial length with choroidal thickening. This makes biometry technically challenging and precise calculation of IOL power less predictable. To the extent possible, the clinician should determine the cause of hypotony and undertake specific treatment before cataract surgery. If the cataract obscures examination of the posterior segment, B-scan ultrasonography is helpful in revealing posterior segment pathology. A cyclodialysis cleft or retinal detachment requires a more extensive procedure combined with cataract surgery. Severe hypotony or pre-phthisis is a poor prognostic indicator for visual improvement after cataract extraction.

Glaucoma and Cataract

Assessment

When cataract surgery is being considered in a patient with glaucoma, assessment of the patient's glaucoma control contributes to the surgical plan. It is challenging to predict the visual outcome in an eye with both cataract and glaucoma because both conditions may contribute to blurred vision, and the patient's visual symptoms may not be directly attributable to one condition or the other exclusively. An advanced visual field defect may limit visual improvement after cataract surgery. In contrast, an advanced cataract may exaggerate a mild visual field abnormality (Fig 9-10). Surgical options include cataract surgery alone, combined cataract/filtering surgery, or staged procedures of filtering surgery followed by cataract surgery at a later time. Uncomplicated phacoemulsification alone may serve to lower the long-term IOP by 10% to 34% in some eyes. Small-incision cataract surgery with a clear corneal approach minimizes conjunctival damage, an essential

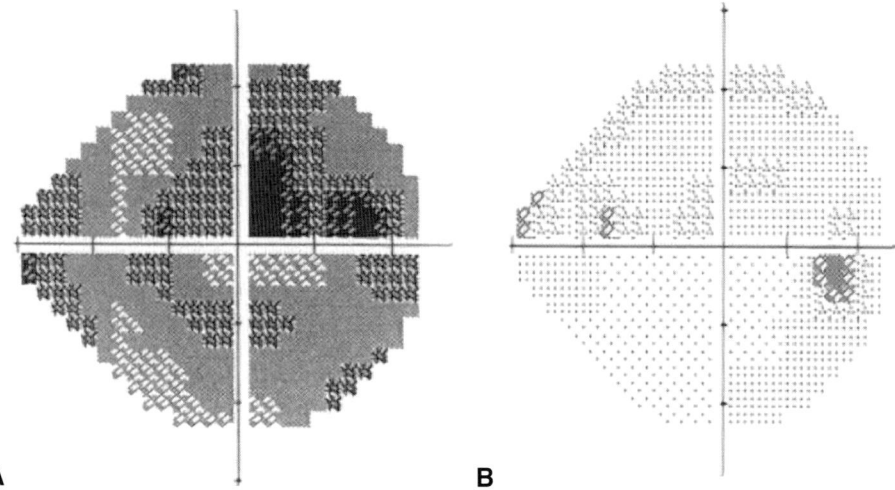

Figure 9-10 Visual field before and after cataract surgery. Media opacity such as cataract can impair the visual field. **A,** An abnormal Humphrey visual field in a glaucoma patient with a dense cataract. **B,** Improved Humphrey visual field following cataract removal and lens implantation. *(Courtesy of Lisa Rosenberg, MD.)*

consideration if filtering surgery is required in the future. In addition, a small incision at a temporal or superotemporal location makes cataract surgery in an eye with a functioning filtering bleb much easier, and it is also less likely to compromise IOP control by an existing functioning bleb. Issues that influence surgical approach include preoperative and desired postoperative IOP level, degree of damage to the optic nerve and visual field, number of medications required to control IOP, patient compliance, side effects of medication, and impact on quality of life. For a comprehensive discussion of surgical decision making in the glaucomatous eye as well as combined cataract and filtering surgery, see BCSC Section 10, *Glaucoma*.

Cataract Surgery in the Glaucoma Patient

Most of the surgical challenges in glaucoma patients are not unique to these eyes. For instance, zonular compromise and phacodonesis may complicate capsulorrhexis and lens removal in an eye with traumatic or exfoliation glaucoma. Uveitic glaucoma and miotic therapy may limit pupillary dilation and increase the risk for postoperative macular edema. Postoperative IOP elevation from retained viscoelastic agent or inflammation occurs more commonly and the pressure rises to a higher level in glaucomatous eyes with reduced outflow capacity through the trabecular meshwork. Management of these operative challenges is discussed in detail elsewhere in this chapter and also in BCSC Section 10, *Glaucoma*.

The use of topical prostaglandin medication has been associated with postoperative cystoid macular edema (CME), although proven cases are few. Because the incidence of clinically significant postoperative CME after uncomplicated phacoemulsification is very rare, it is difficult to attribute macular edema in the early postoperative period to the use of prostaglandin medication. In such cases, discontinuation of the prostaglandin is advisable to determine wheher this medication is contributing to the edema.

> Miyake K, Ibaraki N. Prostaglandins and cystoid macular edema. *Surv Ophthalmol.* 2002;47(suppl 1):S203–S218.

Cataract Surgery in an Eye With a Functioning Filter

Small-incision cataract surgery in the glaucomatous eye provides the surgeon with options that do not interfere with previous filtering surgery. With a temporal corneal incision, the surgeon avoids the superior conjunctiva and site of filtering surgery. If conversion to extracapsular technique is indicated (eg, in the setting of extreme phacodonesis and zonular instability or capsular rupture with vitreous present in the anterior chamber), the surgeon may choose to extend the clear corneal incision to permit delivery of the crystalline lens. Alternatively, closure of the temporal incision and creation of a larger corneoscleral wound at the top of the eye minimizes astigmatism but may also compromise an existing filter positioned centrally at the limbus.

> Balyeat HD. Cataract surgery in the glaucoma patient. Part 1: a cataract surgeon's perspective. *Focal Points: Clinical Modules for Ophthalmologists.* San Francisco: American Academy of Ophthalmology; 1998, module 3.
>
> Heffelfinger BL, Berman MN, Krupin T, Rosenberg LF, Ruderman JM. Surgical management of coexisting glaucoma and cataract. In: *Ophthalmology Clinics of North America, Glaucoma Diagnosis and Management.* Philadelphia: Saunders; 2000:545–552.
>
> Poley BJ, Lindstrom RL, Samuelson TW, Schulze R Jr. Intraocular pressure reduction after phacoemulsification with intraocular lens implantation in glaucomatous and nonglaucomatous eyes: evaluation of a causal relationship between the natural lens and open-angle glaucoma. *J Cataract Refract Surg.* 2009;35(11):1946–1955.
>
> Skuta GL. Cataract surgery in the glaucoma patient. Part 2: a glaucoma surgeon's perspective. *Focal Points: Clinical Modules for Ophthalmologists.* San Francisco: American Academy of Ophthalmology; 1998, module 4.
>
> Verges C, Cazal J, Lavin C. Surgical strategies in patients with cataract and glaucoma. *Curr Opin Ophthalmol.* 2005;16(1):44–52.

Uveitis

Chronic recurring intraocular inflammation and the corticosteroid therapy used to treat it contribute to cataract formation. Decreased vision due to cataract must be differentiated from coexisting macular edema or posterior segment pathology. Fluorescein angiography, angioscopy, or optical coherence tomography should be used preoperatively to identify CME. Complications can be minimized when inflammation has been controlled for several months before surgery and is treated aggressively after surgery. Topical and oral corticosteroids are the mainstay of therapy, and topical NSAIDs and cytotoxic agents may be used to supplement treatment.

Uveitic eyes dilate poorly and require expansion and lysis of iridolenticular adhesions discussed previously for small pupils. A pupillary membrane must be incised and stripped

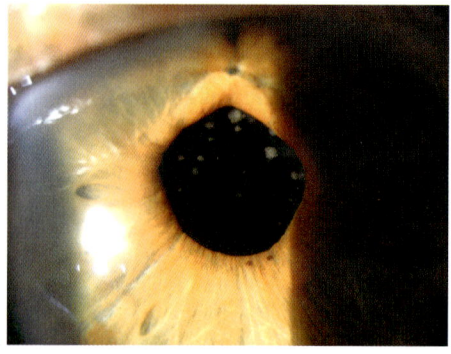 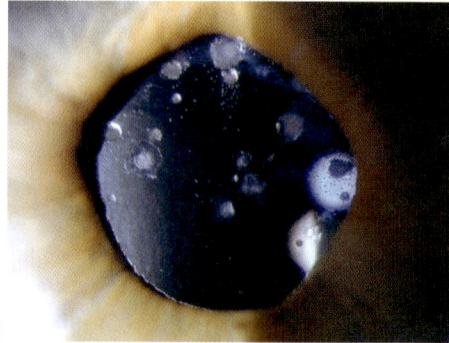

Figure 9-11 Low-power **(A)** and high-power **(B)** views of silicone IOL with keratic precipitates. *(Courtesy of Steven Vold, MD; photography by Matthew Poe.)*

to avoid interfering with the capsulorrhexis. Overly vigorous pupil stretching and manipulation lead to iris bleeding and fibrinous inflammation postoperatively. Meticulous cleanup of cortical material helps prevent exuberant postoperative inflammation.

Insertion of a silicone lens implant is discouraged because inflammatory precipitates collect on the lens surface (Fig 9-11). Acrylic implants are well tolerated and preferred in uveitic eyes. When complications arise during this difficult surgery and a lens cannot be inserted into the capsular bag, it may be advisable to omit placing a lens in the ciliary sulcus or implanting an anterior chamber lens. In types of uveitis associated with membrane formation, repeated Nd:YAG procedures may be necessary to clear the lens surface. (See also BCSC Section 9, *Intraocular Inflammation and Uveitis*.)

> Abela-Formanek C, Amon M, Kahraman G, Schauersberger J, Dunavoelgyi R. Biocompatibility of hydrophilic acrylic, hydrophobic acrylic, and silicone intraocular lenses in eyes with uveitis having cataract surgery: long-term follow-up. *J Cataract Refract Surg.* 2011;37(1):104–112.
>
> Foster CS. Cataract surgery in the patient with uveitis. *Focal Points: Clinical Modules for Ophthalmologists.* San Francisco: American Academy of Ophthalmology; 1994, module 4.
>
> Kawaguchi T, Mochizuki M, Miyata K, Miyata N. Phacoemulsification cataract extraction and intraocular lens implantation in patients with uveitis. *J Cataract Refract Surg.* 2007;33(2):305–309.
>
> Tessler HH, Farber MD. Intraocular lens implantation versus no intraocular lens implantation in patients with chronic iridocyclitis and pars planitis: a randomized prospective study. *Ophthalmology.* 1993;100(8):1206–1209.

Retinal Conditions

Retinal Disease

Review of ocular records may reveal the retina patient's visual acuity before the onset of cataract. Macular function tests, such as the macular photostress test or the potential acuity test (see Chapter 6), may be helpful in determining visual outcome in patients with retinal disease. The clinician must interpret test results with caution because poor or equivocal performance on such tests does not rule out all benefit from cataract removal, while favorable results may be misleading. Optical coherence tomography and fluorescein angiography detect the presence of diabetic or hypertensive retinopathy, degenerative changes, macular distortion, and leakage of fluid into the foveal area. Proper management of patient expectations is essential and especially prudent when eyes have vision-threatening retinal disease.

If diabetic macular edema is present and the view of the retina is adequate, the clinician may consider preoperative focal laser treatment. Studies have shown that preoperative administration of topical NSAIDs can decrease the incidence of postoperative CME and that NSAIDs are beneficial in preventing macular edema in patients with diabetes.

If the patient is known to have peripheral vitreoretinopathy, a retina specialist should examine the patient before surgery to determine whether pretreatment with laser or cryotherapy would help reduce the risk of retinal tears or detachment. After prophylactic treatment, a period of at least 4 weeks should elapse before elective cataract surgery. (See also BCSC Section 12, *Retina and Vitreous*.)

If the view of the retina is restricted by a small pupil preoperatively, cataract surgery provides an opportunity to enlarge the pupil using stretch maneuvers, iris hooks, expansion devices, or multiple sphincterotomies. In addition, a generous anterior capsulotomy and complete cortical cleanup will enhance the view of the retinal periphery after surgery.

Whenever safely possible, a posterior chamber IOL should be inserted. The surgeon should avoid using a silicone IOL in a patient for whom a vitrectomy is a possibility, because condensation on the posterior surface of the implant limits visibility during pars plana vitrectomy.

> Colin J. The role of NSAIDs in the management of postoperative ophthalmic inflammation. *Drugs*. 2007;67(9):1291–1308.
> Eriksson U, Alm A, Björnhall G, Granstam E, Matsson AW. Macular edema and visual outcome following cataract surgery in patients with diabetic retinopathy and controls. *Graefes Arch Clin Exp Ophthalmol*. 2011;249(3):349–359.
> Hong T, Mitchell P, de Loryn T, Rochtchina E, Cugati S, Wang JJ. Development and progression of diabetic retinopathy 12 months after phacoemulsification cataract surgery. *Ophthalmology*. 2009;116(8):1510–1514.
> Shah AS, Chen SH. Cataract surgery and diabetes. *Curr Opin Ophthalmol*. 2010;21(1):4–9.

Cataract Following Pars Plana Vitrectomy

Nuclear cataract formation is common after pars plana vitrectomy, especially in patients older than 50 years. Posterior subcapsular opacification is typical after the use of silicone oil during retinal surgery. In the absence of a vitreous cushion, the posterior capsule becomes more mobile, requiring exquisite attention to chamber fluctuation with fluidics and maneuvers inside the eye during surgery. Lowering the irrigation bottle and fluid-flow rate prior to placing the phaco tip inside the eye is helpful. This maneuver is also recommended when zonular integrity is altered from prior retinal surgery or preexisting ocular disease. The surgeon should beware of overfilling the anterior chamber with OVD in an effort to avoid further zonular stretch and breakage. Extra caution is also advised to avoid losing pieces of the lens during hydrodissection when an inadvertent capsular break may have occurred during retinal surgery. A large capsulorrhexis allows prolapse of the nucleus during hydrodissection for an iris-plane phaco chop. If the surgeon selects an extracapsular surgical technique instead of phacoemulsification, the absence of vitreous reduces posterior pressure to aid lens expression. Alternatively, after capsulorrhexis and mobilization of the nucleus from its cortical attachments, the nucleus can be removed using a lens loop or irrigating vectis.

Cataract With Intraocular Silicone Oil

Cataracts in eyes with silicone oil are usually very soft. Silicone oil can migrate through a break in the zonular fibers if the anterior chamber is overfilled with OVD during surgery. The clinician should use low-flow irrigation or decrease the aspiration rate during surgery to minimize pressure on the zonular fibers and the risk of silicone oil migration into the anterior chamber. Droplets of silicone oil that were not apparent in the anterior chamber during surgery might become visible postoperatively. A few droplets are usually not toxic to the cornea. Silicone lens implants are contraindicated in these eyes because silicone oil adheres to the implant surface. The surgeon should create an inferior iridectomy if a patent one is not already present.

Ocular Trauma

Ocular Assessment

When a patient presents with a history of ocular trauma sufficient to cause a dense cataract, the surgeon should have a high suspicion for damage to other anterior segment structures. Damage to the corneal endothelium, zonular fibers, and anterior chamber angle all demand an adjustment in surgical technique. Gonioscopy is essential when planning IOL placement. The surgeon must be hypervigilant while evaluating ocular findings and determining the potential for visual recovery, as discussed in Chapter 6. Cataract may occur acutely after substantial trauma (see Chapter 4). A slowly progressive cataract after ocular trauma can be monitored while intraocular inflammation and other comorbidities are treated. Special circumstances in the traumatized eye are discussed in the following sections.

Visualization During Surgery

Corneal laceration and edema may impair the view into the eye so that phacoemulsification cannot be performed safely. Instead, an extracapsular approach may be advisable. Hemorrhage during surgery may further interfere with visualization into the anterior segment. Use of OVDs and intracameral air helps occlude vessels and marginalize bleeding. If visualization remains inadequate, then the surgeon should close the wound, with surgery pursued later.

Inflammation

Lens protein may leak into the aqueous and vitreous, inciting glaucoma. When uveitis is severe, it may mimic infectious endophthalmitis. Fibrin membranes on the iris lead to synechiae, pupil seclusion, and miosis. The surgeon should use pupil-enlarging maneuvers as described previously. A peripheral iridectomy is important in the setting of inflammation for prevention of pupillary block glaucoma. Inflamed uveal tissue bleeds with the slightest manipulation. OVDs should be used liberally to protect corneal endothelium and improve the view into the anterior segment. Postoperative IOP elevation is typical and exacerbated by the use of OVD. Control of inflammation warrants cycloplegia and intensive topical and possibly oral corticosteroid therapy.

Retained Foreign Matter

A foreign body in the anterior chamber may be easier to see when the patient is seated upright at the slit lamp rather than positioned supine under the operating microscope. Irrigating solutions may dislodge a foreign body from its preoperative location. When an intraocular foreign body is suspected to reside in the posterior segment, indirect ophthalmoscopy is an excellent method to use if ocular media are sufficiently clear. When the view is obscured by cataract or hemorrhage, a computed tomography scan, x-ray, or ultrasonogram can help the clinician determine the presence and location of the foreign body. When a metallic foreign body is suspected, magnetic resonance imaging is contraindicated because the magnet might dislodge it. A dense cataract may be removed either by a pars plana or an anterior approach, followed by pars plana vitrectomy and removal of the foreign body.

Damage to Other Ocular Tissues

Iris trauma commonly coexists with traumatic cataract (Fig 9-12). Sphincter ruptures cause irregular pupil size and shape. The surgeon can repair iridodialysis at the time of cataract removal by suturing the iris root to the scleral spur. Though not apparent on slit-lamp examination, corneal endothelial damage can be significant and not manifest until after surgery, when severe corneal edema forms. Trauma sufficient to cause iris tears and

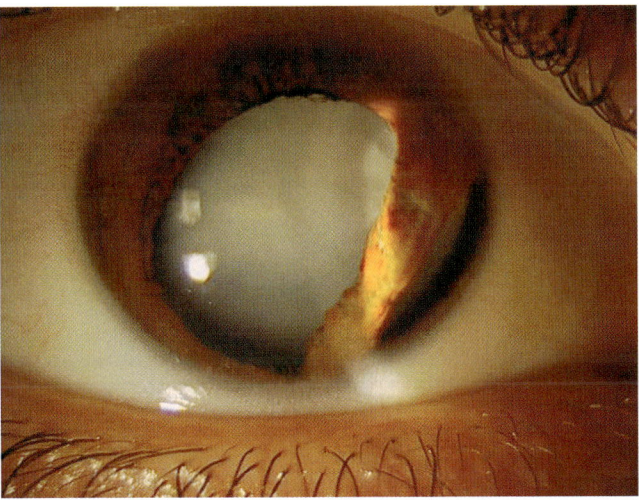

Figure 9-12 Traumatic cataract and iridodialysis secondary to a paintball injury. *(Courtesy of Mark H. Blecher, MD.)*

cataract also warrants careful inspection for zonular damage and posterior segment insult. Surgical planning to manage these findings intraoperatively is discussed in previous sections. If a retinal detachment is present, cataract removal may be necessary to allow adequate visualization for subsequent surgical repair.

Removal of Traumatic Cataract

When the clinician identifies cortical material in the anterior chamber or if a mature cataract interferes with the diagnosis and treatment of injuries in the posterior segment, the cataract should be removed promptly. Rupture of the capsule causes rapid hydration of the lens cortex, leading to formation of a milky-white cataract. This type of cataract is usually soft and can be aspirated through the large port of the irrigating/aspirating handpiece. The surgeon should beware of preexisting capsule rupture that may not be visible on preoperative examination. Hydrodissection should be performed slowly to minimize the possibility of extending a capsular break and causing the lens to fall into the posterior segment.

OVD can be used to tamponade vitreous in areas of zonular incompetence. However, when the nucleus is markedly subluxed and vitreous fills a substantial part of the anterior chamber, the surgeon should consider removing the cataract through a pars plana approach. Referral to a retina specialist is advisable if the surgeon is not skilled in this technique.

If a hard nuclear cataract was present before the trauma, techniques for cataract removal described in the section Zonular Dehiscence With Lens Subluxation or Dislocation should be applied. If vitreous has migrated into the anterior chamber, the surgeon must perform an anterior vitrectomy before starting phacoemulsification or cortical aspiration in order to avoid vitreous aspiration and retinal traction.

Vision Rehabilitation

Primary implantation of a posterior chamber lens after ocular trauma is recommended when intraocular inflammation and hemorrhage are minimal and the view of anterior segment structures is good. An anterior chamber IOL or transsclerally fixated posterior chamber lens may be necessary in case of inadequate capsular support for a posterior chamber IOL. In rare situations, the surgeon may decide against placing an IOL primarily and instead insert an IOL as a secondary procedure later, after sufficient evaluation of the anterior segment and anterior angle anatomy. Scarring resulting from a corneal laceration changes the contour of the cornea and keratometry measurements, and inaccurate biometry increases the risk of postoperative anisometropia. A rigid contact lens may be required to mask irregular astigmatism.

IOL selection after trauma

The clinician should tailor selection of a lens implant to the patient's ocular anatomy and to the desired postoperative outcome. Silicone lens implants should be avoided in patients with a history of uveitis because inflammatory debris is more likely to collect on the surface of the optic and impair vision. Acrylic lenses are preferred in these cases and in eyes that are more likely to undergo vitreoretinal surgery in the future. In eyes that have more than 4 clock-hours of inadequate zonular support but have an intact anterior capsule, a 3-piece posterior chamber lens may be placed in the ciliary sulcus. Alternatively, if there is no capsular support, a 3-piece lens may be sewn to the scleral wall. Finally, the design of current anterior chamber lenses is sufficiently flexible for the open-angle glaucomatous eye to tolerate. Ultimately, the choice of IOL is determined by the surgeon's experience with lens options and implantation methods.

> Hannush SB. Sutured posterior chamber intraocular lenses. *Focal Points: Clinical Modules for Ophthalmologists.* San Francisco: American Academy of Ophthalmology; 2006, module 9.

APPENDIX

Surgical Procedures for Extracapsular and Intracapsular Cataract Extraction

For a more in-depth discussion of the various topics mentioned in the appendix, please see the appropriate sections in Chapter 7.

The Modern Extracapsular Cataract Surgical Procedure

Patient Preparation

After informed consent is obtained, the patient's operative site is marked and the pupil is maximally dilated. Confirmation of the correct patient and the correct surgical site is performed. Neither ocular massage nor hyperosmotics are commonly used for extracapsular cataract extraction (ECCE). Pupillary dilation is critical to the success of ECCE.

The patient should have a chance to void before transport to the operating room.

Incision

Nucleus expression requires a limbal chord length of 8–12 mm, smaller than the incision needed for intracapsular cataract extraction (ICCE). The initial incision usually consists of a limbal groove, fashioned with a round-tipped steel blade, sharp microknife, or diamond knife. Some surgeons prefer a slightly more posterior incision with anterior dissection creating a scleral flap or tunnel. These incisions are typically placed superiorly. A stab incision is made under the flap into the anterior chamber in preparation for an anterior capsulotomy, and the cystitome is inserted to begin the procedure. The anterior chamber depth can be stabilized by ophthalmic viscosurgical devices (OVDs), air bubble, or continuous fluid irrigation.

Anterior Capsulotomy

The main function of the anterior capsulotomy is to permit removal of the cataract while leaving behind the intact capsular bag, which provides stabilization for the IOL that will be implanted. There are many techniques for opening the anterior capsule. A sharp cystitome or bent needle may be used to make a series of connected punctures or small tears in a circle to create the can-opener capsulotomy (see Chapter 7, Fig 7-25A). Alternatively, the surgeon can create a smooth capsulorrhexis by making a puncture or small tear. The edge of this tear is then grasped with the cystitome tip or with forceps and pulled around smoothly, removing a circular portion of anterior capsule (see Chapter 7, Fig 7-25B). This technique provides greater structural integrity for the lens capsule to maintain implant stability and centration. If a small capsulorrhexis is created and manual expression is planned, relaxing incisions are often made in the superior aspect of the capsulorrhexis, or in the 3- and 9-o'clock positions to allow the nucleus adequate room to exit the capsule during expression. After the capsulotomy is completed, the incision is widened to allow safe passage of the nucleus through the incision. Anterior capsulotomy is discussed in greater detail in the section on phacoemulsification.

Nucleus removal

Manual expression involves pressing on the inferior limbus to tip the superior pole of the nucleus up and out of the capsular bag. Additional counterpressure on the globe from an instrument indenting the sclera posterior to the limbus 180° away from the incision will express the nucleus from the chamber. The surgeon removes the nucleus from the eye by loosening and elevating it from the capsule with the use of a hook or irrigating cannula and then supporting it on a lens loop, spoon, or vectis that will slide or irrigate it out of the chamber. Alternatively, the surgeon may fragment the nucleus while it is within the eye, using forceps or nucleus splitters to deliver it for removal in portions through a smaller incision.

The incision is partially sutured to allow deepening of the chamber with irrigation. Using the irrigation/aspiration (I/A) equipment, the surgeon then aspirates the lens cortex under direct visualization in the pupillary space. The posterior capsule may be polished with an abrasive-tipped irrigation cannula, wiped with a silicone-lined "squeegee," or vacuumed clean with low aspiration to remove epithelial and cortical particles from the capsule surface.

IOL Insertion

Prior to IOL insertion, the anterior chamber is usually filled with an OVD. OVDs provide the most reliable anterior chamber maintenance along with protection of the corneal endothelium. A posterior chamber IOL (PCIOL) may be inserted into the sulcus or into the capsular bag. Sulcus fixation usually requires an IOL with a larger overall diameter (at least 13 mm) and a large-diameter optic (at least 6 mm), which is more forgiving in case of postoperative decentration.

If the surgeon wishes to insert the IOL into the capsular bag, an OVD is usually injected into the bag, with care being taken to separate the anterior capsule flap completely from the posterior capsule. Direct visualization of haptic insertion is critical.

Closure

The ECCE incision is typically closed with either multiple interrupted sutures of 10-0 nylon or with one long running suture. Proper suture tension helps reduce postoperative astigmatism: loose sutures cause astigmatism *perpendicular to* the axis of the suture, whereas tight sutures create astigmatism *in* the axis of the suture.

Postoperative Course

Visual acuity on the first postoperative day should be consistent with the refractive state of the eye, the clarity of the cornea and media, and the visual potential of the retina and optic nerve. A mild eyelid reaction with edema and erythema may occur. The conjunctival flap may be injected and boggy, but it should not be elevated by fluid. The cornea may have some mild degree of edema. The anterior chamber should have normal depth, and a mild cellular reaction is typical. The posterior capsule should be clear and intact, and the implant should be well positioned and stable. The red reflex should be bright and clear. IOP elevations may be associated with retained OVD. Topical antibiotic and corticosteroid eyedrops are generally prescribed postoperatively.

The postoperative course should be characterized by steady improvement of vision and comfort, as the inflammatory reaction subsides during the first 2 weeks. The refraction is typically stable by the sixth to eighth postoperative week, and spectacles may then be prescribed. If a significant amount of postoperative astigmatism results along the axis of the sutures, the clinician can selectively remove the sutures as guided by wound stability, keratometry readings, or corneal topography measurements.

The Modern Intracapsular Cataract Surgical Procedure

Patient Preparation

The preparation for planned intracapsular cataract surgery is much like that for ECCE. After informed consent is obtained, the patient's operative site is marked and the pupil is maximally dilated. Confirmation of the correct patient and the correct surgical site is performed. A local anesthetic is administered. Orbital massage by digital pressure or compressive devices may be used to decrease the pressure effect that administration of extra anesthetic can have on the eye. Some surgeons use mannitol to decrease the orbital and vitreous volume. Mannitol should be used with caution in patients with congestive heart failure, diabetes mellitus, or kidney failure. In addition, mannitol must be used with care in geriatric patients to avoid rapid diuresis that may result in subdural hematomas from traction on bridging vessels.

The patient should have a chance to void before transport to the operating room.

Procedure

After the skin and ocular surface have been prepared and draping has been completed, an eyelid speculum is placed between the eyelids. A suture is usually required to hold the eye in a slight downward position. The surgeon can accomplish this step by placing a 6-0 silk suture beneath the superior rectus tendon or within sclera and securing the suture to the superior drape.

Incision

The surgeon creates either a fornix-based or a limbal-based conjunctival flap. Battery-powered or wet-field cautery is typically used for hemostasis. A scleral support ring may be needed in young patients or in those with high myopia to avoid scleral collapse when the lens is extracted; in patients with deep-set eyes, the ring may be needed to improve exposure.

Once 160° to 180° of the corneoscleral limbus has been exposed, incision placement varies according to surgeon preference and patient need. More-anterior or corneal incisions may be of shorter chord length and involve less bleeding. However, their closure induces central corneal steepening in the meridian of the incision. Incisions that are more posterior heal faster and, when covered by a conjunctival flap, are more comfortable to the patient. Posterior incisions induce less astigmatism and are less damaging to the corneal endothelium, but they cause more bleeding.

Sutures are pre-placed across the incision and looped out of the way; their presence allows rapid closure of the eye in case of choroidal hemorrhage, patient valsalva, or other instances of positive posterior pressure. An additional suture may be placed through the anterior wound lip only, allowing the assistant to elevate the cornea to facilitate lens delivery.

Iridectomy and cataract delivery

An iridectomy is performed at this point. If the eye has a small pupil, the surgeon can consider performing sector iridectomy, radial iridotomy, or multiple sphincterotomies or using iris hooks or pupil expanders.

α-Chymotrypsin, if available, can be injected via a cannula through the pupillary space into the posterior chamber. An iris retractor can be used to expose the superior surface of the lens. A cellulose sponge is used to dry the anterior lens capsule. The surgeon positions the cryoprobe on the lens surface and depresses the foot pedal of the cryoprobe. Once an ice ball has formed (see Chapter 7, Fig 7-6), gentle maneuvers are used to deliver the lens. Sometimes the iris retractor or a cellulose sponge can be used to strip the vitreous from the posterior surface of the lens during delivery. Vitreous loss, combined with the larger incision of intracapsular surgery, contributes to posterior scleral collapse. Thus, every cataract surgeon should have as a part of his or her armamentarium—especially for intracapsular surgery—strategies to manage vitreous loss. The anterior vitrectomy apparatus that is part of the phaco machine provides controlled conditions for vitreous removal. Otherwise, aspiration of vitreous through a blunt cannula may be employed.

A lens implant may be inserted at this point. An anterior chamber lens can be selected after instillation of acetylcholine or carbachol. Other lens implant options include posterior chamber lenses with either iris or scleral fixation suture support.

Fine sutures are used to close the incision while an OVD or balanced salt solution is used to keep the anterior chamber formed. The conjunctival flap is secured. Subconjunctival or sub-Tenon antibiotics or steroids can be used at this point. A patch and shield should be applied.

Postoperative Course

As with ECCE, visual acuity on the first postoperative day should be consistent with the refractive state of the eye, the clarity of the cornea and media, and the visual potential of the retina and optic nerve. If the eye has been left aphakic, visual acuity can be estimated with a +10 to +12 D lens, or a +4 D lens can be used as a telescope. The surgeon should evaluate the cornea, the security of the incision, the depth of the anterior chamber, the degree of inflammatory reaction, and the IOP. The posterior segment should be visualized so that vitreous clarity and position can be judged and any retinal or optic nerve pathology noted.

It is not unusual to see a mild eyelid reaction with edema and erythema. The upper eyelid may be moderately ptotic. The conjunctiva is often mildly injected, and subconjunctival hemorrhage may be present. The cornea should be clear, but some superior edema is often present from the bending of the cornea during lens extraction. This edema generally resolves during the first postoperative week. The anterior chamber should have normal depth with mild to moderate cellular reaction. The pupil should be round, and the iridectomy patent. The anterior vitreous face location should be noted. A good red reflex should be present.

The postoperative course should be characterized by steady improvement of vision and comfort. Topical antibiotics and steroids are typically prescribed during the first postoperative weeks. The refraction generally becomes stable 6 to 12 weeks after intracapsular surgery, depending on the wound-closure technique employed. Because ICCE requires a larger incision, achieving a stable refraction usually takes longer than after ECCE or phaco techniques, which require smaller incisions.

Basic Texts

Lens and Cataract

Apple DJ, Auffarth GU, Peng Q, Visessook N. *Foldable Intraocular Lenses: Evolution, Clinicopathologic Correlations, and Complications.* Thorofare, NJ: Slack; 2000.

Bahadur GG, Sinskey RM. *Manual of Cataract Surgery.* 2nd ed. Boston: Butterworth-Heinemann; 1999.

Buratto L, Werner L, Zanini M, Apple DJ. *Phacoemulsification: Principles and Techniques.* 2nd ed. Thorofare, NJ: Slack; 2003.

Chang D. *Phaco Chop: Mastering Techniques, Optimizing Technology, and Avoiding Complications.* Thorofare, NJ: Slack; 2004.

Fine IH. *Clear Corneal Lens Surgery.* Thorofare, NJ: Slack; 1999.

Gills JP, Fenzl R, Martin RG, eds. *Cataract Surgery: The State of the Art.* Thorofare, NJ: Slack; 1998.

Gills JP, Martin RG, Sanders DR, eds. *Sutureless Cataract Surgery: An Evolution Toward Minimally Invasive Technique.* Thorofare, NJ: Slack; 1992.

Harding J. *Cataract: Biochemistry, Epidemiology, and Pharmacology.* New York: Chapman & Hall; 1991.

Jaffe NS, Jaffe MS, Jaffe GF. *Cataract Surgery and Its Complications.* 6th ed. St Louis: Mosby; 1998.

Koch PS, Hoffman J. *Mastering Phacoemulsification: A Simplified Manual of Strategies for the Spring, Crack, and Stop and Chop Technique.* 4th ed. Thorofare, NJ: Slack; 1994.

Kohnen T, Koch DD, eds. *Essentials in Ophthalmology—Cataract and Refractive Surgery.* Germany: Springer-Verlag; 2006.

Pineda R, Espaillat A, Perez VL, Rowe S. *The Complicated Cataract: The Massachusetts Eye and Ear Infirmary Phacoemulsification Practice Handbook.* Thorofare, NJ: Slack; 2001.

Seibel BS. *Phacodynamics: Mastering the Tools and Techniques of Phacoemulsification Surgery.* 4th ed. Thorofare, NJ: Slack; 2005.

Steinert RF, ed. *Cataract Surgery: Techniques, Complications, and Management.* 2nd ed. Philadelphia: Saunders; 2004.

Tasman W, Jaeger EA, eds. *Duane's Ophthalmology on DVD-ROM.* Philadelphia: Lippincott Williams & Wilkins; 2012.

Wilson ME Jr, Trivedi RH, Pandey SK. *Pediatric Cataract Surgery: Techniques, Complications, and Management.* Philadelphia: Lippincott Williams & Wilkins; 2005.

Related Academy Materials

Focal Points: Clinical Modules for Ophthalmologists

Print modules are available through an annual subscription or limited back-year set. Online modules are available through an annual subscription or for individual purchase. For a complete list of back issues, visit www.aao.org/focalpointsarchive.

Arbisser LB. Anterior vitrectomy for the anterior segment surgeon (Module 2, 2009).
Chang DF. Intraoperative floppy iris syndrome (Module 11, 2010).
Devgan U. Basic principles of phacoemulsification and fluid dynamics (Module 8, 2010).
Dorey MW, Condon GP. Management of dislocated intraocular lenses (Module 9, 2009).
Reeves SW, Davis EA. Surgical treatment of presbyopia (Module 7, 2009).
Rosenfeld SI, O'Brien TP. The dissatisfied presbyopia-correcting IOL patient (Module 8, 2011).
Tabin GC, Feilmeier MR. Cataract surgery in the developing world (Module 9, 2011).

Print Publications

Dunn JP, Langer PD, eds. *Basic Techniques of Ophthalmic Surgery* (2009).
Oetting TA, ed. *Basic Principles of Ophthalmic Surgery.* 2nd ed. (2011).
Rockwood EJ, ed. *ProVision: Preferred Responses in Ophthalmology. Series 4.* Self-Assessment Program. 2-vol set (2007).
Wilson FM II, Blomquist PH, eds. *Practical Ophthalmology: A Manual for Beginning Residents.* 6th ed. (2009).

Academy Maintenance of Certification (MOC)

MOC Exam Review Course (2011); www.aao.org/moc

Ophthalmic Technology Assessments

Ophthalmic Technology Assessments are available at www.aao.org/ota and are published in the Academy's journal, *Ophthalmology*.

Ophthalmic Technology Assessment Committee. *Capsule Staining as an Adjunct to Cataract Surgery* (2006).
Ophthalmic Technology Assessment Committee. *Intracameral Anesthesia* (2001; reviewed for currency 2006).
Ophthalmic Technology Assessment Committee. *Intraocular Lens Implantation in the Absence of Ocular Support* (2003; reviewed for currency 2008).

Preferred Practice Patterns

Preferred Practice Patterns are available at www.aao.org/ppp.

Preferred Practice Patterns Committee, Cataract and Anterior Segment Panel. *Cataract in the Adult Eye* (2011).

DVDs

Henderson BA, Afshari NA, eds. *Challenging Cases in Cataract Surgery* (2009).
Osher RH. *Complications During Cataract Surgery: Anterior Capsule* (2009).
Osher RH. *Complications During Cataract Surgery: Posterior Capsule* (2010).
Osher RH. *Complications During Cataract Surgery: Thermal Injury, Iris Prolapse, Choroidal Hemorrhage, and Dropped Nucleus* (2011).

Online Materials

Focal Points modules; www.aao.org/focalpointsarchive
ONE Network, Academy Grand Rounds, Cataract and Anterior Segment; www.aao.org/cases
ONE Network, Online Courses, Cataract and Anterior Segment; www.aao.org/courses
Ophthalmic Technology Assessments; www.aao.org/ota
Practicing Ophthalmologists Learning System (2011); www.aao.org/learningsystem
Preferred Practice Patterns; www.aao.org/ppp
Rockwood EJ, ed. *ProVision: Preferred Responses in Ophthalmology. Series 4. Self-Assessment Program.* 2-vol set (2007); www.aao.org/provision

---

To order any of these materials, please order online at www.aao.org/store, or call the Academy's Customer Service toll-free number, 866-561-8558, in the U.S. If outside the U.S., call 415-561-8540 between 8:00 AM and 5:00 PM PST.

Requesting Continuing Medical Education Credit

The American Academy of Ophthalmology is accredited by the Accreditation Council for Continuing Medical Education to provide continuing medical education for physicians.

The American Academy of Ophthalmology designates this enduring material for a maximum of 10 *AMA PRA Category 1 Credits*™. Physicians should claim only the credit commensurate with the extent of their participation in the activity.

The American Medical Association requires that all learners participating in activities involving enduring materials complete a formal assessment before claiming continuing medical education (CME) credit. To assess your achievement in this activity and ensure that a specified level of knowledge has been reached, a posttest for this Section of the Basic and Clinical Science Course is provided. A minimum score of 80% must be obtained to pass the test and claim CME credit.

To take the posttest and request CME credit online:

1. Go to www.aao.org/cme and log in.
2. Click on "Review or claim CME online" and then "Report AAO credits."
3. Select the appropriate Academy activity. You will be directed to the posttest.
4. Once you have passed the test with a score of 80% or higher, you will be directed to your transcript. *If you are not an Academy member, you will be able to print out a certificate of participation once you have passed the test.*

To take the posttest and request CME credit using a paper form:

1. Complete the CME Posttest Request Form on page 223 and return it to the address provided. *Please note that there is a $20.00 processing fee for all paper requests.* The posttest will be mailed to you.
2. Return the completed test as directed. Once you have passed the test with a score of 80% or higher, your transcript will be updated automatically. To receive verification of your CME credits, be sure to check the appropriate box on the posttest.

   Please note that test results will not be provided. If you do not achieve a minimum score of 80%, another test will be sent to you automatically, at no charge. If you do not reach the specified level of knowledge (80%) on your second attempt, you will need to pay an additional processing fee to receive the third test.

Note: Submission of the CME Posttest Request Form does not represent claiming CME credit.

• **Credit must be claimed by June 1, 2015** •

For assistance, contact the Academy's Customer Service department at 866-561-8558 (US only) or 415-561-8540 between 8:00 AM and 5:00 PM (PST), Monday through Friday, or send an e-mail to customer_service@aao.org.

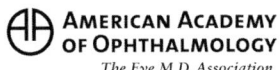

CME Posttest Request Form
Basic and Clinical Science Course, 2012–2013
Section 11

Please note that requesting CME credit with this form will incur a fee of $20.00. (Prepayment required.)

☐ Yes, please send me the posttest for BCSC Section 11. I choose not to report my CME credit online for free. I have enclosed a payment of **$20.00** for processing.

Academy Member ID Number (if known): _____

Name: _____
     First   Last

Address: _____

_____
    City   State/Province   ZIP/Postal Code   Country

Phone Number: _____ Fax Number: _____

E-mail Address: _____

Method of Payment: ☐ Check   ☐ Credit Card   Make checks payable to AAO.

Credit Card Type: ☐ Visa   ☐ MasterCard   ☐ American Express   ☐ Discover

Card Number: _____ Expiration Date: _____

Credit must be claimed by June 1, 2015. Please note that submission of this form does not represent claiming CME credits.

Test results will not be sent. If a participant does not achieve an 80% pass rate, one new posttest will be sent at no charge. Additional processing fees are incurred thereafter.

Please mail completed form to:
American Academy of Ophthalmology, CME Posttest
Dept. 34051
PO Box 39000
San Francisco, CA 94139

Please allow 3 weeks for delivery of the posttest.

Academy use only:

PN: _____   MC: _____

Study Questions

Please note that these questions are *not* part of your CME reporting process. They are provided here for self-assessment and identification of personal professional practice gaps. The required CME posttest is available online or by request (see "Requesting CME Credit"). Following the questions are a blank answer sheet and answers with discussions. Although a concerted effort has been made to avoid ambiguity and redundancy in these questions, the authors recognize that differences of opinion may occur regarding the "best" answer. The discussions are provided to demonstrate the rationale used to derive the answer. They may also be helpful in confirming that your approach to the problem was correct or, if necessary, in fixing the principle in your memory. The Section 11 faculty would like to thank the Self-Assessment Committee for working with them to provide these self-assessment questions and discussions.

1. Which of the following is *not* a function of the crystalline lens?
   a. maintaining clarity
   b. providing accommodation
   c. metabolizing toxins
   d. refracting light

2. What is a normal change in the normal human crystalline lens as it ages?
   a. It develops an increasingly curved shape, resulting in more refractive power.
   b. It develops an increasingly flatter shape, resulting in less refractive power.
   c. It undergoes an increase in the index of refraction as a result of the decreasing presence of insoluble protein particles.
   d. It undergoes a decrease in the index of refraction as a result of the decreasing presence of insoluble protein particles.

3. What occurs during terminal differentiation?
   a. Lens epithelial cells elongate into lens fibers.
   b. The mass of cellular proteins is decreased.
   c. Glycolysis assumes a lesser role in metabolism.
   d. Cell organelles increase their metabolic activity.

4. What is the first presenting sign of Marfan syndrome in the eye?
   a. pupillary block glaucoma
   b. monocular diplopia
   c. the need for aphakic correction
   d. inferonasal subluxation

5. Why are glutathione and vitamins A and C present in the anterior chamber?
   a. to adjust the pH and act as a buffer
   b. to protect the corneal endothelium
   c. to scavenge free radicals
   d. to induce DNA damage

6. What occurs when the ciliary muscle contracts?
   a. The diameter of the muscle ring is reduced, thereby increasing tension on the zonular fibers, allowing the lens to become more spherical.
   b. The diameter of the muscle ring is increased, thereby increasing tension on the zonular fibers, allowing the lens to become more spherical.
   c. The diameter of the muscle ring is reduced, thereby relaxing tension on the zonular fibers, allowing the lens to become more spherical.
   d. The diameter of the muscle ring is increased, thereby relaxing tension on the zonular fibers, allowing the lens to become more spherical.

7. The Y-sutures seen in the adult lens are the result of which of the following?
   a. the junction of the adult nucleus with the surrounding cortex
   b. scarring from the tunica vasculosa lentis
   c. the elaboration of the adult nucleus around the fetal nucleus
   d. fusion of the embryonic cells within the fetal nucleus

8. Which of the following systemic diseases is *not* associated with ectopia lentis?
   a. homocystinuria
   b. Ehlers-Danlos syndrome
   c. Marfan syndrome
   d. myotonic dystrophy

9. What is a typical characteristic of a lens coloboma?
   a. usually associated with previous lens trauma
   b. typically located superiorly
   c. typically associated with normal zonular attachments
   d. often associated with cortical lens opacification

10. Which of the following is seen in Peters anomaly?
    a. treatment with rigid gas-permeable contact lenses
    b. defects in the corneal endothelium and Descemet membrane
    c. identification of *PAX6* mutation in all cases
    d. bilaterality in 10% of cases

11. "Oil droplet," crystalline, and "snowflake" cataracts are characteristic of which diseases, respectively?
    a. diabetes, myotonic dystrophy, galactosemia
    b. myotonic dystrophy, galactosemia, diabetes
    c. galactosemia, diabetes, myotonic dystrophy
    d. galactosemia, myotonic dystrophy, diabetes

12. A patient presents with a mature lens and secondary glaucoma without evidence of pupillary block. What is the most likely diagnosis?
    a. phacomorphic glaucoma
    b. phacolytic glaucoma
    c. phacoantigenic uveitis
    d. lens particle glaucoma

13. Which change is most characteristic of exfoliation syndrome?
    a. exfoliative material confined to the lens capsule
    b. strong zonular fibers
    c. increased pigmentation of the trabecular meshwork
    d. hypotony

14. A 65-year-old patient presents with a gradual reduction in vision 1 year after vitrectomy to repair a retinal detachment. What is the most likely explanation?
    a. redetachment of the retina
    b. posterior subcapsular cataract from intensive steroid therapy
    c. nuclear cataract after vitrectomy to repair the retinal detachment
    d. phacoantigenic uveitis from leakage of lens protein

15. Which of the following is true regarding the epidemiology of cataracts?
    a. They are more prevalent in persons younger than 65 years.
    b. They are more prevalent in men.
    c. They occur only as a consequence of age.
    d. They are the leading cause of reversible blindness.

16. In the developing world, which of the following could apply to a patient who develops a visually significant cataract?
    a. An additional person may be removed from the workforce for care of the patient.
    b. The patient must receive prompt attention to have the cataract removed.
    c. The patient is at lower risk for falls.
    d. The patient is older than 65 years.

17. What did the Beaver Dam Eye Study determine regarding visually significant cataracts?
    a. They occur earlier in men than in women.
    b. They interfere with vision only after patients are older than 75 years.
    c. They are more likely to be cortical than nuclear.
    d. The incidence of visually significant cataract increases slowly from age 54 to 75.

18. If the best-corrected visual acuity for a patient with cataract is 20/100, a surgeon would be most likely to recommend surgery if
    a. pinhole acuity is also 20/100
    b. potential acuity meter (PAM) acuity is 20/25
    c. laser interferometry reveals that the patient has no ability to recognize the orientation of the diffraction pattern
    d. a Maddox rod test shows multiple interruptions in the red light streak

19. If a patient has a dense white cataract and the posterior pole is not visible, which of the following would be most helpful for the clinician in deciding whether to perform surgery?
    a. specular microscopy
    b. B-scan ultrasonography
    c. laser interferometry
    d. Maddox rod test

20. If a patient is found to have a best-corrected visual acuity of 20/40 in each eye but reports that vision is adequate for his needs, which factor would cause the ophthalmologist to consider cataract surgery?
    a. The level of lens opacity equals the level of vision loss.
    b. The patient has no medical problems that would contraindicate surgery.
    c. The ophthalmologist is unable to see the patient's retina well enough to evaluate it.
    d. The patient would be able to perform his activities of daily living more easily with better vision.

21. In a highly myopic patient, which of the following best describes an appropriate step in decreasing operative risks?
    a. raising the height of the irrigating bottle
    b. maintaining a loose incision to allow for increased leakage
    c. carefully examining the peripheral retina preoperatively
    d. warning the patient of blurred vision from postoperative anisometropia

22. Which of the following is a source of potential complications during cataract surgery in a uveitis patient?
    a. shallow anterior chamber
    b. zonular laxity
    c. endogenous endophthalmitis
    d. phacolytic glaucoma

23. Which one of the following steps would reduce the operative risks of surgery for a mature, white cataract?
    a. placing a small initial incision in the anterior capsule and injecting sufficient viscoelastic into the lens to expel liquid cortex prior to completing the capsulorrhexis
    b. steepening the dome of the anterior capsule by removing the viscoelastic after the initial capsule puncture
    c. staining the capsule with trypan blue or indocyanine green dye
    d. creating numerous radial relaxing incisions in the anterior capsule with long Vannas scissors

24. A patient with visually significant cataract is found to dilate poorly on preoperative examination. Which of the following is the most likely cause of this poor dilation?
    a. pigment dispersion syndrome
    b. atopic dermatitis
    c. exfoliation syndrome
    d. hypertension

25. Which of the following would be the best initial treatment of a postoperative shallow anterior chamber caused by ciliary block glaucoma?
    a. miotics and peripheral iridotomy
    b. cycloplegia and aqueous suppressants
    c. emergent vitrectomy
    d. cyclophotocoagulation

26. In operating on a patient with exfoliation syndrome, a surgeon chooses to make a large anterior continuous curvilinear capsulorrhexis (CCC). What postoperative complication will most likely be avoided?
    a. opacification of the posterior lens capsule
    b. postoperative phimosis of the anterior capsule
    c. postoperative spike in intraocular pressure
    d. glare and halos

27. In cataract surgery in which the posterior lens capsule ruptures and vitreous presents in the anterior chamber, when is anterior vitrectomy complete?
    a. when vitreous is removed from the wound
    b. when a posterior chamber intraocular lens (IOL) can be placed
    c. when the surgeon can see the retina
    d. when vitreous is removed anterior to the posterior lens capsule

Answer Sheet for Section 11 Study Questions

Question	Answer	Question	Answer
1	a b c d	15	a b c d
2	a b c d	16	a b c d
3	a b c d	17	a b c d
4	a b c d	18	a b c d
5	a b c d	19	a b c d
6	a b c d	20	a b c d
7	a b c d	21	a b c d
8	a b c d	22	a b c d
9	a b c d	23	a b c d
10	a b c d	24	a b c d
11	a b c d	25	a b c d
12	a b c d	26	a b c d
13	a b c d	27	a b c d
14	a b c d		

Answers

1. **c.** Lens cells have no mechanism for metabolizing toxins. The lens remains clear because the lens fibers contain no nuclei or organelles that would scatter light. The lens refracts light because the relative density of the lens is greater than that of the fluids (aqueous and vitreous) surrounding it. The lens, until the onset of presbyopia, remains flexible to provide accommodation in response to the tension placed on the capsule from the ciliary muscle and zonular fibers.

2. **a.** With age, the human lens develops an increasingly curved shape, which results in more refractive power. This change may be accompanied by—and sometimes offset by—a decrease in the index of refraction of the lens, probably resulting from an increase in water-insoluble proteins.

3. **a.** Terminal differentiation involves elongation of the lens epithelial cells into lens fibers. This change is associated with a tremendous increase in the mass of cellular proteins in each cell. The cells lose organelles, including nuclei, mitochondria, and ribosomes. The loss of cell organelles is optically advantageous; however, the cells then become more dependent on glycolysis for energy production and less active metabolically.

4. **b.** Monocular diplopia occurs when the lens is partially dislocated, and light can pass both through and around the edge of the lens. Pupillary block glaucoma from anterior dislocation of the lens is a rare event. Aphakic correction is required when the lens is totally subluxed into the vitreous. When the lens subluxates, it usually does so superotemporally.

5. **c.** Glutathione and vitamins A and C are powerful free radical scavengers. They have no effect on the pH or the corneal endothelium. They actually protect DNA from being damaged by free radicals.

6. **c.** The ciliary muscle is a ring, but upon contraction it does not have the effect that one would intuitively expect of a sphincter. When it contracts, the diameter of the muscle ring is reduced, thereby relaxing tension on the zonular fibers, allowing the lens to become more spherical.

7. **d.** The Y-sutures represent the edges of the secondary lens fibers of the fetal nucleus. The anterior Y is erect and the posterior one is inverted. They can be seen in the center of the adult nucleus in a clear lens. The junction of the adult nucleus and surrounding cortex is invisible until the nucleus develops sclerosis. The tunica vasculosa lentis surrounds the lens as it grows. The Y-sutures are within the fetal nucleus, not around it.

8. **d.** Myotonic dystrophy is not associated with ectopia lentis.

9. **d.** A lens coloboma is a wedge-shaped defect or indentation of the lens periphery that occurs as an isolated anomaly or is secondary to the lack of ciliary body or zonular development. Cortical lens opacification or thickening of the lens capsule may appear adjacent to the defect. Lens colobomas are typically located inferiorly and may be associated with colobomas of the uvea.

10. **b.** Peters anomaly is bilateral in 80% of cases. *PAX6* mutations occur in patients with Peters anomaly, but many cases are associated with mutations in other alleles. Treatment usually involves sector iridectomy and/or penetrating keratoplasty as well as management of coexisting glaucoma. Rigid gas-permeable contact lenses would be ineffective since they do not address the effects of the central corneal opacity.

11. **d.** Galactosemia produces an "oil droplet" cataract that appears within the first few weeks of life. Untreated, galactosemia is rapidly fatal. Crystalline cataracts in myotonic dystrophy develop a Christmas tree–appearing cortical cataract as well as posterior subcapsular changes that will lead to complete opacification. The acute cataract of uncontrolled diabetes has a snowflake appearance in the anterior and posterior subcapsular region.

12. **b.** Phacolytic glaucoma occurs when denatured lens protein leaks through an intact but permeable capsule. In phacomorphic glaucoma, the mature lens causes pupillary block and secondary angle closure. In phacoantigenic uveitis, leaking of lens protein produces a granulomatous inflammatory reaction. Lens particle glaucoma is associated with penetrating lens injury or surgery.

13. **c.** Increased pigmentation of the trabeculum and reduced outflow occur frequently in exfoliation syndrome. Exfoliative material has been found in many bodily organs as well as on the iris and corneal endothelium. Intraocular pressure may rise as a result of the obstruction of the trabecular meshwork by the exfoliative material.

14. **c.** Nuclear cataract is common in patients older than 50 years if vitrectomy has been used to repair a retinal detachment. Redetachment of the retina is an acute phenomenon and unlikely 1 year after repair. Steroid therapy after retinal detachment is usually brief and unlikely to cause nuclear cataract. Phacoantigenic uveitis produces an inflammatory reaction and is extremely rare.

15. **d.** Census data confirm that cataracts are the leading cause of reversible blindness. Cataracts increase in prevalence with increasing age and are a leading cause of blindness worldwide. They can occur as a congenital condition or as a result of trauma, metabolic diseases, or medications. Major epidemiologic studies confirm an increased prevalence in women.

16. **a.** When 1 individual is incapacitated by blindness, the care that is required to provide for that person may remove the caregiver from the workforce as well. The ratio of surgeries to population in the developing world is as low as 50 per million. Reduced vision is a primary factor in decreasing mobility and increasing the risk of falls. Cataracts form earlier in life in populations in which nutrition is not optimal.

17. **d.** Cataracts begin to interfere with vision in persons aged 43–54 years, and, from that age range, the incidence increases 13-fold in those aged 75 years or older. The overall incidence of cataract is greater in women than in men. Nuclear cataracts are more frequent than cortical cataracts at all ages.

18. **b.** The potential acuity meter (PAM) projects the equivalent of a Snellen visual acuity chart into the eye, specifically through clear spaces in the lens, by means of a beam of light to allow an estimate of macular function. The pinhole test approximates the PAM; a reduced acuity would signal other ocular conditions that cataract surgery might not improve. Laser interferometry usually is beneficial in denser cataracts: the patient's failure to discern the orientation of the diffraction pattern would indicate reduced visual potential. The patient's inability to see a continuous red line on a Maddox rod test would suggest areas of decreased retinal sensitivity in the macula.

19. **b.** B-scan ultrasonography is indicated to evaluate for occult tumors, retinal detachment, and posterior staphyloma or other posterior pathology that could affect the visual outcome. Laser interferometry and Maddox rod testing are not reliable with such a dense cataract. Specular microscopy would be indicated only if signs of corneal endothelial dysfunction were present.

20. **c.** The only consideration that would prompt the surgeon to consider operating would be the inability to evaluate the patient's retina. This would be the case even if the cataract explained the vision loss and the patient appeared well enough to undergo surgery. If the patient reports that his vision is adequate for his needs, surgery should be postponed.

21. **c.** Careful examination of the retinal periphery may reveal the presence of lattice degeneration, retinal holes, and other abnormalities that warrant consideration of preoperative treatment and/or diligent postoperative evaluation. Lowering the height of the irrigating bottle produces less stress on the zonular fibers and reduces the risk of posterior capsule tears. All incisions should be carefully closed to reduce the risk of infection. Myopic patients do need to be cautioned about anisometropia, and intolerable imbalances may prompt consideration of second-eye surgery.

22. **b.** Chronic ciliary body inflammation at the zonular fibers may lead to zonular laxity similar to that seen in exfoliation syndrome. The technical aspects of cataract surgery can be more difficult in patients with uveitis. There may be limited access to the lens because of posterior synechiae, a pupillary membrane, pupillary sphincter fibrosis, and a floppy iris. Lysing synechiae, excising pupillary membranes, and using pupil expanders and viscoelastics can counteract and overcome the effects of an abnormal iris. Rupture of the capsulorrhexis with extension to the zonular fibers can further complicate the procedure, and capsular dyes may be necessary to maintain a continuous capsular tear during the rhexis.

23. **c.** When cataract surgery is performed on a patient with a white lens, there is little or no red reflection. This makes it difficult to perform a circular capsulorrhexis. Utilizing a capsular dye improves visualization of the capsule, facilitating the creation of an anterior capsulorrhexis. The other methods described increase the operative risks. Steepening the dome of the anterior capsule increases the propensity for radial anterior capsule tearing and therefore should be avoided. Maximally filling the anterior chamber with viscoelastic during the capsulorrhexis can reduce leakage of white lens material into the anterior chamber, improving the view of the anterior capsule. Creation of numerous radial relaxing incisions is a method used when the initial capsulorrhexis is unsuccessful; it would not be the primary step in creation of a capsulorrhexis. A small puncture in the anterior capsule with injection of viscoelastic to expel liquid cortex prior to the completion of the capsulorrhexis can be used initially but is not considered necessary with the advent of capsular dyes.

24. **c.** Exfoliation syndrome is a common disorder associated with the deposition of a fibrillogranular material on the anterior surface of the lens and elsewhere in the anterior segment. With respect to cataract surgery, patients with this condition may have zonular laxity, capsular fragility, and poor pupillary dilation.

25. **b.** Causes of a shallow chamber postoperatively include wound leak, pupillary block, suprachoroidal effusion or hemorrhage, and ciliary block glaucoma with aqueous misdirection into the vitreous cavity. If the cause is known to be ciliary block glaucoma, initial treatment with cycloplegia and aqueous suppressants may relieve the condition. Surgical disruption of the vitreous face by YAG laser or a vitrectomy may be necessary at a later time to permanently restore normal aqueous circulation and anterior chamber depth if the initial treatment fails.

26. **b.** A large capsulorrhexis will reduce the risk of phimosis and increased tension on the weakened zonular fibers of the patient, also reducing the risk of late posterior dislocation

of the intraocular lens. Opacification of the posterior lens capsule is dependent not on the size of the capsulorrhexis but rather on the anterior capsule overlapping the edge of the intraocular lens. Postoperative pressure spikes are not dependent on capsulorrhexis size, although they are more common in patients with exfoliation. Glare and halos are also not caused by a large anterior capsulorrhexis.

27. **d.** Loss of vitreous is not a problem for the eye; vitreous traction is. The goal of vitreous removal is to reduce the possibility of traction. The clinician may prevent traction by removing enough vitreous to keep it away from the incision. Therefore, a vitrectomy is not complete until all vitreous is removed anterior to the posterior capsule. This ensures a lower risk of traction, and it is also the best way to decrease the risk of postoperative cystoid macular edema (CME).

Index

(f = figure; t = table)

A constant, in IOL power determination/power prediction formulas, 84
A-scan ultrasonography, for axial length measurement, 82–83, 83f, 84, 84–85
Ab externo/ab interno approaches, for IOL dislocation repair, 164–165, 165f
Accommodation, 19–20, 19t
  aging affecting, 19–20
  amplitude of, 19–20
  changes with, 19, 19f
  Helmholtz theory of, 19
Accommodative intraocular lenses, 137
  complications associated with, 169
Acid, ocular injuries caused by, cataract and, 53
ACIOL. See Intraocular lenses (IOLs), anterior chamber
Acne rosacea. See Rosacea
Acrylic, for intraocular lenses, 135–136. See also Foldable intraocular lens
  capsular opacification and, 170
  glistenings and, 169
  instrumentation for handling, 138
  uveitis and, 204
Active transport/secretion, in lens
  epithelium as site of, 17–18
  pump–leak theory and, 18–19, 18f
Activities of Daily Vision Scale (ADVS), 71
ADVS. See Activities of Daily Vision Scale
Affinity constant (K_m), "sugar" cataract development and, 15
Age/aging
  accommodative response/presbyopia and, 19–20
  cataracts related to, 39–47. See also Age-related cataracts
  lens changes associated with, 7, 20, 39–47, 40f
  lens proteins affected by, 13, 39
Age-related cataracts, 39–47. See also specific type
  cortical, 41–42, 42f, 43f, 44f, 45f
  in diabetes, 55
  epidemiology of, 65–68
  genetic contributions to, 37–38
  nuclear, 39–40, 41f
  nutritional deficiency and, 57–58
  posterior subcapsular, 42–44, 47f
Age-Related Eye Disease Study (AREDS), 66
AK. See Astigmatic keratotomy
AL. See Axial length
Alcohol use/abuse, cataract formation and, 58–59
Aldose reductase
  in cataract formation, 15
  in lens glucose/carbohydrate metabolism, 14f, 15
Aldose reductase inhibitors, cataract prevention/management and, 72–73
Alfuzosin, intraoperative floppy iris syndrome and, 155

Alkalis (alkaline solutions), ocular injuries caused by, cataract and, 53
Alpha (α)-blockers, intraoperative floppy iris syndrome and, 74, 154–155
Alpha (α)-chymotrypsin, for ICCE, 93, 214
Alpha (α)-crystallins, 11–12, 11f
Alport syndrome, lenticonus in, 26
Amikacin, for postoperative endophthalmitis, 181
Amiodarone, lens changes caused by, 49
Amniotic membrane transplantation, for corneal edema after cataract surgery, 148
Amplitude of accommodation, 19–20
Anaerobic glycolysis, in lens glucose/carbohydrate metabolism, 13–15, 14f
Anesthesia, for cataract surgery, 98–102, 99f, 100f, 101f
Angiographic cystoid macular edema, after cataract surgery, 182
Angle closure/angle-closure glaucoma
  ciliary block (malignant), cataract surgery and, 153, 157–158
  microspherophakia and, 29
  secondary, with pupillary block
    microspherophakia and, 29
    phacomorphic glaucoma and, 63, 64f
Aniridia, 29–30, 29f
  cataract surgery in patient with, 200
Anisometropia
  asymmetric lens-induced myopia causing, 70
  second-eye cataract surgery for, 73
Ankylosing spondylitis, cataract surgery in patient with, 188, 189f
Anomalies, congenital. See specific type and Congenital anomalies
Anterior capsule fibrosis and phimosis, 171
  Nd:YAG laser capsulotomy for, 171, 171–175, 172f, 199. See also Nd:YAG laser therapy, capsulotomy
Anterior capsule opacity, 169, 170
Anterior capsulotomy. See Capsulotomy, anterior
Anterior chamber
  flat or shallow
    cataract surgery and, 152–154
      intraoperative complications, 152–153
      posterior fluid misdirection and, 152–153
      postoperative complications, 153–154
      preoperative considerations/IOL power determination and, 79, 84
  gonioscopy/evaluation of, before cataract surgery, 79
  phacoemulsification in, 119
  vitreous prolapse in, 162
Anterior chamber intraocular lenses. See Intraocular lenses
Anterior lenticonus/lentiglobus, 26

Anterior polar cataract (APC), 30–31, 32f
Anterior pole, 5, 6f
Anterior pupillary membrane, 25, 25f
Anterior segment
　disorders of, cataract surgery complications causing, 151–162. *See also specific type*
　trauma to, 206
Anterior segment dysgenesis syndrome, Peters anomaly and, 27–28
Anterior sutures, 9
Antibiotics
　for postoperative endophthalmitis, 181
　prophylactic, cataract surgery and, 127–129, 128f, 180
　　corneal melting and, 150
Anticholinesterase agents. *See* Cholinesterase/acetylcholinesterase inhibitors
Anticoagulant therapy, cataract surgery and, 74, 175–176, 189–190
Antimicrobial prophylaxis, cataract surgery and, 127–129, 128f
　corneal melting and, 150
Antiplatelet therapy, cataract surgery and, 175–176
Aphakia
　congenital, 26
　intraocular lenses for correction of, 132–141. *See also* Intraocular lenses
　　secondary anterior chamber IOL implantation and, 140
Applanation ultrasonography, for axial length measurement, 82
AquaLase Liquefaction Device, 127
Aquaporin 0 (major intrinsic protein/MIP), 12, 17
Aquaporins (water channels), 12, 17
Aqueous misdirection (malignant/ciliary block glaucoma), cataract surgery and, 153, 157–158
Arachnodactyly, in Marfan syndrome, 36, 36f
AREDS (Age-Related Eye Disease Study), 66
Arterial retrobulbar hemorrhage, cataract surgery and, 176
Arthritis
　cataract surgery in patients with, 188
　rheumatoid, cataract surgery in patient with, corneal melting/keratolysis and, 150
Aspiration, in phacoemulsification, 104, 108–109, 108f, 109f, 110f
　strategies for, 125–126
Aspiration flow rate, in phacoemulsification, 104
　setting, 119
　vacuum rise time and, 109, 110f
Aspirin, cataract surgery in patient taking, 189
Astigmatic keratotomy, cataract surgery and, 130
Astigmatism
　in cataract patient
　　modification during surgery and, 130–131
　　toric intraocular lenses for, 131
　after cataract surgery, 150, 213
　irregular, refractive surgery and, cataract surgery outcome and, 193, 193f
　　limbal relaxing incisions for, 130–131
　　suture-induced, cataract surgery and, 150, 212–213
Atopic dermatitis, cataracts associated with, 62
Atropine, accommodation affected by, 19
Axes, optic, 5, 6f
Axial length
　extremes in, cataract surgery in patient with, 200–201
　in IOL power determination, 82–83, 84, 84–85
　　optical measurement of, 83
　　ultrasound measurement of, 82–83, 83f, 84, 84–85
　unexpected refractive results after surgery and, 168

B-scan ultrasonography, before cataract surgery, 80–81, 84, 84–85
Balanced salt solution (BSS)
　in ECCE, 94
　in phacoemulsification, 108
Baltimore Eye Survey, 67
Barbados Eye Study, 67
Barraquer erysiphake, 92, 92f
Basement membrane dystrophy, epithelial, cataract surgery in patient with, 191, 192f
Beaded filaments, 12
Beaver Dam Eye Study, 67
Behavioral/psychiatric disorders, cataract surgery in patient with, 187
Benign prostatic hypertrophy, α-blockers/tamsulosin for, intraoperative floppy iris syndrome and, 74, 154–155
Beta (β)-crystallins, 12
Betagamma (β,γ)-crystallins, 11f, 12
Biometry/biometrics
　before cataract surgery, 82–83, 83f
　in IOL power determination/selection, 82–83, 83f, 84
Biomicroscopy, slit-lamp. *See* Slit-lamp biomicroscopy/examination
Bladder (Wedl) cells, 44, 170
Bleeding diathesis, cataract surgery in patient with, 189–190
Blepharitis, cataract surgery in patient with, 77, 190
Blindness, cataract causing, 65, 65t
Blue-blocking intraocular lenses, 138
Blue-dot (cerulean) cataract, 33, 34f
Blunt trauma, lens injury/cataract caused by, 50–51, 50f. *See also* Trauma
BMI. *See* Body mass index
BMP. *See* Bone morphogenetic protein
Body mass index (BMI), cataract risk and, 67
Bone morphogenetic protein, lens placode formation and, 21
Brown-McLean syndrome, 148
Brunescent cataract, 40
　lens proteins in, 13
　surgery for removal of, 195–196
BSS. *See* Balanced salt solution

Bullous keratopathy, after cataract surgery, 147, 147*f*, 167
   IOL design and, 167
Burns, thermal, cataract surgery incision, 149
Burst-mode phacoemulsification, 107

Calcium deposits, on intraocular lenses, 169
Can-opener capsulotomy
   for ECCE, 212
   for phacoemulsification, 115, 116*f*
Cannulas, for ECCE, 95–96, 95*f*
Cantholysis, lateral, bulbar hemorrhage release and, 99
Capsular block syndrome, 166–167
Capsular cataracts, 33–34
Capsular fibrosis, 171
   IOL decentration/dislocation and, 164
   Nd:YAG laser capsulotomy for, 171, 171–175, 172*f*, 199. *See also* Nd:YAG laser therapy, capsulotomy
Capsular hooks, 198, 198*f*, 199
Capsular opacification, 169–171
   IOL design/material and, 170
   Nd:YAG laser capsulotomy for, 169, 171–175, 174*f*. *See also* Nd:YAG laser therapy, capsulotomy
Capsular phimosis, 171
   in exfoliation syndrome, 199
   Nd:YAG laser capsulotomy for, 171, 172*f*, 199. *See also* Nd:YAG laser therapy, capsulotomy
Capsular rupture, cataract surgery and, 144*t*, 160–162
Capsular tension rings, for zonular incompetence, 198, 199
Capsule, lens. *See* Lens capsule
Capsule staining, for cataract surgery, 195, 195*f*
Capsulorrhexis
   advanced cataract and, 195
   capsule staining for, 195, 195*f*
   continuous curvilinear, 115–117, 116*f*
      capsule staining for, 195, 195*f*
      for ECCE, 212
      loose zonules and, 117
         in glaucoma patient, 202
   for ECCE, 211
   loose zonules and, 117
      in glaucoma patient, 202
   for phacoemulsification, 115–117, 116*f*
Capsulotomy
   anterior
      for ECCE, 211
      for phacoemulsification, 115, 116*f*
   can-opener, 115, 116*f*
   Nd:YAG laser, 171–175, 172*f*, 174*f*
      for capsular block syndrome, 166–167
      for capsule opacification, 169, 171–175, 174*f*
      complications of, 173–175
      contraindications to, 172
      indications for, 171–172
      lens particle glaucoma and, 63

      procedure for, 172–173, 174*f*
      retinal detachment and, 175, 184
Carbohydrate metabolism, in lens, 13–15, 14*f*
Carotenoids, cataract risk affected by, 58
Catalase, in lens, 16
Cataract
   advanced, surgery for extraction of, 195–196
   age-related, 39–47. *See also* Age-related cataracts
      epidemiology of, 65–68
      genetic contributions to, 37–38
   alcohol use/abuse and, 58–59
   atopic dermatitis and, 62
   brunescent, 40
      lens proteins in, 13
      surgery for removal of, 195–196
   capsular, 33–34
   cerulean, 33, 34*f*
   chemical injuries causing, 53
   in children, 30–35, 31*t*. *See also* Cataract, congenital
   clinical studies of, 66–68
   complete (total), 34
   congenital, 30–35, 31*t*
      aniridia and, 29*f*, 30
      bilateral, 31*t*
      genetic contributions to, 37–38
      unilateral, 31*t*
   contrast sensitivity affected by, 70, 76–77
   contusion, 50, 50*f*
   coronary, 33
   cortical, 41–42, 42*f*, 43*f*, 44*f*, 45*f*
      uveitis and, 59, 60*f*
      visual acuity and, 70*t*
   degenerative ocular disorders and, 64
   diabetic, 55, 56*f*
      "sugar," aldose reductase in development of, 15
      surgery for, 188
         preoperative evaluation and, 80
   drug-induced, 47–49
   electrical injury causing, 54, 55*f*
   epidemiology of, 65–68, 65*t*
   evaluation of, 69–88, 70*t*
   fundus evaluation in patient with, 80–81
   in galactosemia, 56–57, 56*f*
   glassblowers', 52–53
   glaucoma and, 63, 64*f*, 201–203, 202*f*
      management of, 201–203, 202*f*
      preoperative evaluation/management and, 75, 201–202, 202*f*
   history in, 69–71, 70*t*
      surgery evaluation and, 73–75
   hypermature, 42, 45*f*
      phacolytic glaucoma and, 63
   hypocalcemia and, 57
   infantile, 30–35, 31*t*. *See also* Cataract, congenital
   intralenticular foreign-body causing, 51
   intumescent, 42
      phacomorphic glaucoma and, 63, 64*f*
      surgery for removal of, 196
   ischemia causing, 64

after keratoplasty, 193
lamellar (zonular), 30, 32f
lens proteins and, 13
management of, 71–88. *See also* Cataract surgery
   in glaucoma patient, 201–203, 202f
   low vision aids in, 71
   nonsurgical, 71–72
   pharmacologic, 71–72
mature, 42, 44f
   phacolytic glaucoma and, 63
membranous, 34, 35f
metabolic, 55–57, 56f
morgagnian, 42, 46f
in myotonic dystrophy, 57
nuclear, 39–40, 41f
   in children/congenital, 33, 34f
   genetic contributions to, 37–38
   hyperbaric oxygen therapy and, 60–61
   visual acuity and, 39, 70t
   vitrectomy and, 16, 60, 205–206
nutritional disease and, 57–58
oxidative damage and, 16
pediatric, 30–35, 31t. *See also* Cataract, congenital
perforating/penetrating injuries causing, 51, 51f, 52f
persistent fetal vasculature (persistent hyperplastic primary vitreous) and, 38
phacolytic glaucoma and, 63
phacomorphic glaucoma and, 63, 64f
polar, 30–31, 32f
   surgery for removal of, 196–197
posterior lenticonus/lentiglobus and, 26
postvitrectomy, 16, 60, 205–206
radiation-induced, 51–53
after refractive surgery, 193–194, 193f
rosette, 50, 50f
rubella, 35
in siderosis bulbi, 53, 54f
smoking/tobacco use and, 58–59, 67–68
snowflake, 55, 56f
socioeconomic impact of, 66
steroid-induced, 47–48, 203
subcapsular, posterior, 42–44, 47f
   corticosteroids causing, 47–48
   ischemia causing, 64
   in myotonic dystrophy, 57
   silicone oil use and, 205
   uveitis and, 59
   visual acuity and, 43, 70, 70t
"sugar," aldose reductase in development of, 15
sunflower, in chalcosis/Wilson disease, 54, 57
sutural (stellate), 33, 33f
tetanic, 57
total (complete), 34
traumatic, 50–54, 50f, 51f, 52f, 55f, 206–209, 207f
   surgery for, 206–209
treatment-induced, 60. *See also* Cataract, drug-induced
uveitis and, 59, 60f, 203–204

visual acuity and, 39, 43, 70, 70t
   preoperative evaluation and, 75, 76
in Wilson disease, 57
zonular (lamellar), 30, 32f
Cataract surgery, 89–142. *See also specific procedure and* Phacoemulsification
in acne rosacea, 77, 190
in α-blocker patients, 74, 154–155
ancient/medieval techniques for, 89–90, 89f, 90f
anesthesia for, 98–102, 99f, 100f, 101f
aniridia and, 200
anterior capsule fibrosis and phimosis and, 171, 172f
in anticoagulated patients, 74, 175–176, 189–190
antimicrobial prophylaxis for, 127–129, 128f
   corneal melting and, 150
astigmatism and
   modification of preexisting, 130–131
   suture-induced, 150, 212–213
   toric IOLs for, 131
axial length extremes and, 200–201
biometry before, 82–83, 83f
in bleeding diathesis, 189–190
in blepharitis patients, 190
Brown-McLean syndrome after, 148
bullous keratopathy after, 147, 147f, 167
   IOL design and, 167
capsular block syndrome and, 166–167
capsular opacification and contraction and, 169–175, 172f, 174f
   Nd:YAG laser capsulotomy for, 169, 171–175, 174f. *See also* Nd:YAG laser therapy, capsulotomy
capsular rupture and, 144t, 160–162
capsule staining and, 195, 195f
capsulorrhexis in, 115–117, 116f
   capsule staining for, 195, 195f
   loose zonules and, 117
choroidal hemorrhage and. *See* Cataract surgery, suprachoroidal hemorrhage/effusion and
chronic uveitis after, 158–159
ciliary block (malignant) glaucoma and, 153, 157–158
in claustrophobic patient, 187
clear corneal incision for, 113–115, 113f, 115f
   glaucoma and, 201–202
communication with patient and, 188
complications of, 143–185, 144t. *See also specific type*
   anterior segment, 151–162
   antimicrobial prophylaxis in prevention of, 127–129, 128f, 180
   capsular opacification and contraction and, 169–175, 172f, 174f
   corneal, 146–150
   endophthalmitis, 143, 144t, 179–181, 179f
   hemorrhage, 175–179
   IOL implantation and, 133, 144t, 162–169

needle penetration of globe and, 185
retinal, 181–185, 182f
conjunctival evaluation before, 78
corneal conditions and, 191–194, 192f, 193f
corneal edema and, 143, 144t, 146–148, 146t, 147f
corneal evaluation before, 78, 83–84
pachymetry, 84
topography, 83–84
corneal melting/keratolysis after, 150
in patient with dry eye, 150, 191
cyclodialysis and, 157
cystoid macular edema and, 143, 144t
in glaucoma patient, 202–203
after Nd:YAG capsulotomy, 175
vitreous prolapse and, 162
in dementia/mentally disabled patient, 187
Descemet membrane detachment and, 149
with Descemet membrane–stripping automated
endothelial keratoplasty and intraocular lens
insertion (triple procedure), 141, 192
in diabetic patients, 188
preoperative evaluation and, 80
economics of, 66
elevated intraocular pressure after, 154. See also
Elevated intraocular pressure
in glaucoma patient, 202
endophthalmitis after, 143, 144t, 179–181, 179f
prevention of, 127–129, 128f, 180
endothelial keratoplasty and, 141, 192
epithelial downgrowth and, 151
in exfoliation syndrome, 199
external eye examination before, 77–78
external ocular abnormalities and, 190–191
extracapsular cataract extraction (ECCE),
211–213. See also Extracapsular cataract
extraction
early techniques for, 90–92, 91f
modern procedure for, 94–96, 95f, 211–213
renaissance/rediscovery of, 94
filtering bleb (inadvertent) after, 148–149
filtering surgery before, 203
flat or shallow anterior chamber and, 152–154
intraoperative complications, 152–153
postoperative complications, 153–154
preoperative considerations/IOL power
determination and, 79, 84
Fuchs heterochromic uveitis and, 59
fundus evaluation before, 80–81
in glaucoma patient, 201–203, 202f
filtering surgery before, 203
preoperative evaluation and, 75, 201–202, 202f
globe exposure for, 110
hemorrhage and, 175–179, 189–190
high hyperopia and, 200–201
high myopia and, 200
history of use of
in recent past, 93–96, 93f, 95f
in remote past, 89–92, 89f, 91f, 92f
hyphema after, 167, 177

hypotony/flat anterior chamber after, 153
in hypotony patients, 201
incisions for. See also Incisions, for cataract
surgery
complications related to, 148–149
for ECCE, 211
glaucoma and, 201–202
for ICCE, 214
intraocular lens implantation and, 138
leaking, 144t, 148–149
flat anterior chamber and, 153
modification of preexisting astigmatism
and, 130
for phacoemulsification
clear corneal, 113–115, 113f, 115f
scleral tunnel, 111–113, 111f, 112f
indications for, 72–73
informed consent for, 88
intracapsular cataract extraction (ICCE), 93–94,
93f, 213–215. See also Intracapsular cataract
extraction
early techniques for, 92, 92f
modern advances/procedure for, 93–94, 93f,
213–215
intraocular lens implantation and, 132–141. See
also Intraocular lenses
complications of, 162–169
intraoperative floppy iris syndrome and, 74,
154–155, 156f
iridodialysis and, 157
iris trauma during, 144t, 157
in iris trauma patient, 207–208, 207f
in keratoconjunctivitis sicca, 190–191
after keratoplasty, 193
lens anatomy alterations and, 195–200
lens–iris diaphragm retropulsion syndrome
and, 156
lens visualization and, 194–195, 194f, 195f
trauma affecting, 206
loose zonules and, 117, 118
in glaucoma patient, 202
macular function evaluation before, 82
retinal disease and, 204–205
manual small-incision, 96
measurements taken before, 82–84, 83f
nanophthalmos and, 200–201
nucleus removal in
femtosecond laser for, 127
fluid-based phacolysis for, 127
laser photolysis for, 127
phacoemulsification for, 102–126. See also
Phacoemulsification
ocular hypotension after, 153
ophthalmic viscosurgical devices (viscoelastic
agents) in, 96–98, 97t. See also Ophthalmic
viscosurgical devices
outcomes of, 141–142
improving, 86
paracentesis for, 110

pars plana lensectomy, 132
patient preparation for, 88
in patient unable to communicate, 188
in pemphigoid patients, 191
with penetrating keratoplasty and intraocular lens
    insertion (triple procedure), 141, 192
phacoemulsification, 102–126. See also
    Phacoemulsification
posterior capsule opacification and, 143, 169–171
    Nd:YAG laser capsulotomy for, 169, 171–175,
    174f. See also Nd:YAG laser therapy,
    capsulotomy
posterior capsule rupture and, 144t, 160–162
posterior misdirection of irrigation fluid and,
    152–153
postoperative care and
    after ECCE, 213
    after ICCE, 215
potential acuity estimation before, 81
preoperative evaluation/preparation for, 73–75
pseudophakic bullous keratopathy after, 147,
    147f, 167
    IOL design and, 167
psychosocial considerations in, 72, 75, 187–188
pupil expansion and, 194, 194f
    in uveitis, 203–204
pupillary capture and, 166, 167f
    IOL decentration and, 163
rate of, 65
refraction before, 76
refractive errors after, 168
after refractive surgery, 75, 78, 193–194
    IOL power calculation and, 86–88, 193
with refractive surgery, 130–131. See also Cataract
    surgery, astigmatism and
retained foreign matter and, 207
retained lens material and, 143, 147, 159–160
retinal complications and, 181–185, 182f
retinal detachment after, 143, 144t, 184–185
    family history as risk factor and, 75
    Nd:YAG laser capsulotomy and, 175, 184
in retinal disease, 75, 204–205
retinal light toxicity and, 183–184
retrobulbar hemorrhage and, 144t, 176–177, 189
scleral tunnel incisions for, 111–113, 111f, 112f
slit-lamp examination before, 78–80
specular microscopy before, 84
stromal/epithelial edema after, 146–148
suprachoroidal hemorrhage/effusion and, 144t,
    177–179, 189
    delayed, 178–179
    expulsive, 178
    flat anterior chamber and, 152
systemic conditions and, 188–190, 189f
in tamsulosin patient, 74, 154, 155
toxic anterior segment syndrome and, 151–152
after trauma, 206–209, 207f
in triple procedure, 141, 192
uveitis and, 158–159, 203–204
in uveitis patient, 75, 158, 203–204

visual function evaluation after, 141
visual function evaluation before, 71, 76–77
vitreal complications/vitreous abnormalities and
    with ICCE, 214
    posterior vitreous detachment, 184
    prolapse, 162
    vitreocorneal adherence, 148
wound closure for
    complications associated with, 148–149
    after ECCE, 212–213
    postoperative endophthalmitis and, 180
    for scleral tunnel incisions, 112–113, 112f
wound dehiscence/rupture and, 149
zonular abnormalities and, 195–200
    iris coloboma/corectopia and, 196, 197f
    zonular dehiscence/lens subluxation or dislocation
        and, 197–199, 198f
Cation balance, in lens, maintenance of, 17–19, 18f
Cavitation, 102, 105, 105f, 107
CCC. See Continuous curvilinear capsulorrhexis
Ceftazidime, for endophthalmitis, after cataract
    surgery, 181
Cerulean cataract, 33, 34f
Chalcosis, 54
Chatter, 103, 107
Chemical injury (burns), cataracts caused by, 53
Children, cataract in, 30–35, 31t
    genetic contributions to, 37–38
Chlorpromazine, lens changes caused by, 49
Cholinesterase/acetylcholinesterase inhibitors
    (anticholinesterase agents)
    in cataract surgery, traumatic cataract, 208
    cataracts caused by, 49
Chondroitin sulfate, as viscoelastic, 96
Chopping techniques, in phacoemulsification,
    122–124, 124f
    instrument settings for, 118–119
Choroidal/suprachoroidal hemorrhage, cataract
    surgery and, 144t, 177–179, 189
    delayed, 178–179
    expulsive, 178
    flat or shallow anterior chamber and, 152
Chromophores, ultraviolet, intraocular lenses
    with, 138
Chymotrypsin (α-chymotrypsin), for ICCE, 93, 214
Cicatricial pemphigoid, cataract surgery in patient
    with, 191
Cigarette smoking, cataract development and, 58–59,
    67–68
Ciliary block, after cataract surgery, flat or shallow
    anterior chamber and, 153
Ciliary block (malignant) glaucoma, cataract surgery
    and, 153, 157–158
Ciliary body, injury of in cataract surgery, 144t
Ciliary muscle, in accommodation, 19, 19t
Claustrophobia, cataract surgery in patient with, 187
Clear corneal incision, 113–115, 113f, 115f
    in glaucoma patients, 201–202
Closed-loop intraocular lenses, pseudophakic
    bullous keratopathy and, 167

CME. *See* Cystoid macular edema
Coagulation
  disorders of, cataract surgery in patient with, 189–190
  laboratory evaluation of, before cataract surgery, 189–190
Cohesive ophthalmic viscosurgical devices, 97, 97*t*
Colobomas
  iris, cataract surgery in patient with, 196, 197*f*
  lens, 26–27, 27*f*
Color vision defects, nuclear cataract and, 40
Communication, between clinician and patient, cataract surgery and, 188
Complete cataract, 34
Confrontation testing, before cataract surgery, 81–82
Congenital anomalies. *See also specific type*
  of lens, 26–35
Congenital aphakia, 26. *See also* Aphakia
Congenital cataract, 30–35. *See also specific type and* Cataract, congenital
  genetic contributions to, 37–38
Congenital rubella syndrome, cataracts and, 35
Conjunctiva, examination of, before cataract surgery, 78
Conjunctival flaps
  for corneal edema after cataract surgery, 147–148
  for ICCE, 214
  wound leak under, inadvertent filtering bleb and, 148–149
Connective tissue disorders, cataract surgery in patient with, 188, 191
Consent, informed, for cataract surgery, 88
Contact lens method, for IOL power calculation after refractive surgery, 87
Continuous curvilinear capsulorrhexis, 115–117, 116*f*. *See also* Capsulorrhexis
  capsule staining for, 195, 195*f*
  for ECCE, 212
  loose zonules and, 117
  for manual small-incision cataract surgery, 96
  for phacoemulsification, 115–117, 116*f*
Continuous phacoemulsification, 106–107
Contrast sensitivity testing, in cataract patient, 70, 76–77
Contusion cataract, 50, 50*f*
Contusion injury, lens damage caused by, 50–51, 50*f*
Copper
  foreign body of, 54
  sunflower cataract in chalcosis/Wilson disease and, 54, 57
Corectopia, cataract surgery in patient with, 196
Cornea
  deposits in, copper/Wilson disease causing, 54, 57
  disorders of
    as cataract surgery complication, 146–150
    cataract surgery in patient with, 191–194, 192*f*, 193*f*
  edema of, after cataract surgery, 143, 144*t*, 146–148, 146*t*, 147*f*
    persistent, with vitreocorneal adherence, 148
  epithelium of, defects/persistent defects of, after cataract surgery, 150
  examination of, before cataract surgery, 78, 83–84
  guttae/guttata
    Brown-McLean syndrome and, 148
    cataract surgery and, 78
  melting of (keratolysis), cataract surgery and, 150
    in patient with dry eye, 150, 191
  opacification of
    cataract/cataract surgery and, 191–192
    in Peters anomaly, 27
  thickness/rigidity of, measurement of, before cataract surgery, 78, 84
  topography of
    cataract surgery and, 83–84
    IOL power determination/selection and, after refractive surgery, 86, 87
  transplantation of
    cataract/cataract surgery following, 193
    in triple procedure, 141, 192
Corneal dystrophies, cataract/cataract surgery in patient with, 191–192, 192*f*
Corneal incision, clear, for cataract surgery, 113–115, 113*f*, 115*f*
Corneal melting (keratolysis), cataract surgery and, 150
  in patient with dry eye, 150, 191
Coronary cataract, 33
Cortex, lens, 6*f*, 8–9
Cortical cataracts, 41–42, 42*f*, 43*f*, 44*f*, 45*f*
  uveitis and, 59, 60*f*
  visual acuity and, 70*t*
Cortical spokes, 42, 43*f*
Corticosteroids (steroids)
  cataracts caused by, 47–48, 203
  for postoperative cystoid macular edema, 183
Couching, 89–90, 89*f*, 90*f*
Cough, cataract surgery in patient with, 188
Coumadin. *See* Warfarin
Coupling, astigmatic keratotomy and, 130
Cranial nerve III (oculomotor nerve), in accommodation, 19
Cryoprobe, for lens extraction, 93, 93*f*
Crystallins, 11–12, 11*f*
  aging affecting, 39
  α, 11–12, 11*f*
  β, 12
  β,γ, 11*f*, 12
  γ, 12
CTRs. *See* Capsular tension rings
Cuneiform opacities, 42, 43*f*
Cyclodialysis, after cataract surgery, 157
Cycloplegia/cycloplegics, 19
Cystitome, for ECCE, 95
Cystoid macular edema, postoperative, 143, 144*t*, 181–183, 182*f*
  in glaucoma patient, 202–203
  after Nd:YAG capsulotomy, 175
  vitreous prolapse and, 162
Cytoskeletal (urea-soluble) lens proteins, 11*f*, 12

Deafness (hearing loss), cataract surgery in patient with, 188
Decentration/dislocation (intraocular lens), 143, 144*t*, 162–166, 163*f*, 164*f*, 165*f*
Degenerations, cataracts associated with, 64
Delayed suprachoroidal hemorrhage, after cataract surgery, 178–179
Dementia, cataract surgery in patient with, 187
Dermatitis, atopic, cataracts associated with, 62
Descemet membrane, detachment of, after cataract surgery, 149
Descemet membrane–stripping automated endothelial keratoplasty (DSAEK), in triple procedure, 141
Developmental defects of lens, 35–38. *See also specific type*
Diabetes mellitus, cataracts associated with, 55, 56*f*
  "sugar," aldose reductase in development of, 15
  surgery for, 188
    preoperative evaluation and, 80
Diabetic macular edema, cataract surgery and, 205
Dialing, for posterior chamber IOL implantation, 139
Diaphragm pump, for phacoemulsification aspiration, 109, 109*f*
  vacuum rise time for, 109, 110*f*
Diffusion, glucose transport into lens and, 13
Diplopia, monocular, in cataracts, 40, 41, 43, 70
DisCoVisc, 98
Dislocated lens, 35. *See also* Ectopia lentis
  cataract surgery in patient with, 197–199, 198*f*
  traumatic, 36, 50–51, 50*f*
Dislocation/decentration, intraocular lens, 143, 144*t*, 162–166, 163*f*, 164*f*, 165*f*
Dispersive ophthalmic viscosurgical devices, 97, 97*t*
Doxazosin, intraoperative floppy iris syndrome and, 74, 155
Drugs, lens changes caused by, 47–49
Dry-eye syndrome, cataract surgery in patient with, 190–191
  corneal melting/keratolysis and, 150, 191
DSAEK. *See* Descemet membrane–stripping automated endothelial keratoplasty
Dulcitol (galactitol), in cataract formation, 56
Duty cycle, in phacoemulsification, 103
Dysphotopsias, intraocular lenses and, 168
Dystrophies, corneal, cataract/cataract surgery in patient with, 191–192, 192*f*

ECCE. *See* Extracapsular cataract extraction
Echothiophate, cataract and, 49
Ectoderm, in lens development, 21, 22*f*
Ectopia lentis, 35–37, 36*f*
  cataract surgery in patient with, 197–199, 198*f*
  et pupillae, 38
  in homocystinuria, 37
  in hyperlysinemia, 37
  in Marfan syndrome, 36–37, 36*f*
  simple, 36
  traumatic, 36, 50–51, 50*f*

Edema, corneal. *See* Cornea, edema of
Effusion, suprachoroidal, cataract surgery and, 177–178
  flat or shallow anterior chamber and, 152
Electrical injury, lens damage/cataracts caused by, 54, 55*f*
Electrolytes, in lens, maintenance of balance of, 17–19, 18*f*
Elevated intraocular pressure
  cataract surgery and, 154
    epithelial downgrowth and, 151
    expulsive suprachoroidal hemorrhage and, 178
    flat or shallow anterior chamber and, 152, 153–154, 154
    in glaucoma patients, 75, 201, 202
    retrobulbar hemorrhage and, 176
    stromal/epithelial corneal edema and, 147
  in glaucoma
    cataract surgery and, 75, 201, 202
    phacolytic glaucoma and, 63
  Nd:YAG laser capsulotomy and, 173–175
Elschnig pearls, 170
Embryonic lens nucleus, 9, 22–23, 23*f*
  opacification of (congenital nuclear cataract), 33, 34*f*
Emulsification. *See also* Phacoemulsification
  locations of, 119–120, 120*f*, 121*f*
Endophthalmitis, postoperative, 143, 144*t*, 179–181, 179*f*
  prevention of, 127–129, 128*f*, 180
Endophthalmitis Vitrectomy Study (EVS), 179, 180
Endothelial dystrophy, cataract surgery in patient with, 192
Endothelial keratoplasty
  cataract surgery and, 141, 192
  for corneal edema after cataract surgery, 147
Energy, phaco, 103, 126. *See also* Power
  advances in, 126
Enophthalmos, cataract surgery in patient with, 77
Enterococcus, postoperative endophthalmitis caused by, 180
EPHA2 gene, in age-related cataracts, 37
Epicapsular star, 27, 28*f*
Epimerase deficiency, galactosemia/cataract formation and, 57
Epithelial basement membrane dystrophy, cataract surgery in patient with, 191, 192*f*
Epithelial defects, corneal/persistent corneal, after cataract surgery, 150
Epithelial downgrowth, cataract surgery and, 151
Epithelium, lens, 6*f*, 8, 8*f*
  active transport and, 17–18
  development of, 23, 23*f*
  opacification of (capsular cataract), 33–34
Equator (lens), 5, 6*f*
Erysiphakes, 92, 92*f*
EVS (Endophthalmitis Vitrectomy Study), 179, 180
Exfoliation. *See also* Exfoliation syndrome
  true, infrared radiation/heat causing, 52–53

Exfoliation syndrome (pseudoexfoliation), 61–62, 61f
  cataract surgery in patient with, 199
  postoperative hyphema and, 177
  zonular incompetence and, 197, 198f, 199
Expulsive choroidal/suprachoroidal hemorrhage, cataract surgery and, 178
External (outer) eye
  cataract surgery in patient with abnormalities of, 190–191
  examination of, before cataract surgery, 77–78
Extracapsular cataract extraction (ECCE), 94–96, 95f, 211–213. See also Cataract surgery
  for advanced cataract, 196
  advantages of, 95
  anterior capsulotomy in, 211
  in anticoagulated patient, 189
  capsular opacification and, 169–171
    Nd:YAG laser capsulotomy for, 169, 171–175, 174f. See also Nd:YAG laser therapy, capsulotomy
  cystoid macular edema and, 182
  early techniques for, 90–92, 91f
  equipment for, 95–96, 95f
  flat or shallow anterior chamber and, 152–154
    intraoperative complications, 152–153
    postoperative complications, 153–154
  incisions for, 211
  intraocular lenses for, 133, 133–136, 136f, 212
  lens particle glaucoma and, 63
  manual small-incision cataract surgery and, 96
  nucleus removal in, 95, 212
  ocular trauma affecting visualization and, 206
  patient preparation for, 211
  postoperative course and, 213
  procedure for, 94–96, 95f, 211–213
  renaissance/rediscovery of, 94
  retained lens fragments after, 159
  retinal detachment and, 184
  after vitrectomy, 206
  vitreocorneal adherence/persistent corneal edema and, 148
  wound closure and, 212–213
Extracapsular IOL dislocation, 162, 163f
Eye
  axial length of
    extremes of, cataract surgery in patient with, 200–201
    in IOL power determination, 82–83, 83f, 84, 84–85, 168
  external
    cataract surgery in patient with abnormalities of, 190–191
    examination of, before cataract surgery, 77–78
Eyedrops (topical medications), after cataract surgery, 129
  corneal melting and, 150, 191

Facial nerve block, for cataract surgery, 101, 101f
Facilitated diffusion, glucose transport into lens and, 13

Feiz and Mannis formula, for IOL power determination/selection, 87
Femtosecond laser, for cataract extraction, 127
Fetal lens nucleus, 9, 23f, 24–25, 24f
  opacification of (congenital nuclear cataract), 33, 34f
Fetal vasculature, persistent. See Persistent fetal vasculature
Fibrillin defects, in Marfan syndrome, 36
Filensin, 12
Filtering bleb, inadvertent, after cataract surgery, 148–149
Filtering procedures, cataract surgery after, 203
Flaps, conjunctival
  for corneal edema after cataract surgery, 147–148
  for ICCE, 214
  wound leak under, inadvertent filtering bleb and, 148–149
Flat anterior chamber. See Anterior chamber, flat or shallow
Flexible-loop anterior chamber intraocular lenses, 133, 135f
Flomax. See Tamsulosin
Floppy iris syndrome, intraoperative, 74, 154–155, 156f
Fluid-based phacolysis, 127
Fluorescein angiography, in cataract surgery evaluation, 82
Foldable intraocular lenses, 135–136, 136f
  implantation procedure for, 138, 139
Followability, in phacoemulsification, 104
Foot-pedal controls, phaco machine, 104–105
Foreign bodies
  intralenticular, 51
  intraocular, retained
    cataract surgery and, 207
    siderosis and, 53, 54f
Fornices, sterilization of during cataract surgery, 128
FOXC1 gene, in Peters anomaly, 28
Free radicals, in lens, 16–17
Frequency, in phacoemulsification, 103
Fuchs heterochromic uveitis, cataracts/cataract surgery in, 59, 60f
Fundus, evaluation of, before cataract surgery, 80–81

G6P. See Glucose-6-phosphate
Galactitol (dulcitol), in cataract formation, 56
Galactokinase deficiency, galactosemia/cataract formation and, 56, 57
Galactose, in cataract formation, 56
Galactose 1-phosphate uridyltransferase (Gal-1-PUT), galactosemia caused by defects in, 56
Galactosemia, 56–57, 56f
Gamma (γ)-crystallins, 12
Gap junctions, in lens, 17
General anesthesia, for cataract surgery, 101
  in arthritis patients, 188
Genetic/hereditary factors, in age-related cataracts, 37–38
Geometric optics, intraocular lenses and, 136

Germinative zone, 8
Glare
  cataracts and, 41, 43, 70, 70t, 76
  with intraocular lenses, 168
Glare testing, in cataract evaluation, 76
Glassblowers' cataract, 52–53
Glaucoma
  cataracts and, 63, 64f, 201–203, 202f
    management of, 201–203, 202f
      preoperative evaluation/management and, 75, 201–202, 202f
  ciliary block (malignant), cataract surgery and, 153, 157–158
  lens-induced, 63–64, 64f
  lens particle, 63
  microspherophakia and, 29
  phacolytic, 63
  phacomorphic, 63, 64f
Glaukomflecken, 64
Glistenings, intraocular lens, 169
Globe
  exposure of for phacoemulsification, 110
  needle penetration/perforation of, 185
  stabilization of for clear corneal incision, 113
Glucose
  in cataract formation, 15, 55. *See also* Diabetes mellitus
  metabolism of in lens, 13–15, 14f
Glucose-6-phosphate, in lens glucose/carbohydrate metabolism, 13, 14f
Glutathione, in lens, oxidative changes and, 13, 16
Glutathione peroxidase, in lens, 16
Glycolysis, in lens glucose/carbohydrate metabolism, 13–15, 14f
"Golden ring" sign, 118
Gonioscopy
  before cataract surgery, 79
  in trauma evaluation, 206
Gundersen flap, 147–148

Haigis formula, for IOL power determination/selection, 85
Handpiece, phaco, 105–106, 105f, 106f, 107f
Haptic, insertion of intraocular lens with, 139
Healon 5, 98
Hearing loss (deafness), cataract surgery in patient with, 188
Helmholtz theory of accommodation, 19
Hemorrhages, cataract surgery and, 144t, 175–179, 189–190
  flat anterior chamber and, 152
  patient receiving anticoagulation therapy and, 74, 175–176, 189–190
  retrobulbar, 144t, 176–177, 189
  suprachoroidal/choroidal, 144t, 177–179, 189
    delayed, 178–179
    expulsive, 178
    flat anterior chamber and, 152
Hemostasis disorders, cataract surgery in patient with, 189–190

Heparin therapy, cataract surgery and, 189
Hepatolenticular degeneration (Wilson disease), 57
Heterochromia iridis, in siderosis bulbi, 54f
Hexokinase, in lens glucose/carbohydrate metabolism, 13, 14f, 15
Hexose monophosphate shunt, in lens glucose/carbohydrate metabolism, 14f, 15
High hyperopia, cataract surgery in patient with, 200–201
High myopia, cataract surgery in patient with, 200
Historical methods, for IOL power calculation after refractive surgery, 87–88
History, in cataract, 69–71, 70t
  evaluation for surgery and, 73–75
HMG-CoA (3-hydroxy-3-methylglutaryl coenzyme-A) reductase inhibitors, cataracts and, 49
HMP shunt. *See* Hexose monophosphate shunt
Hoffer Q formula, for IOL power determination/selection, 85, 87
Holladay 2 formula, for IOL power determination, 85
Homocystinuria, 37
  ectopia lentis in, 37
Horizontal phaco chop techniques, 122–123, 124f
HPMC. *See* Hydroxypropyl methylcellulose
Hyaloid artery/system, tunica vasculosa lentis development and, 25, 25f
Hyaluronate/sodium hyaluronate, as viscoelastic, 96
Hydrodelineation, in phacoemulsification, 118
  for advanced cataract, 195
Hydrodissection, in phacoemulsification, 117–118
  for advanced cataract, 195
Hydrogel polymers, for intraocular lenses, capsular opacification and, 170
3-Hydroxy-3-methylglutaryl coenzyme-A (HMG-CoA) reductase inhibitors, cataracts and, 49
Hydroxypropyl methylcellulose (HPMC), as viscoelastic, 97
Hyperbaric oxygen therapy, oxidative lens damage/cataracts and, 16, 60–61
Hyperlysinemia, 37
Hypermature cataract, 42, 45f
  phacolytic glaucoma and, 63
Hyperopia
  after cataract surgery, prior refractive surgery and, 193–194
  cataract surgery in patient with, 200–201
Hyphema, after cataract surgery, 167, 177
Hypocalcemia, cataracts associated with, 57
Hypopyon, chronic uveitis after cataract surgery and, 158
Hypotony
  cataract surgery in patient with, 201
  during/after surgery, flat anterior chamber and, 153

IAPB (International Agency for the Prevention of Blindness), 65
ICCE. *See* Intracapsular cataract extraction
IFIS. *See* Intraoperative floppy iris syndrome

Immersion ultrasonography, for axial length
    measurement, 82, 83f
Incision leaks, after cataract surgery, 144t,
    148–149
  flat anterior chamber and, 153
Incisions, for cataract surgery
  clear corneal, 113–115, 113f, 115f
  closure of
    complications associated with, 148–149
    after ECCE, 212–213
    postoperative endophthalmitis and, 180
    for scleral tunnel incisions, 112–113, 112f
  complications associated with, 148–149
    flat or shallow anterior chamber, 152
  dehiscence/rupture of, 149
  for ECCE, 211
    wound closure and, 212–213
  glaucoma and, 201–202
  for ICCE, 214
    problems associated with, 94
  induced astigmatism and, 150, 213
  intraocular lens implantation and, 138
  modification of preexisting astigmatism
    and, 130
  for phacoemulsification
    clear corneal, 113–115, 113f, 115f
    scleral tunnel, 111–113, 111f, 112f
  postoperative leaking and, 144t, 148–149
    flat anterior chamber and, 153
  scleral tunnel, 111–113, 111f, 112f
    wound closure and, 112–113, 112f
  self-sealing
    beveled/biplanar, clear corneal incisions and,
      114, 115f
    scleral tunnel incisions and, 112, 113
  thermal wounds of, 149
Index of refraction. See Refractive index
Infantile cataract. See Cataract, congenital
Inflammation (ocular), cataracts/cataract surgery
    and, 59, 60f, 75, 158, 188
  postoperative, 158–159
  trauma and, 206–207
Inflow, in phacoemulsification, 103
Informed consent, for cataract surgery, 88
Infrared radiation, lens affected by, 52–53
Instrumentation. See Ophthalmic instrumentation;
    Surgical instruments
Interferometry, laser, before cataract surgery, 81
Interlenticular opacifications, IOL, 169
International Agency for the Prevention of Blindness
    (IAPB), 65
Intracameral injections, lidocaine, for cataract
    surgery, 99–100
Intracapsular cataract extraction (ICCE), 93–94, 93f,
    213–215. See also Cataract surgery
  advantages of, 93
  in anticoagulated patient, 189
  contraindications to, 94
  cystoid macular edema and, 182
  disadvantages of, 94
  early techniques for, 92, 92f
  intraocular lenses for, 94, 133, 135f
    limitations and, 94
  modern advances in, 93–94, 93f
  patient preparation for, 213
  postoperative course for, 215
  postoperative flat or shallow anterior chamber
    and, 153–154
  procedure for, 213–214
  retinal detachment and, 184
  vitreocorneal adherence/persistent corneal edema
    and, 148
Intracapsular IOL dislocation, 163, 163f
Intralenticular foreign bodies, 51
Intraocular lenses (IOLs), 132–141. See also Cataract
    surgery
  accommodative, 137
    complications associated with, 169
  anterior chamber, 133, 135f
    after capsular rupture, 161
    closed-loop, pseudophakic bullous keratopathy
      and, 167
    complications associated with, 133
    contraindications to, 140–141
    flexible-loop, 133, 135f
    history of development of, 133, 135f
    after ICCE, 94, 133, 134f, 214
    implantation procedure for
      primary, 139–140
      secondary, 140
    preoperative gonioscopy and, 79
  biometry in power calculation/selection of, 82–83,
    83f, 84
  blue-blocking, 138
  capsular block syndrome and, 166–167
  closed-loop, pseudophakic bullous keratopathy
    and, 167
  complications of, 133, 144t, 162–169
  contraindications to, 140–141
  corneal disease and, 191
  cystoid macular edema and, 183
  decentration and dislocation of, 143, 144t,
    162–166, 163f, 164f, 165f
    laser capsulotomy and, 173
  flexible-loop, 133, 135f
  foldable, 135–136, 136f
    implantation procedure for, 138, 139
  glare and, 168
  history of, 132–133, 132f, 134f, 135f
  implantation of, 132–141
    anterior chamber, 139–140
    after capsular rupture, 161
    complications of, 133, 144t, 162–169
    contraindications to, 140–141
    after ECCE, 133, 133–136, 136f, 212
    after ICCE, 94, 133, 214
      limitations and, 94
    posterior chamber, 138–139
    procedure for, 138–140
    techniques of, 138

multifocal, 136–137
  complications associated with, 169
  after ocular trauma, 208–209
  opacification of, 168–169
  with penetrating/Descemet membrane–stripping automated endothelial keratoplasty and cataract surgery (triple procedure), 141, 192
  posterior chamber, 133–136, 136f
    capsular block syndrome and, 166–167
    after capsular rupture, 161
    contraindications to, 140–141
    after ECCE, 133, 133–136, 136f, 212
    history of development of, 133
    implantation procedure for, 138–139
    after keratoplasty, 193
    pupillary capture caused by anterior displacement of, 166, 167f
    in retinal disease patient, 205
    sutured, 139
  power determination for, 84–88
    biometry in, 82–83, 83f, 84
    contact lens method for, 87
    formulas for, 85, 87
    historical methods for, 87
    improving outcomes of surgery and, 86
    incorrect, 168
    preventing errors in, 84–85
    refraction and, 76
    refractive surgery and, 86–88, 193
    regression formulas for, 85, 87
    topographical method for, 87
    triple procedure and, 192
    unexpected refractive results after surgery and, 168
  pseudoaccommodative, 137
  pseudophakic bullous keratopathy and, 167
  pupil evaluation and, 78
  pupillary capture of, 166, 167f
  in retinal disease patient, 205
  toric, 131
    complications associated with, 169
  traumatic cataract and, 208–209
  with UV chromophores, 138
  in uveitic eye, 204
  uveitis-glaucoma-hyphema (UGH) syndrome and, 167
    decentration and, 163
Intraocular pressure
  decreased, after cataract surgery, flat anterior chamber and, 153
  elevated/increased. *See* Elevated intraocular pressure
Intraoperative floppy iris syndrome, 74, 154–155, 156f
Intravitreal corticosteroids, for cystoid macular edema, 183
Intumescent cortical cataract, 42
  phacomorphic glaucoma and, 63, 64f
  surgery for removal of, 196

Ionizing radiation, cataracts caused by, 51–52
Iridectomy
  for ICCE, 214
  peripheral, cataract surgery on inflamed eye and, 207
Iridodialysis
  during cataract surgery, 157
  cataract surgery in patient with, 207–208, 207f
Iridodonesis, cataract surgery and, 79, 197
Iris
  absence of (aniridia), 29–30, 29f
    cataract surgery in patient with, 200
  coloboma of, cataract surgery in patient with, 196, 197f
  evaluation of, before cataract surgery, 79
  heterochromia of (heterochromia iridis), in siderosis bulbi, 54f
  traumatic damage to
    during cataract surgery, 144t, 157
    cataract surgery in patient with, 207–208, 207f
Iris clip intraocular lenses, pseudophakic bullous keratopathy and, 167
Iris hooks
  for pupil expansion, 194, 194f
  for zonular incompetence, 199
Iris plane, phacoemulsification at, 119–120, 120f
Iris retractor, for intraoperative floppy iris syndrome, 155
Iris sphincter. *See* Sphincter muscle
Iris suture fixation, peripheral, for intraocular lens decentration, 163–164, 164f
Iron, foreign body of, siderosis caused by, 53, 54f
Irrigation, in phacoemulsification, 108
  posterior fluid misdirection and, 152–153
  strategies for, 125–126
  with toxic solutions, corneal edema caused by, 147, 151–152
Irvine-Gass syndrome, 162, 181. *See also* Cystoid macular edema
Ischemia, cataracts caused by, 64

K_m (Michaelis/affinity constant), "sugar" cataract development and, 15
Kalt forceps, 92, 92f
Kayser-Fleischer ring, 57
Kelman phaco tip, 105, 105f
Keratectomy, photorefractive (PRK). *See* Photorefractive keratectomy
Keratoconjunctivitis sicca, cataract surgery in patient with, 190–191
  corneal melting/keratolysis and, 150, 191
Keratolysis (corneal melting), cataract surgery and, 150
  in patient with dry eye, 150, 191
Keratometry, in IOL power determination/selection, 84
  corneal irregularities and, 191
  refractive surgery and, 86
  unexpected refractive results after surgery and, 168

Keratopathy, bullous, after cataract surgery, 147, 147f, 167
    IOL design and, 167
Keratoplasty
    for corneal edema after cataract surgery, 147
    endothelial
        cataract surgery and, 141, 192
        for corneal edema after cataract surgery, 147
        Descemet membrane–stripping automated (DSAEK), in triple procedure, 141
    penetrating (PK)
        cataract/cataract surgery following, 193
        cataract surgery and IOL implantation combined with (triple procedure), 141, 192
        for corneal edema after cataract surgery, 147
Keratorefractive surgery (KRS), cataract/cataract surgery and, 130–131, 193–194, 193f
    IOL power calculation and, 86–88, 193
    preoperative evaluation/planning and, 75, 78
Keratotomy
    astigmatic, cataract surgery and, 130
    radial, cataract surgery after, 78
        hyperopia and, 193–194
        IOL power calculation and, 86
Ketorolac, for postoperative cystoid macular edema, 183
Kuglen hook, for pupil expansion, 194

Labetalol, intraoperative floppy iris syndrome and, 155
Lamellae, zonular, 7
Lamellar (zonular) cataracts, 30, 32f
Laser capsulotomy (Nd:YAG), 171–175, 172f, 174f
    for anterior capsule fibrosis and phimosis, 171, 171–175, 172f, 199
    for capsular block syndrome, 166–167
    for capsule opacification, 169, 171–175, 174f
    complications of, 173–175
    contraindications to, 172
    indications for, 171–172
    lens particle glaucoma and, 63
    procedure for, 172–173, 174f
    retinal detachment and, 175, 184
Laser in situ keratomileusis. See LASIK
Laser interferometry, before cataract surgery, 81
Laser photolysis, 127
Laser pupilloplasty, for cataracts, 71
LASIK (laser in situ keratomileusis), cataract surgery after, 194
    IOL power calculation and, 86
Lateral cantholysis, bulbar hemorrhage release and, 99
Lens (crystalline)
    absence of, 26. See also Aphakia
    aging changes in, 7, 20, 39–47, 40f. See also Age-related cataracts
    alcohol use/abuse and, 58–59
    anatomy of, 5–9, 5f, 6f, 7f, 8f
        altered, cataract surgery and, 195–200
    biochemistry and metabolism of, 11–17
    capsule of. See Lens capsule
    carbohydrate metabolism in, 13–15, 14f
    changing shape of. See Accommodation
    chemical injuries affecting, 53
    colobomas of, 26–27, 27f
    coloration change in, 39, 40f
    congenital anomalies and abnormalities of, 26–35
    cortex of, 6f, 8–9
    degenerative ocular disorders and, 64
    development/embryology of, 21–38
        congenital anomalies and abnormalities and, 26–35
        developmental defects and, 35–38
        normal, 21–25, 22–23f, 24f, 25f
    diabetes mellitus affecting, 55, 56f
    dislocated, 35. See also Ectopia lentis
        cataract surgery in patient with, 197–199, 198f
        traumatic, 36, 50–51, 50f
    disorders of, 39–64. See also specific disorder and Cataract
    drug-induced changes in, 47–49
    electrical injury of, 54, 55f
    epithelium of, 6f, 8, 8f
        active transport and, 17–18
        development of, 23, 23f
        opacification of (capsular cataract), 33–34
    evaluation of, before cataract surgery, 79
    exfoliation syndrome/pseudoexfoliation and, 61–62, 61f
    foreign body in, 51
    free radicals affecting, 16–17
    glaucoma and, 63–64, 64f
    in homocystinuria, 37
    in hyperlysinemia, 37
    ischemic damage to, 64
    luxed/luxated, 35. See also Ectopia lentis
        cataract surgery in patient with, 197–199, 198f
        traumatic, 36, 50–51, 50f
    in Marfan syndrome, 36–37, 36f
    metabolic diseases affecting, 55–57, 56f
    molecular biology of, 11–13, 11f
    nucleus of, 6f, 8–9
        congenital cataract of, 33, 34f
        embryonic, 9, 22–23, 23f
            opacification of (congenital nuclear cataract), 33, 34f
        fetal, 9, 23f, 24–25, 24f
            opacification of (congenital nuclear cataract), 33, 34f
        opacification of. See Nuclear cataract
    removal/disassembly of
        in ECCE, 95, 212
        femtosecond laser for, 127
        fluid-based phacolysis for, 127
        laser photolysis for, 127
        in manual small-incision cataract surgery, 96
        in phacoemulsification
            locations for, 119–120, 120f, 121f
            techniques of, 121–125, 122f, 123f, 124f, 125f
    rotation of in phacoemulsification, 118, 125f

nutritional diseases affecting, 57–58
oxidative damage to, 16–17
perforating and penetrating injury of, 51, 51*f*, 52*f*
 glaucoma and, 63
physiology of, 17–19, 19*f*
radiation affecting, 51–53
removal of. *See also* Cataract surgery; Lensectomy;
 Phacoemulsification
 in early cataract surgery, 91–92, 91*f*, 92, 92*f*
retained, cataract surgery and, 143, 147, 159–160
size of, 7
smoking/tobacco use and, 58–59, 67–68
subluxed/subluxated, 35, 36*f*. *See also* Ectopia
 lentis
 cataract surgery in patient with, 197–199, 198*f*
 traumatic, 36, 50–51, 50*f*
sutures of, 9
 development of, 23*f*, 24–25, 24*f*
 opacification of (sutural/stellate cataract),
  33, 33*f*
transport functions in, 17–19, 18*f*
traumatic damage to, 50–54, 50*f*, 51*f*, 52*f*, 54*f*, 55*f*,
 206–209, 207*f*
 glaucoma and, 63
 phacoantigenic uveitis and, 62
 surgery and, 206–209, 207*f*
uveitis and, 59, 60*f*. *See also* Phacoantigenic
 (phacoanaphylactic) uveitis
water and cation balance in, maintenance of,
 17–19, 18*f*
zonular fibers/zonules of, 5, 6*f*, 7–8
 absent/abnormal, cataract surgery and, 117, 118
  in glaucoma patient, 202
  iris coloboma/corectopia and, 196, 197*f*
 development of, 25
 evaluation of before cataract surgery, 79
Lens capsule, 6*f*, 7, 7*f*
 development of, 21, 22*f*, 23, 23*f*
 exfoliation of, infrared radiation/heat causing,
  52–53
 rupture of, cataract surgery and, 144*t*, 160–162
 staining, in cataract surgery, 195, 195*f*
Lens crystallins, 11–12, 11*f*. *See also* Crystallins
Lens fibers
 accommodation and, 19
 development of, 8, 8*f*
  primary fibers, 22, 23*f*
  secondary fibers, 23–24, 23*f*
   microspherophakia and, 29
 zonular (zonules of Zinn), 5, 6*f*, 7–8
  absent/abnormal, cataract surgery and, 117, 118
   in glaucoma patient, 202
   iris coloboma/corectopia and, 196, 197*f*
  development of, 25
  evaluation of before cataract surgery, 79
Lens-induced glaucoma, 63–64, 64*f*
Lens–iris diaphragm retropulsion syndrome, 156
Lens Opacities Classification System III
 (LOCS III), 67
Lens particle glaucoma, 63

Lens pit, 21
Lens placode, 21, 22*f*
Lens proteins, 11–12, 11*f*
 aging affecting, 13, 39
 crystallins, 11–12, 11*f*. *See also* Crystallins
 cytoskeletal and membrane, 11*f*, 12
 in phacoantigenic uveitis/endophthalmitis, 62
 in phacolytic glaucoma, 63
 urea-insoluble (membrane structural), 11*f*, 12
 urea-soluble (cytoskeletal), 11*f*, 12
 water-insoluble, 11, 11*f*, 12
  age affecting, 13
 water-soluble, 11, 11*f*. *See also* Crystallins
  conversion of to water-insoluble, 13
Lens vesicle, formation of, 21, 22*f*
Lensectomy
 in Marfan syndrome, 37
 pars plana, 132
Lenticonus/lentiglobus, 26, 26*f*
 anterior, 26
 posterior, 26, 26*f*
Lenticular myopia (myopic shift), 39, 70
Lentiglobus. *See* Lenticonus/lentiglobus
Lester hooks, for pupil expansion, 194
Leukomas, in Peters anomaly, 27
Lidocaine, for cataract surgery, 99–101, 101*f*
LIDRS. *See* Lens–iris diaphragm retropulsion
 syndrome
Light toxicity/photic damage, cataract surgery and,
 183–184
Limbal groove, for ECCE, 211
Limbal relaxing incisions, cataract surgery and,
 130–131
 manual small-incision, 96
Lipid peroxidation, in lens opacification, 16
Load, in phacoemulsification, 103
Local anesthesia. *See* Anesthesia
LOCS III (Lens Opacities Classification
 System III), 67
LogMAR, cystoid macular edema after cataract
 surgery and, 182
Longitudinal Study of Cataract, 67
Low vision aids, for cataract, 71
LRI. *See* Limbal relaxing incisions
LSC (Longitudinal Study of Cataract), 67
Lutein, cataract risk affected by, 58
Luxed/luxated lens, 35. *See also* Ectopia lentis
 cataract surgery in patient with, 197–199, 198*f*
 traumatic, 36, 50–51, 50*f*

Macula, evaluation of before cataract surgery,
 80, 82
Macular degeneration, cataract surgery in patient
 with, 80
Macular edema
 cystoid, postoperative, 143, 144*t*, 181–183, 182*f*
  in glaucoma patient, 202–203
  after Nd:YAG capsulotomy, 175
  vitreous prolapse and, 162
 diabetic, cataract surgery and, 205

Macular function testing, before cataract surgery, 82
    retinal disease and, 204–205
Major intrinsic protein (MIP/aquaporin 0), 12, 17
Malignant (ciliary block) glaucoma, cataract surgery
    and, 153, 157–158
Malondialdehyde (MDA), oxidative lens damage
    and, 16
Malyugin ring, for pupil expansion, 194f
Manual small-incision cataract surgery, 96
MAR (minimum angle of resolution/recognition),
    logarithm of (logMAR), cystoid macular edema
    after cataract surgery and, 182
Marcus Gunn pupil (relative afferent pupillary
    defect), cataract surgery on patient with, 77
Marfan syndrome, 36–37, 36f
Mature cataract, 42, 44f
    phacolytic glaucoma and, 63
Mazzocco foldable intraocular lens, 135, 136f
McCannel sutures, for intraocular lens decentration,
    163–164, 164f
Medical history, cataract surgery evaluation and,
    73–74, 188, 189f
Meibomian gland dysfunction, blepharitis in,
    cataract surgery and, 190
Membrane structural (urea-insoluble) lens proteins,
    11f, 12
Membranous cataract, 34, 35f
Meridians, 5
Mesodermal dysgenesis, Peters anomaly and, 27–28
Metabolic disorders, cataracts and, 55–57, 56f
Metallosis, lens damage/cataracts caused by,
    53–54, 54f
Methionine, in homocystinuria, 37
Methylcellulose
    hydroxypropyl (HPMC), as viscoelastic, 97
    as viscoelastic, 97
Michaelis constant (K_m), "sugar" cataract
    development and, 15
Microscope
    operating, phototoxicity and, 183–184
    specular, examination before cataract surgery
    and, 84
Microspherophakia, 28–29, 28f
Microwave radiation, cataract development and, 53
MICS. See Manual small-incision cataract surgery
Minimum angle of resolution/recognition (MAR),
    logarithm of (logMAR), cystoid macular edema
    after cataract surgery and, 182
Miosis/miotic agents
    cataracts caused by, 49
    for glaucoma, cataract/cataract surgery and, 202
MIP. See Major intrinsic protein
Mittendorf dot, 25, 27
Monocular diplopia, in cataracts, 40, 41, 43, 70
Morgagnian cataract, 42, 46f
Morgagnian globules, 42
Motility examination. See Ocular motility,
    assessment of
Multifocal lenses, intraocular, 136–137
    complications associated with, 169

Multiplanar incisions, clear corneal, 113–114, 114f
Mydriasis/mydriatics, for pupillary capture, 166
Myopia
    cataract surgery in patient with, 200
    lenticular (myopic shift), 39, 70
Myopic shift, in cataracts (lenticular myopia), 39, 70
Myotonic dystrophy, lens disorders/cataracts in,
    57, 58f

Na^+,K^+-ATPase (sodium-potassium pump), in lens
    active transport, 18
    pump–leak theory and, 18–19, 18f
NADP, in lens glucose/carbohydrate metabolism,
    14f, 15
NADPH, in lens glucose/carbohydrate metabolism,
    14f, 15
Nanophthalmos, cataract surgery in patient with,
    200–201
National Eye Institute Visual Function Questionnaire
    (NEI-VFQ), 71
Nd:YAG laser therapy
    capsulotomy, 171–175, 172f, 174f
        for anterior capsule fibrosis and phimosis, 171,
            171–175, 172f, 199
        for capsular block syndrome, 166–167
        for capsule opacification, 169, 171–175, 174f
        complications of, 173–175
        contraindications to, 172
        indications for, 171–172
        lens particle glaucoma and, 63
        procedure for, 172–173, 174f
        retinal detachment and, 175, 184
    photolysis, 127
    vitreolysis, for vitreous prolapse in anterior
        chamber, 162
"Near clear" incision, for cataract surgery, 114
Near visual acuity, age-related loss of, 20
Needle penetration/perforation of globe, 185
Negative dysphotopsias, intraocular lenses and, 168
NEI-VFQ (National Eye Institute Visual Function
    Questionnaire), 71
Nerve block, facial, for cataract surgery, 101, 101f
Neurocristopathy, Peters anomaly and, 27–28
Nicotinamide adenine dinucleotide phosphate
    (NADPH), in lens glucose/carbohydrate
    metabolism, 14f, 15
Nonsteroidal anti-inflammatory drugs (NSAIDs),
    corneal melting after cataract surgery associated
    with, 150, 191
Nuclear cataracts, 39–40, 41f
    congenital, 33, 34f
    genetic contributions to, 37–38
    hyperbaric oxygen therapy and, 60–61
    visual acuity and, 39, 70t
    vitrectomy and, 16, 60, 205–206
Nuclear disassembly techniques, 121–125, 122f, 123f,
    124f, 125f
    chopping techniques, 122–124, 124f
    one-handed, 124–125, 125f
    phaco fracture, 121–122, 122f, 123f

Nuclear sclerosis, 39
Nucleus (lens). *See* Lens (crystalline), nucleus of
Nutritional deficiency, cataract formation and, 57–58

Occlusion, in phacoemulsification, 104
OCT. *See* Optical coherence tomography/biometry
Ocular history, in cataract, 69–71, 70t
  evaluation for surgery and, 75
Ocular hypotension. *See* Hypotony
Ocular motility, assessment of before cataract
    surgery, 77
Ocular trauma
  assessment of, 206
  cataract surgery after, 206–209, 207f
  ectopia lentis caused by, 36
  lens damage/cataracts caused by, 50–54, 50f, 51f,
      52f, 54f, 55f, 206–209, 207f
    glaucoma and, 63
    phacoantigenic uveitis and, 62
    surgery for, 206–209, 207f
Oculomotor nerve. *See* Cranial nerve III
Oil droplet appearance
  in galactosemia, 56, 56f
  in lenticonus/lentiglobus, 26
  visual acuity and, 70
One-handed nucleus disassembly, 124–125, 125f
Opacities
  fundus evaluation with, 80–81
  intraocular lens, 168–169
Operating microscope, phototoxicity and, 183–184
Ophthalmic instrumentation, phototoxicity from,
    cataract surgery and, 183–184
Ophthalmic viscosurgical devices (viscoelastic
    agents), 96–98, 97t
  for advanced cataract extraction, 196
  for capsular rupture during surgery, 160, 161
  for cataract surgery in aniridia, 200
  for cataract surgery in high hyperopia, 200–201
  for cataract surgery in traumatic cataract, 208
  characteristics of, 98
  in ECCE, 94, 212
  elevated intraocular pressure and, 154
  for inflamed eye, 207
  for intraoperative floppy iris syndrome, 155
  for intumescent cataract extraction, 196
  IOL implantation and, 138, 139, 140, 141
  in phacoemulsification, 102, 110, 117, 126
  physical properties of, 97–98, 97t
  for pupil expansion, 98, 194
Ophthalmoscopy, before cataract surgery, 80
Optic axis, 5, 6f
Optic cup, development of, 21
Optic nerve (cranial nerve II), evaluation of, before
    cataract surgery, 80
Optic vesicle, lens development and, 21, 22f
Optical clarity, of ophthalmic viscosurgical
    device, 98
Optical coherence tomography/biometry
  before cataract surgery, 82, 84
  in IOL power determination, 84

OVDs. *See* Ophthalmic viscosurgical devices
Overrefraction, cataract surgery evaluation and, 76
Oxygen therapy, hyperbaric, oxidative lens damage
    and, 16, 60–61

Pachymetry, before cataract surgery, 84
PAM. *See* Potential acuity meter
Panel control ultrasound, for phacoemulsification, 106
Paracentesis, in phacoemulsification, 110
Parasympatholytic agents, accommodation affected
    by, 19
Parasympathomimetic agents, accommodation
    affected by, 19
Pars plana lensectomy, 132
Pars plana vitrectomy
  for capsular rupture during cataract surgery,
      160–161
  cataract/cataract surgery after, 205–206
  pars plana lensectomy and, 132
  for postoperative endophthalmitis, 181
  for retained lens fragments after
      phacoemulsification, 159–160
PAX6 gene mutation
  in aniridia, 29
  in Peters anomaly, 28
PCIOL. *See* Intraocular lenses (IOLs), posterior
    chamber
PCO. *See* Posterior capsular opacification
Pemphigoid, cicatricial, cataract surgery in patient
    with, 191
Penetrating injuries, lens damage caused by, 51,
    51f, 52f
  glaucoma and, 63
Penetrating keratoplasty. *See* Keratoplasty,
    penetrating
Pentose phosphate pathway (hexose monophosphate
    shunt), in lens glucose/carbohydrate metabolism,
    14f, 15
Perforating injuries, lens damage caused by, 51, 51f, 52f
  glaucoma and, 63
Peribulbar anesthesia, for cataract surgery, 99, 100f
Peripheral iris suture fixation, for intraocular lens
    decentration, 163–164, 164f
Peristaltic pump, for phacoemulsification aspiration,
    108, 108f
  vacuum rise time for, 108, 110f
Peroxidation, lipid, in lens opacification, 16
Persistent corneal epithelial defects, after cataract
    surgery, 150
Persistent fetal vasculature (persistent hyperplastic
    primary vitreous), 38
Peters anomaly, 27–28
PFV. *See* Persistent fetal vasculature
Phaco chop technique, 122–124, 124f
Phaco fracture technique, 121–122, 122f, 123f
Phaco handpiece, 105–106, 105f, 106f, 107f
Phaco tip, 105–106, 105f, 106f, 107f
Phacoantigenic (phacoanaphylactic) uveitis, 62
Phacodonesis, cataract surgery and, 197
  in glaucoma patient, 202

Phacoemulsification, 102–126. *See also* Cataract surgery
  for advanced cataract, 195–196
  anterior capsulotomy for, 115, 116*f*
  in anterior chamber, 119
  in anticoagulated patient, 189
  aspiration system for, 108–109, 108*f*, 109*f*, 110*f*
    strategies for use of, 125–126
  burst-mode, 107
  capsular opacification and, 169–171
    Nd:YAG laser capsulotomy for, 169, 171–175, 174*f*. *See also* Nd:YAG laser therapy, capsulotomy
  capsular rupture during, 144*t*, 160–162
  capsulorrhexis in, 115–117, 116*f*
    loose zonules and, 117
  clear corneal incision for, 113–115, 113*f*, 115*f*
  continuous, 106–107
  cystoid macular edema after, 182
  flat or shallow anterior chamber and, 152–154
    intraoperative complications, 152–153
    postoperative complications, 153–154
  foldable intraocular lenses for, 135–136, 136*f*. *See also* Foldable intraocular lenses
  in glaucoma patient, 201–203
    after filtering surgery, 203
    intraocular pressure lowered by, 201
  globe exposure for, 110
  high myopia and, 200
  hydrodelineation in, 118
  hydrodissection in, 117–118
  incisions for
    clear corneal incisions, 113–115, 113*f*, 115*f*
    scleral tunnel incisions, 111–113, 111*f*, 112*f*
  instrumentation for, 104–106, 105*f*, 106*f*, 107*f*
    settings for, 118–119
  for intumescent cataract extraction, 196
  at iris plane, 119–120, 120*f*
  irrigation in, 108
    posterior fluid misdirection and, 152–153
    strategies for, 125–126
    toxic solutions exposure and, corneal edema caused by, 147, 151–152
  lens particle glaucoma and, 63
  linear ultrasound, 106
  locations of, 119–120, 120*f*, 121*f*
  nuclear rotation in, 118, 125*f*
  nucleus disassembly/removal in
    locations for emulsification and, 119–120, 120*f*, 121*f*
    techniques of, 121–125, 122*f*, 123*f*, 124*f*, 125*f*
      chopping techniques, 122–124, 124*f*
      one-handed, 124–125, 125*f*
      phaco fracture, 121–122, 122*f*, 123*f*
  ocular trauma affecting visualization and, 206
  panel control ultrasound and, 106
  paracentesis for, 110
  after pars plana vitrectomy, 205–206
  in posterior chamber, 120, 121*f*
  for posterior polar cataract, 196–197
  power delivery and, 106–108
    advances in, 126
  procedure for, 110–126
  pulsed, 107
  retained lens fragments after, 143, 147, 159–160
  retinal detachment and, 143, 144*t*, 184
  scleral tunnel incisions for, 111–113, 111*f*, 112*f*
  supracapsular, 121
  suprachoroidal effusion/hemorrhage risk and, 177
  in triple procedure, 141
  ultrasonics terminology and, 102–104
  vacuum terminology and, 104
  after vitrectomy, 205–206
  vitreocorneal adherence/persistent corneal edema and, 148
  in zonular dehiscence/lens subluxation or dislocation, 197–199, 198*f*
Phacolysis, fluid-based, 127
Phacolytic glaucoma, 63
Phacomorphic glaucoma, 63, 64*f*
Phakinin, 12
Phenothiazines, lens changes caused by, 48–49, 48*f*
Phosphofructokinase, in lens glucose/carbohydrate metabolism, 13, 14*f*
Phospholine. *See* Echothiophate
Photic damage/light toxicity, cataract surgery and, 183–184
Photolysis, laser, 127
Photorefractive keratectomy (PRK), cataract surgery after, 194
  IOL power calculation and, 86
Phototherapeutic keratectomy (PTK), for corneal/epithelial erosions, 147
PHPV (persistent hyperplastic primary vitreous). *See* Persistent fetal vasculature
Piezoelectric crystal, in phacoemulsification handpiece, 103
Pigmentations/pigment deposits, lens
  aging and, 39, 40*f*
  drugs causing, 48, 48*f*, 49
Pilocarpine
  accommodation affected by, 19
  cataracts caused by, 49
Pits, lens, 21, 22*f*
PITX2 gene, in Peters anomaly, 28
Placode, lens, 21, 22*f*
Plate-haptic IOLs, implantation of, 139
Pleomorphism, specular photomicroscopy in evaluation of, before cataract surgery, 84
PMMA. *See* Polymethylmethacrylate
Polar cataracts, 30–31, 32*f*
  surgery for removal of, 196–197
Polymegethism, specular photomicroscopy in evaluation of, before cataract surgery, 84
Polymethylmethacrylate (PMMA), intraocular lenses made from, 132–133, 133*f*
  capsular opacification and, 170
  implantation procedure for, 138
  instrumentation for handling, 138

Polyol (sorbitol) pathway
   in cataract formation, 15
   in lens glucose/carbohydrate metabolism, 14f, 15
Polyopia, in cataracts, 70
Positive dysphotopsias, intraocular lenses and, 168
"Positive vitreous pressure," flat or shallow anterior chamber and, 152
Posterior capsular opacification (PCO)
   cataract surgery and, 143, 169–171
   Nd:YAG laser capsulotomy for, 169, 171–175, 174f. See also Nd:YAG laser therapy, capsulotomy
Posterior capsular rupture, cataract surgery and, 144t, 160–162
Posterior chamber, phacoemulsification in, 120, 121f
Posterior chamber intraocular lenses. See Intraocular lenses
Posterior fluid misdirection, flat or shallow anterior chamber and, 152–153
Posterior lenticonus/lentiglobus, 26, 26f
Posterior polar cataract, 31
   surgery for removal of, 196–197
Posterior pole, 5, 6f
Posterior subcapsular cataract, 42–44, 47f
   corticosteroids causing, 47–48
   ischemia causing, 64
   in myotonic dystrophy, 57
   silicone oil use and, 205
   uveitis and, 59
   visual acuity and, 43, 70, 70t
Posterior sutures, 9
Posterior synechiae, in uveitis, lens changes/cataract and, 59
Posterior vitreous detachment, retinal detachment after cataract surgery and, 184
Postoperative care
   after ECCE, 213
   after ICCE, 215
Postoperative endophthalmitis, 143, 144t, 179–181, 179f
   prevention of, 127–129, 128f, 180
Postvitrectomy cataract, 16, 60, 205–206
Potassium balance, in lens, pump-leak theory of maintenance of, 18–19, 18f
Potential acuity meter (PAM), in cataract surgery evaluation, 81
Power, in phacoemulsification, 103
   delivery of, 106–108
   advances in, 126
Power (optical), intraocular lens, determination of, 84–88
   biometry in, 82–83, 83f, 84
   contact lens method for, 87
   formulas for, 85, 87
   historical methods for, 87
   improving outcomes of surgery and, 86
   incorrect, 168
   preventing errors in, 84–85
   refraction and, 76
   refractive surgery and, 86–88, 193
   regression formulas for, 85, 87
   topographical method for, 87
   triple procedure and, 192
   unexpected refractive results after surgery and, 168
Power prediction formulas, for IOLs, 85, 87
Prazosin, intraoperative floppy iris syndrome and, 74, 155
Preoperative assessment/preparation, 73–88
   antimicrobial prophylaxis and, 127–128
   in diabetic patient, 80
   ECCE, 211
   ICCE, 213
   ocular trauma and, 206
Presbyopia, 20
Primary aphakia, 26. See also Aphakia
Primary coloboma, 26. See also Coloboma
Primary lens fibers, development of, 22, 23f
Primary vitreous, persistent hyperplasia of. See Persistent fetal vasculature
PRK. See Photorefractive keratectomy
Proparacaine, for cataract surgery, 99
Propionibacterium acnes, chronic uveitis after cataract surgery caused by, 158
Prostaglandins, cystoid macular edema after cataract surgery and, 202–203
PSC. See Posterior subcapsular cataract
Pseudoaccommodative intraocular lenses, 137
Pseudoexfoliation (exfoliation syndrome), 61–62, 61f
   cataract surgery in patient with, 199
   postoperative hyphema and, 177
   zonular incompetence and, 197, 198f, 199
Pseudophakic bullous edema/keratopathy, after cataract surgery, 147, 147f, 167
   IOL design and, 167
Pseudophakodonesis, IOL dislocation and, 164–165, 166
Pseudoplasticity, of ophthalmic viscosurgical device, 97
Pulsed phacoemulsification, 107
Pump-leak theory, 18–19, 18f
Pupil expansion rings, for intraoperative floppy iris syndrome, 155, 156f
Pupillary block
   after cataract surgery, flat or shallow anterior chamber and, 153–154
   intumescent cataract causing, phacomorphic glaucoma and, 63, 64f
   microspherophakia causing, 29
Pupillary capture, after cataract surgery, 166, 167f
   IOL decentration and, 163
Pupillary light reflex (pupillary response to light), evaluation of, before cataract surgery, 77
Pupillary membrane, anterior, 25, 25f
Pupillary rings, 194, 194f
Pupilloplasty, for cataracts, 71
Pupils
   in ectopia lentis et pupillae, 38
   examination of, before cataract surgery, 77–78
   Marcus Gunn (relative afferent pupillary defect), cataract surgery on patient with, 77

size of, cataract surgery and, 78, 194–195, 194f
   IOL selection and, 78
   trauma and, 206–207
   uveitis and, 203–204
   in uveitic eye, cataract surgery and, 203–204
PVD. *See* Posterior vitreous detachment
Pyridoxine (vitamin B_6), for homocystinuria, 37

Q formula, Hoffer, for IOL power determination/selection, 85, 87

Race, cataract development and, 67
Radial keratotomy (RK), cataract surgery after, 78
   hyperopia and, 193–194
   IOL power calculation and, 86
Radiation, cataracts caused by, 51–53
RAM. *See* Retinal Acuity Meter
RAPD. *See* Relative afferent pupillary defect
Red reflex
   in complete cataract, 34
   in lenticonus/lentiglobus, 26
   poor, cataract surgery and, 195, 195f
Refracting power, in IOL power determination, 84
Refraction, clinical, in cataract patients
   nonsurgical management and, 71
   before surgery/IOL power determination and, 76
Refractive errors, unexpected, after cataract surgery, 168
Refractive index, of lens, 7
Refractive surgery, cataract/cataract surgery and, 130–131
   IOL power calculation and, 86–88, 193
   preoperative evaluation/planning and, 75, 78
Regression formulas, for IOL power determination, 85, 87
Relative afferent pupillary defect (Marcus Gunn pupil), cataract surgery on patient with, 77
Relaxing incisions
   for anterior capsule contraction, 172f, 173
   limbal, 130–131
      manual small-incision, 96
Resolution, minimum angle of (MAR), logarithm of (logMAR), cystoid macular edema after cataract surgery and, 182
Retained lens material, cataract surgery and, 143, 147, 159–160
Retina
   disorders of. *See* Retinal disease
   examination of before cataract surgery, 80
   oxidative lens damage during surgery on, 16
   photic injury of during cataract surgery, 183–184
Retinal Acuity Meter (RAM), in cataract surgery evaluation, 81
Retinal detachment, after cataract surgery, 143, 144t, 184–185
   family history as risk factor and, 75
   Nd:YAG laser capsulotomy and, 175, 184
Retinal disease
   after cataract surgery, 181–185, 182f
   cataract surgery in patient with, 75, 204–205

Retinal pigment epithelium (RPE), burns of, during cataract surgery, 183–184
Retinoscopy, before cataract surgery, 80
Retrobulbar anesthesia, 98–99, 99f
   hemorrhage and, 176, 189
Retrobulbar hemorrhage, cataract surgery and, 144t, 176–177, 189
Rhegmatogenous retinal detachment. *See* Retinal detachment
Rheumatoid arthritis, cataract surgery in patient with, corneal melting/keratolysis and, 150
Riders, 30
Ridley lens, 132–133, 132f
Right to Sight, 65
Rise time, in phacoemulsification, 104, 109, 110f
RK. *See* Radial keratotomy
Rosacea, cataract surgery in patient with, 77, 190
Rosette cataract, 50, 50f
RRD (rhegmatogenous retinal detachment). *See* Retinal detachment
Rubella, congenital, cataracts and, 35

Scleral support ring, for ICCE, 214
Scleral tunnel incisions, 111–113, 111f, 112f
   closure of, 112–113, 112f
Sclerosis, nuclear, 39
Sculpting, instrument settings for, 118–119
Second sight, 39, 70
Secondary aphakia, 26. *See also* Aphakia
Secondary coloboma, 26. *See also* Coloboma
Secondary lens fibers, development of, 23–24, 23f
   microspherophakia and, 29
Self-sealing incision
   beveled/biplanar, clear corneal incision and, 114, 115f
   scleral tunnel incisions and, 112, 113
Shallow anterior chamber. *See* Anterior chamber, flat or shallow
Siderosis bulbi, 53, 54f
Siepser slipknot technique, for intraocular lens decentration, 163, 164f
Silicone foldable intraocular lenses, 135–136. *See also* Foldable intraocular lenses
   capsular opacification and, 170
   instrumentation for handling, 138
   in uveitic eye, 204
Silicone oil, cataract/cataract surgery with, 205, 206
Silodosin, intraoperative floppy iris syndrome and, 155
Simple diffusion, glucose transport into lens and, 13
Simvastatin, cataract risk and, 49
Sjögren syndrome, postoperative corneal melting/keratolysis and, 150
Slit-lamp biomicroscopy/examination, before cataract surgery, 78–80
   limitations of, 80
Small-incision cataract surgery, manual, 96
SmartSight patient handout/website, 71
Smith-Indian operation, 92
Smoking, cataract development and, 58–59, 67–68

Snellen acuity. *See* Visual acuity
Snowflake cataract, 55, 56*f*
Social history, cataract surgery evaluation and, 75
Sodium balance, in lens, pump–leak theory of maintenance of, 18–19, 18*f*
Sodium hyaluronate, as viscoelastic, 96
Sodium-potassium pump (Na+,K+-ATPase), in lens active transport, 18
pump–leak theory and, 18–19, 18*f*
Soemmering ring, 170
Sorbitol/sorbitol pathway
in cataract formation, 15
in lens glucose/carbohydrate metabolism, 14*f*, 15
Space maintenance, by ophthalmic viscosurgical device, 98
Specular microscopy, before cataract surgery, 84
Sphincter muscle, damage to, cataract surgery in patient with, 207–208
Spondylitis, ankylosing, cataract surgery in patient with, 188, 189*f*
SRK formulas, for IOL power selection, 85
Staphylococcus
aureus, postoperative endophthalmitis caused by, 180
epidermidis
chronic uveitis after cataract surgery caused by, 158
postoperative endophthalmitis caused by, 180
Statins, cataracts and, 49
Stellate (sutural) cataracts, 33, 33*f*
Steroids. *See* Corticosteroids
"Stop and chop" phaco, 122–123, 124*f*
Streptococcus, postoperative endophthalmitis caused by, 180
Stroke (phacoemulsification), 103
Stromal edema, after cataract surgery, 146–148
Subcapsular cataract, posterior, 42–44, 47*f*
corticosteroids causing, 47–48
ischemia causing, 64
in myotonic dystrophy, 57
silicone oil use and, 205
uveitis and, 59
visual acuity and, 43, 70, 70*t*
Subconjunctival lidocaine, for cataract surgery, 101
Subluxation, intraocular lens, 143, 144*t*, 162–166, 163*f*, 164*f*, 165*f*
Subluxed/subluxated lens, 35, 36*f*. *See also* Ectopia lentis
cataract surgery in patient with, 197–199, 198*f*
traumatic, 36, 50–51, 50*f*
Sub-Tenon drug administration
corticosteroid, postoperative cystoid macular edema and, 183
lidocaine, for cataract surgery, 101, 101*f*
"Sugar" cataracts, aldose reductase in development of, 15
Sunflower cataract, in chalcosis/Wilson disease, 54, 57
Sunglasses, ultraviolet-absorbing, cataract prevention and, 53

Sunlight. *See* Ultraviolet light
Superoxide dismutase, in lens, 16
Supracapsular phacoemulsification, 121
Suprachoroidal/choroidal hemorrhage, 144*t*, 177–179, 189
delayed, 178–179
expulsive, 178
flat or shallow anterior chamber and, 152
Suprachoroidal effusion, 177–178
flat or shallow anterior chamber and, 152
Surface ectoderm, lens development and, 21, 22*f*
Surface tension, of ophthalmic viscosurgical device, 97
Surge, in phacoemulsification, 104
Surgical instruments, for phacoemulsification, 104–106, 105*f*, 106*f*, 107*f*
settings for, 118–119
Sutural cataracts, 33, 33*f*
Sutures (lens), 9
development of, 23*f*, 24–25, 24*f*
opacification of (sutural/stellate cataract), 33, 33*f*
Sutures (surgical), for cataract surgery
astigmatism and, 150, 212–213
manual small-incision cataract surgery and, 96
posterior chamber IOL implantation and, 139
Swinging flashlight test, for relative afferent pupillary defect, before cataract surgery, 77
Synechiae, posterior, in uveitis, lens changes/cataract and, 59

Tamoxifen, cataract risk and, 49
Tamsulosin, intraoperative floppy iris syndrome and, 74, 154, 155
TASS. *See* Toxic anterior segment syndrome
Temporal approach clear/"near clear" technique, for cataract surgery, 114
Tension rings, capsular, for zonular incompetence, 198, 199
Terazosin, intraoperative floppy iris syndrome and, 74, 155
Tetanic cataract, 57
Tetracaine, for cataract surgery, 99
TGF-β. *See* Transforming growth factor β
Thermal injury (burns), cataract surgery incision, 149
Thioridazine, lens changes caused by, 49
Tobacco use, cataract development and, 58–59, 67–68
Topical anesthesia, for cataract surgery, 99–100
Topographical method, for IOL power calculation after refractive surgery, 87
Toric intraocular lenses, 131
complications associated with, 169
Total cataract, 34
Toxic anterior segment syndrome (TASS), 147, 151–152
Toxic solutions, exposure to during cataract surgery, corneal edema caused by, 147, 151–152
Transforming growth factor β, in exfoliation syndrome/pseudoexfoliation, 61–62

Transplantation, corneal
    cataract/cataract surgery following, 193
    in triple procedure, 141, 192
Transport mechanisms, lens, 17–19, 18f
Trauma
    cataract surgery after, 206–209, 207f
    ectopia lentis caused by, 36
    lens damage/cataracts caused by, 50–54, 50f, 51f,
        52f, 54f, 55f, 206–209, 207f
        glaucoma and, 63
        phacoantigenic uveitis and, 62
        surgery for, 206–209, 207f
    patient evaluation after, 206
Triple procedure, 141, 192
Trypan blue dye, for capsule staining, 195, 195f, 196
Tunica vasculosa lentis, 25, 25f
    remnant of
        epicapsular star, 27, 28f
        Mittendorf dot, 25, 27
Tuning, in phacoemulsification, 103
Twin studies, in age-related cataract, 37–38

UDP galactose 4-epimerase deficiency, galactosemia/
    cataract formation and, 56
UGH syndrome. See Uveitis-glaucoma-hyphema
    (UGH) syndrome
Ultrasonic, definition of, 104
Ultrasonography/ultrasound
    before cataract surgery, 80–81, 82–83, 83f
    in IOL power determination/selection, 82–83, 83f,
        84, 84–85
    for phacoemulsification
        linear, 106
        panel control, 106
        terminology related to, 102–104
Ultraviolet-absorbing lenses, cataract prevention
    and, 53
Ultraviolet chromophores/filters, intraocular lenses
    with, 138
Ultraviolet light (ultraviolet radiation)
    cataracts associated with, 53
    lenses absorbing, cataract prevention and, 53
Urea-insoluble (membrane structural) lens proteins,
    11f, 12
Urea-soluble (cytoskeletal) lens proteins, 11f, 12
Uveitis
    cataracts and, 59, 60f, 203–204
        after cataract surgery, 158–159
        surgery in patient with, 75, 158, 203–204, 206–207
        Fuchs heterochromic, cataracts/cataract surgery
            in, 59, 60f
        phacoantigenic/phacoanaphylactic, 62
Uveitis-glaucoma-hyphema (UGH) syndrome,
    intraocular lens implantation and, 167
    decentration and, 163

Vacuum (phacoemulsification)
    definition of, 104
    settings for, 118, 119
    terminology related to, 104

Vacuum rise time (phacoemulsification), 104,
    109, 110f
Vancomycin, for postoperative endophthalmitis, 181
VDA (Visual Disability Assessment), 71
Venous retrobulbar hemorrhage, cataract surgery
    and, 176
Venting, in phacoemulsification, 104
Venturi pump, for phacoemulsification aspiration,
    109, 109f
    vacuum rise time for, 109, 110f
Vertical chopping techniques, in
    phacoemulsification, 123
Vesicle
    lens, formation of, 21, 22f
    optic, lens development and, 21, 22f
VF-14. See Visual Function Index
Videokeratography, IOL power determination/
    selection after refractive surgery and, 86
Vimentin, 12
Viscodissection. See Ophthalmic viscosurgical
    devices
Viscoelastic agents. See Ophthalmic viscosurgical
    devices
Viscoelasticity, of ophthalmic viscosurgical device, 97
Viscomydriasis, 98
Viscosity, of ophthalmic viscosurgical device, 97
Viscosurgical devices, ophthalmic (viscoelastic
    agents). See Ophthalmic viscosurgical devices
VISION 2020, 65
Vision rehabilitation, for cataract patient, 71
    ocular trauma and, 208
Visual acuity
    in cataract, 69–70, 70t
        preoperative evaluation and, 75, 76
    after cataract surgery, 141
        cystoid macular edema and, 182
        with ECCE, 213
        endophthalmitis and, 181
        with ICCE, 215
        incorrect lens power and, 168
Visual axis, Nd:YAG laser capsulotomy location
    and, 172
Visual Disability Assessment (VDA), 71
Visual field defects, in glaucoma, cataract/media
    opacities and, 201, 202f
Visual field testing, before cataract surgery, 81–82
Visual function, measuring, in cataract evaluation, 71
    after surgery, 141
    before surgery, 71, 76–77
Visual Function Index (VF-14), 71
Visual loss/impairment. See also Visual acuity
    cataract and, 65, 65t, 71
Vitamin B_6 (pyridoxine), for homocystinuria, 37
Vitamins
    deficiencies of, cataracts caused by, 57–58
    supplementary, cataract prevention and, 58
Vitrectomy
    anterior
        for capsular rupture during cataract surgery, 160
        for vitreous prolapse, 162

for capsular rupture during cataract surgery, 160–161, 161
cataract/cataract surgery after, 16, 60, 75, 205–206
for cystoid macular edema, postoperative, 183
for endophthalmitis, postoperative, 181
oxidative lens damage and, 16
pars plana. *See* Pars plana vitrectomy
for retained lens fragments after phacoemulsification, 159–160
for vitreocorneal adherence/persistent corneal edema, 148
for vitreous prolapse, 162
Vitreocorneal adherence, after cataract surgery, 148
Vitreolysis, Nd:YAG laser, for vitreous prolapse in anterior chamber, 162
Vitreoretinopathies, cataract surgery in patient with, 205
Vitreous
   cataract surgery complications and, 144*t*
     with ICCE, 214
     posterior vitreous detachment, 184
     prolapse, 162
     vitreocorneal adherence, 148
   primary, persistent hyperplasia of. *See* Persistent fetal vasculature
Vitreous biopsy, in infectious endophthalmitis, after cataract surgery, 181
Vitreous detachment, posterior, retinal detachment after cataract surgery and, 184
Vitreous pressure, positive, flat or shallow anterior chamber and, 152
Vitreous wick syndrome, 162
von Graefe knife, 92
Vossius ring, 50

WAGR syndrome, 29
Warfarin/warfarin derivatives, cataract surgery in patient taking, 189
Water and electrolyte balance, in lens, maintenance of, 17–19, 18*f*
Water channels (aquaporins), 12, 17
Water-insoluble lens proteins, 11, 11*f*, 12
   aging affecting, 13

Water-soluble lens proteins, 11, 11*f*. *See also* Crystallins
   conversion of to water-insoluble, 13
Wedl (bladder) cells, 44, 170
Weill-Marchesani syndrome, microspherophakia in, 29
WHO (World Health Organization), cataract epidemiology and, 65, 65*t*
Wilms tumor, aniridia and, 29
Wilson disease (hepatolenticular degeneration), 57
World Health Organization (WHO), cataract epidemiology and, 65, 65*t*
Wound closure
   complications associated with, 148–149
   after ECCE, 212–213
   postoperative endophthalmitis and, 180
   scleral tunnel incisions and, 112–113, 112*f*
Wound dehiscence/rupture, 149
Wound leaks, 144*t*, 148–149
   flat anterior chamber and, 153

Xylocaine. *See* Lidocaine

Y-sutures, lens, 9
   development of, 24–25, 24*f*
   opacification of (sutural/stellate cataract), 33, 33*f*

Z syndrome, 169
Zeaxanthin, cataract risk affected by, 58
Zinn, zonules of (zonular fibers). *See* Zonular fibers, lens
Zonular (lamellar) cataracts, 30, 32*f*
Zonular dehiscence, cataract surgery and, 197–199, 198*f*
   in glaucoma patient, 202
   iris coloboma/corectopia and, 196, 197*f*
Zonular fibers, lens (zonules of Zinn), 5, 6*f*, 7–8
   absent/abnormal, cataract surgery and, 117, 118
     in glaucoma patient, 202
     iris coloboma/corectopia and, 196, 197*f*
   development of, 25
   evaluation of, before cataract surgery, 79
Zonular lamella, 7
Zonular rupture, cataract surgery and, 144*t*
Zonules, of Zinn (zonular fibers). *See* Zonular fibers, lens